Ashtanga Yoga

The Practice Manual

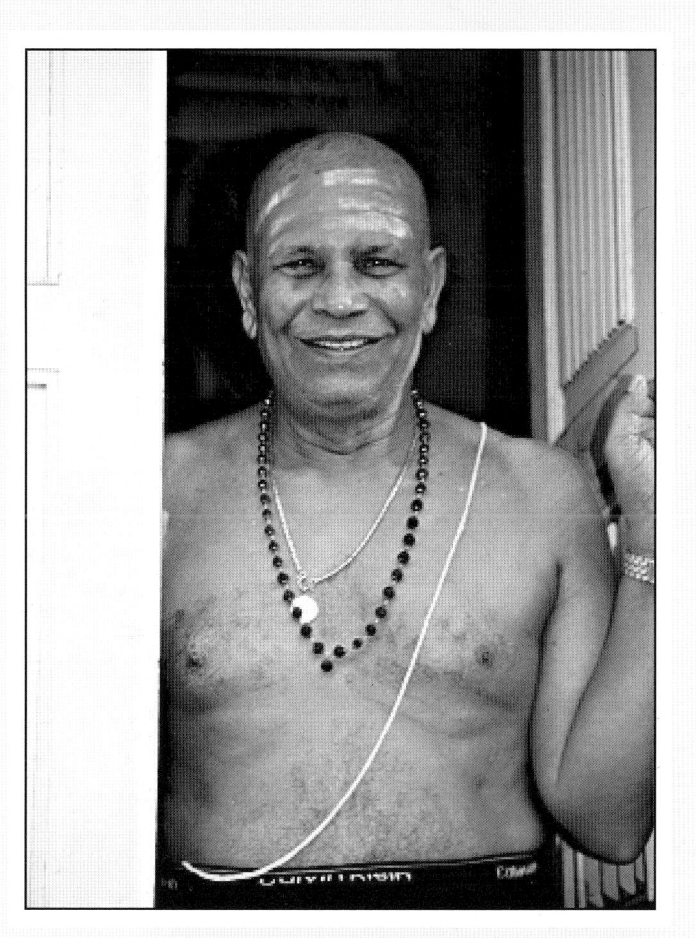

K. Pattabhi Jois

Founder / Director of the Ashtanga Yoga Research Institute
Mysore, India

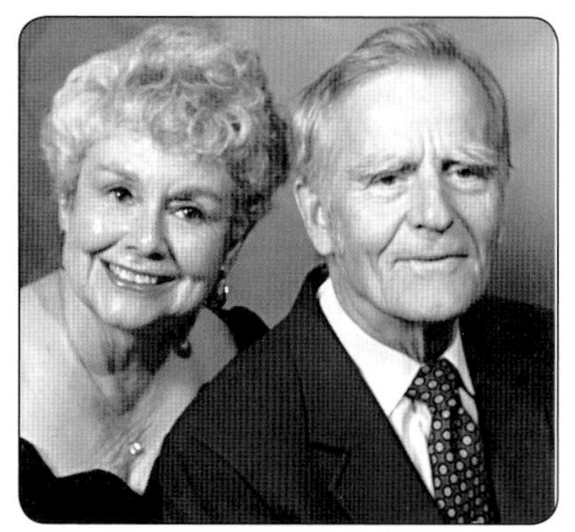

Violet and Stanley Swenson
Houston, TX 1993

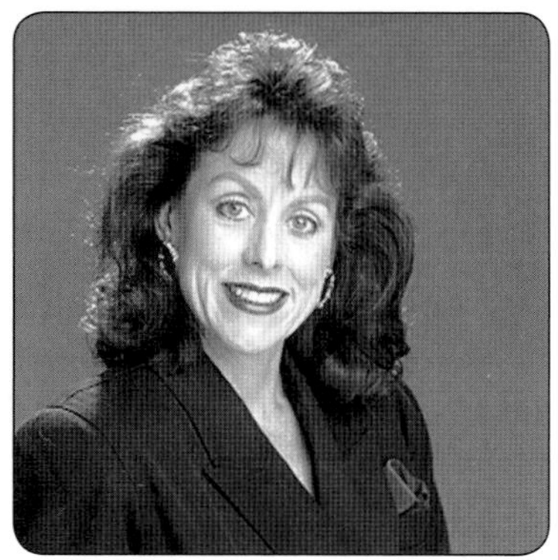

Diana Swenson-Halberdier
Houston, TX 1997

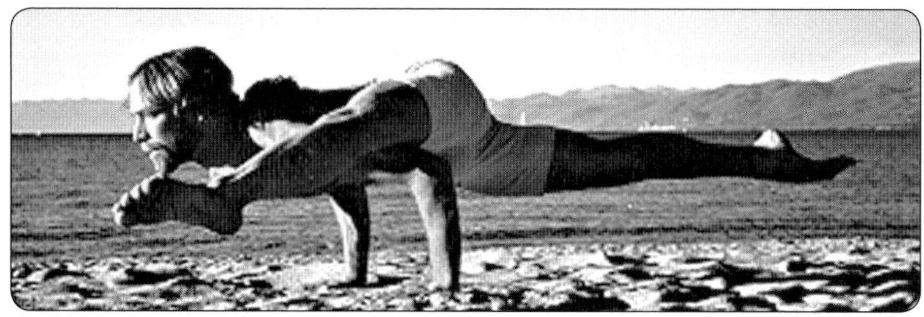

Doug Swenson
Lake Tahoe, CA 1996

What Does A Yogi Look Like?

My biological family has been one of the greatest sources for support and example in my life. From my earliest memories my parents have demonstrated benevolent qualities of compassion, patience and openmindedness. They have exhibited unconditional love by offering full acceptance of whatever bizarre and exotic paths I have chosen to traverse. My brother introduced me to yoga and healthy living when I was 13 years old. His gifts continue to be the most valuable of tools imaginable and I cherish them daily. My sister carries a glowing spark of enthusiasm and determination into every aspect of life and her positive outlook is contagious and inspiring.

The learned sage draped in robes, residing in a cave or mystical temple is the image of spirituality which is sometimes sought by the western student. There are certainly saintly persons residing in such abodes yet it is not the only place to look. In my quest for knowledge I have felt at times to be like a fish swimming in the ocean looking here and there for the ocean itself. All knowledge is available to us within each breath if we are but aware enough to recognize it. I thank my family for exhibiting the qualities of a yogi in their daily life and interactions.

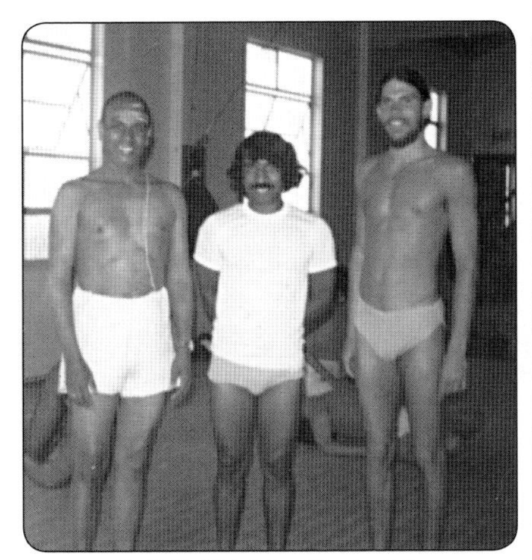

K. Pattabhi Jois, Manju Jois and David Williams
Encinitas, CA 1975

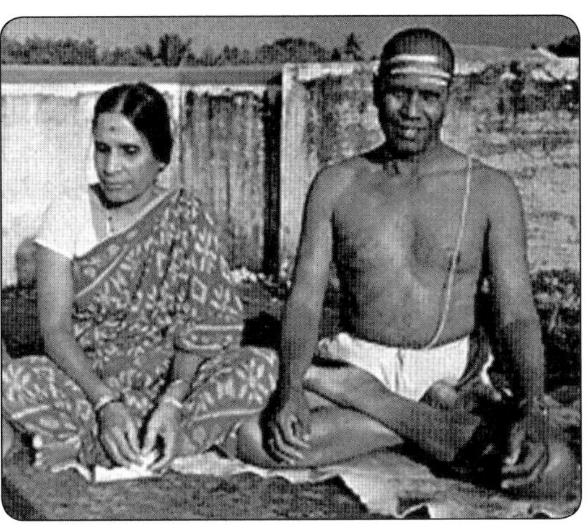

Amma and K. Pattabhi Jois
Mysore, India 1977

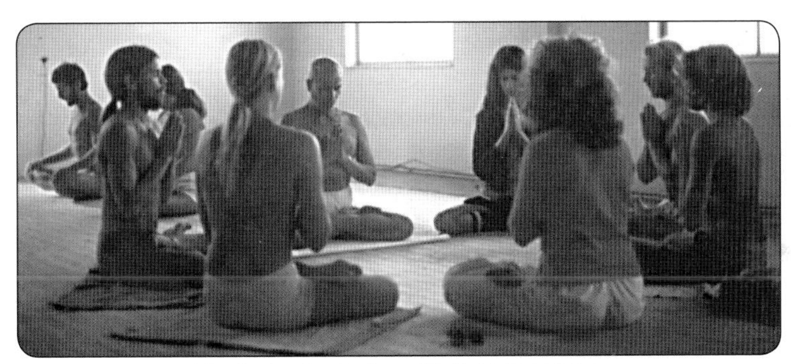

Clockwise beginning with K. Pattabhi Jois
K. Pattabhi Jois, Nancy Gilgoff, Brad Ramsey, Paul Dunaway, Sally Walker, David Swenson and David Williams
Encinitas, CA 1975

A Living Tradition

In addition to my biological family I have a yoga family as well. My brother became my first teacher when he introduced me to hatha yoga in 1969. In 1973 Paul Dunaway brought me to my first Ashtanga class where I met David Williams and Nancy Gilgoff. In 1975 David brought K. Pattabhi Jois and his son Manju to the U. S. and I was able to initiate studies with them.

This method of sharing yoga is the same system which has kept it alive for thousands of years as it passes from one generation to the next. We are all part of a living tradition which connects us to an ancient lineage. I offer respect and obeisances to all of my teachers past, present and future.

Ashtanga Yoga Productions
PO Box 5099, Austin, TX 78763

Website: www.ashtanga.net

First Published 1999
Thirty-second Printing 2019

Design and Layout by David Swenson and Eric Sod

Printed in Korea

ISBN 978-1-891252-08-2 : U.S. $29.95, EU €25

All Studio Photographs by Raul Marroquin

Editing by J. Copeland Woodruff

Contents

Ashtanga Yoga

Ashta = Eight   Anga = Limb   Yoga = Union

"The Eight Limbs of Yoga"

Patanjali, the author of the Yoga Sutras, described the eight aspects of yoga as limbs of a tree.

Patanjali's analogy is the perfect image. Wisdom and spirituality unfold in the same manner as a tree grows. Nature is steady and gradual. The world of yoga, with its myriad styles and approaches, may be likened to a forest filled with variety and color. Every tree in a forest has the same goal: to reach toward the light. One tree's method is not better than another's. Each species has individual characteristics which enable it to grow to its greatest potential. The various yogic systems are unique, yet all have the same purpose: to grow toward enlightenment.

The Eight Limbs of Yoga

Yama - Ethical disciplines
Niyama - Self observation
Asana - Posture
Pranayama - Breath control
Pratyahara - Sense withdrawal
Dharana - Concentration
Dhyana - Meditation
Samadhi - A state of joy and peace

The particular system of yoga described in this manual is derived from the teachings of K. Pattabhi Jois. He is the director and founder of the Ashtanga Yoga Research Institute in Mysore, India. He learned this dynamic method from his teacher, Krishnamacharya, and in turn has handed it down to thousands of students around the world. The approach is based on a specialized sequencing of postures and focused breathing techniques.

When practiced with regulation and awareness, the tree described by Patanjali begins to sprout. Practice is the only means of feeding it. K. Pattabhi Jois is fond of saying, "**99% Practice and 1% Theory**". I have grown to appreciate the depth of this simple statement. Only through practice may we taste the fruits of the yoga tree. Without it we are left to speculate or theorize. If one wants to know the qualities of an apple, it would do no good to draw diagrams and look at apples in a jar. But to bite into the fruit itself, one would gain an immediate experience of its essence. The nutritious effects of the apple would also be readily absorbed and assimilated as we enjoy its qualities. To know Ashtanga Yoga, it must be tasted through practice.

Through **regulation** of practice, the eight limbs are nourished. Personal insights begin to manifest. We become aware of what we put in our bodies and how we interact with the world around us. From this type of introspection, the qualities of **Yama** and **Niyama** begin to develop. **Asanas** and **Pranayama** grow when focused awareness of the breath is applied while practicing each posture. As we keep the mind fixed on the sound and quality of our breath, the senses are encouraged to turn inward and the element of **Pratyahara** manifests. As we improve our abilities of controlling the senses from wandering during practice, the subtle quality of concentration deepens in the form of **Dharana**. In time, the practice moves further internally and refinement of concentration develops as our ability to remain present is enhanced. The practice then grows into a deep resounding meditative experience known as **Dhyana**. At this stage, we are creating greater potential to explore the finest realms of yoga known as **Samadhi**, in which we realize the pure essence of all that exists.

The development of these limbs does not unfold in a linear fashion. They sprout when the time is appropriate. There is no way to rush the growth of a tree. It will expand as our understanding of the depths of yoga matures. Patience may be the greatest tool to assist in our journey down the scenic path of Ashtanga Yoga. It winds through all facets of life. Ashtanga may be utilized as a method of keeping physically fit or it may be traversed as a pathway to explore the subtle realms of spirituality. Whatever purpose we choose, there is only one method to reap its benefits: **Practice!**

Ashtanga Yoga

"The Practice Manual"

This manual is designed as a streamlined tool to give practical guidelines for developing a personal practice. It begins with a basic exploration of the foundations inherent within the Ashtanga Yoga system. Next, in the asana section, you will find alternative versions for every posture. This will provide safe and effective methods of approach while learning the routine. In addition, you will find a brief commentary at the bottom of the page giving helpful hints to remember during practice. The specific point of gaze, known as drishti, will also be found there. Each asana is accompanied by its traditional Sanskrit name with the literal English translation below. So as not to list the translation of **asana** on every page I am including it here. **Asana means Posture**.

In the back of this manual there is a section entitled "The Full Flow". It contains a complete representation of each series. They are laid out in sequences of photos with the Sanskrit name of the asana under each. "The Full Flow" is designed as an easy visual reference to utilize during practice. The asanas are arranged in the traditional sequence, as taught by K. Pattabhi Jois, with the exception of the "Short Forms" in which I have taken liberties to adjust the practice. The "Short Forms" are designed for those new to Ashtanga Yoga or practitioners requiring a less lengthy approach than the full Primary or Intermediate Series.

The manual is equipped with a spiral binding and a hard cover. The spiral will allow you to place it on the floor as a visual reference without it flopping closed and the hard cover will enhance its durability. You may use the manual by itself or in conjunction with our CDs, which are coordinated with all of the routines, including the "Short Forms".

I have done everything possible to make this book both user-friendly and informative. It is best to learn under the guidance of a qualified Ashtanga Yoga instructor. We all do not have the luxury of living near a teacher, so sometimes it is necessary to use whatever means is necessary or available. Ashtanga Yoga ultimately promotes independence. Once you have learned the routine fully, and the flow begins to unfold naturally, you will require less external input from teachers and books and your personal practice will become your greatest guide.

Each practice session is a journey. Endeavor to move with awareness and enjoy the experience. Allow it to unfold as a flower opens. There is no benefit in hurrying. Yoga grows with time. Some days are easy and the mind is calm and the physical body is light and responsive. Other days you may find that the mind is running wild and the body feels like wet cement. We must breathe deeply and remain detached. Asanas are not the goal. They are a vehicle to access a deeper internal awareness. Create a practice that best suits your personal needs so that it is something that you look forward to. Yoga is a place of refuge and a soothing balm for the stresses of modern life. Within each practice find ways to refine your existing understanding so that you continue to grow. Rather than simply moving from asana to asana, ***feel*** that action from deep within. Listen to your breath. Can you ride the breath like a bird on a breeze? Where is the mind? Can you maintain your focus and remain calm even when approaching a posture that you dread? Enjoy yourself. I have never had a practice that I regreted. Not once have I finished a routine and thought, "Oh, I wish I hadn't done that." But there have been days that I didn't practice and later I wished I had. Keep it fun. Take just a few minutes and spend it with yoga. The rest of your day will be better. Yoga is a scenic journey to our deepest spirit. Do as much or as little as feels correct. This manual will achieve its purpose if it somehow encourages you to practice. That is its name, "The Practice Manual". It is always better to do a little than none at all. Use the "Short Forms" or just practice a few sun salutations when time is limited.

"Practice and all is coming!"

K. Pattabhi Jois

Breath, Locks, Flow & Gaze

"The Internal World"

Before beginning to practice, it is necessary to discuss some of the fundamental aspects of Ashtanga Yoga. These elements exist within an unseen world. Without them yoga becomes nothing more than an outward expression of physical movement. When performed correctly these subtle tools allow the practitioner to enter into the mystical realms of prana and experience the subtle wonders of Ashtanga Yoga. These invisible tools are "**Ujjayi Breath**", "**Bandhas**", "**Vinyasa**" and "**Drishti**".

Breath

Ujjayi is a specialized breathing technique which means victorious. This unique form of breathing is performed by creating a soft sound in the back of the throat while inhaling and exhaling through the nose. It is helpful to gently smile while breathing to allow the air to swirl around the back of the throat before continuing its journey to the lungs. This swirling action is what creates the unique sound which has been described as wind in the trees, a distant ocean, a cobra snake or, for the less poetic, Darth Vader from "Star Wars".

To assist those of you who are new to this type of breathing I have an exercise called the "Hhhaaa Method". You must sit up straight and take a full inhale through the nose and then let it out through the mouth with the soft sound of "Hhhaaa" as though you are whispering. Feel the air swirl in the back of the throat. Take a few breaths in this way and then **midway** through an exhale, close your mouth and let the air continue exiting through the nose instead of the mouth. Practice it a few times. Once you can create the sound in the back of the throat while exhaling, you are halfway to the full ujjayi breath. The second step is to gently smile while inhaling and create the same swirling sound as on the exhale. With practice it will become more familiar and soon you'll be able to utilize the ujjayi sound without any effort at all.

The main idea is to create a rhythm in the breath and ride it gracefully throughout the practice. This sound becomes a mantra to set the mind in focus. We must learn to listen to the breath. It is the guide which will tell us the quality of our practice. If we apply too much effort, the breath will become constricted or forced. With too little focus, the ujjayi breath may be drowned out by the sound of our own thoughts. Maintain awareness upon your breath and every moment becomes a meditation.

Breath, Locks, Flow & Gaze

"The World"

Bandhas

Bandhas are a series of internal energy gates within the subtle body which assist in the regulation of pranic flow. There are three which I will discuss. They are "**Mulabandha**", "**Uddiyana Bandha**" and "**Jalandhara Bandha**". You may think of them as valves which work similarly to the valves within the circulatory system. When the heart beats, the blood surges through arteries and veins. Valves keep the blood from sloshing back toward the heart. In this way, when the heart beats, the blood continues its forward movement. **Bandhas** regulate the flow of **prana** (life-force) in a similar way within subtle energy channels known as **nadis**. When engaging the locks, energy is forced to spread throughout these pathways. We are then able to assimilate this energy on a cellular level as the prana bathes and feeds our subtle body and balances the gross nervous system.

Mulabandha

Mulabandha is the root lock. It so called because of its location at the base of our nerve tree, the spinal column. There is a difference of location for this bandha in males and in females. In males the seat of **Mulabandha** is the perineal muscle which is located in front of the anus and behind the genitals. In females the location is near the top of the cervix.

A good way to understand its location is to imagine that you have a need to go to the toilet and there is none in sight. Which muscles would you use to resist this urge? In the beginning one may contract the anus in order to engage the appropriate area, but it is not necessary to be a "tight ass" in order to engage **Mulabandha**. It is more subtle than that. You may utilize a technique given to women to assist in the toning of the pelvic floor after childbirth. It is called the Keigel technique. While urinating, engage the muscles of the pelvic floor and stop the flow of urine and then release the contraction and let it flow again. This contraction will engage more muscles than necessary but over time you may learn to refine the action so that it is more specifically focused. In the beginning these locks may waver. With practice it will become possible to hold them for the entire duration of each yoga session. For more details you may refer to a book entitled, **"Moola Bandha, The Master Key"**.

Breath, Locks, Flow & Gaze

"The Internal World"

Uddiyana Bandha

The second lock is **Uddiyana Bandha** which means flying upward. In its complete expression, **Uddiyana Bandha** is performed by exhaling fully and then drawing the lower belly inward and upward while simultaneously lifting the diaphragm. This level of **Uddiyana** is primarily utilized during the exhale retention phase of specialized breath control methods known as pranayama. This full level of engagement is not possible to maintain throughout practice due to the inability to inhale while total uddiyana bandha is engaged. The level of Uddiyana we should hold for the duration of our practice is more subtle. Rather than sucking in the belly fully, we must instead simply maintain a stillness located three fingers below the navel. This will allow space for the diaphragm to drop during each inhale and the lung's expansion will find its way into the side ribs, back, and chest. The upper portions of the torso must remain soft and pliable so that the inhale expansion may occur to its fullest expression. Upon each exhale the lower abdominal muscles may contract to encourage a total emptying of the lungs. This contraction must then be released in order for the inhale to repeat fully, yet not relaxed so much that the lower belly rises with the incoming breath. The action is subtle. Too much effort and the breath is hindered rather than enhanced. Do not harden the belly as though someone is about to punch you in the stomach. That is over-doing it.

I like to use a visualization to assist in further understanding this bandha. Imagine that you have a string which is attached two inches below the navel. Take that string and draw it straight through the body and tie it around the spine. Now when you inhale the lower belly will remain still and you will maintain freedom in the upper torso. These bandhas are a subtle dynamic that may take many years to understand. Be patient. Don't worry if you don't get it right away. In time they will come. Just as mulabandha, uddiyana bandha should eventually be held for the duration of practice.

Jalandhara Bandha

Jalandhara Bandha is the third lock to discuss. It is the chin-lock. This lock is not utilized as frequently as the other two. It occurs spontaneously in some asanas such as shoulder stand and is prescribed for use in others. It is, however, used extensively for pranayama. To engage jalandhara bandha you may extend the chin forward and then draw it back into the notch which is formed where the two clavicle bones meet, at the bony protrusions below your Adam's apple. When engaging all three bandhas simultaneously it is called "mahabandha" or the great lock. Bandhas are an integral part of Ashtanga Yoga but they cannot be understood through mental powers. Understanding of the them will grow from these early seeds of awareness as personal practice develops.

Vinyasa

"The Marriage of Breath & Movement"

Vinyasa is the unique linking of one asana to the next in a serpentine flow. It is more than a simple set of physical maneuvers. It is a dynamic marriage of our internal and external worlds. Vinyasa is an outward expression of the subtle movement of life force. It is a manifestation of prana. Vinyasa orchestrates balance. A balance of strength and flexibility, lightness and heaviness, movement and stillness. Through vinyasa one may know the vibration of life. This integration manifests when the act of breathing and movement cease to be separate entities. The two actions converge to create a symphony of seamless unity. Each action encourages the other. They exist as one. The mind is then set free and the practice may become a rhythmic dance.

In order to understand vinyasa we must start with the gross aspects and through refinement we may gain knowledge of its subtleties. Vinyasa begins with an understanding of the physical set of movements prescribed as links between asanas. Through repetition this action becomes familiar to the body on a cellular level. Vinyasa assists in creating heat which allows more freedom of exploration within the asanas. It also brings the body back to a neutral position between postures. Vinyasa is like an "etch-a-sketch". After exiting from one asana, the body's screen is cleared and prepared for entry into the next. Without linking this movement with breath, the action remains within the physical realm. There is joy in developing our physical bodies, yet to discover vinyasa's magic we must explore the breath simultaneously. When this marriage is successfully achieved, the action becomes one of spirit and the physical practice acts as a conduit for a deeper exploration of our core identity.

At the end of the standing sequence I have inserted a section called, "**Applying the Physics of Flight**". This is a detailed description of the dynamics required for transporting ourselves from **Downward Dog** into a seated position. After **Paschimottanasana C**, I have included a section entitled "**Dancing With Prana**". It encompasses a description for the first jumping-back vinyasa from a seated position. Within each section I will give a variety of vinyasa options to choose from. Utilize the one which most suits your needs. Enjoy the flow and keep your breath full!

Weave the Tapestry of Vinyasa
From the Threads of Breath and Movement

Drishti

"Looking Out / Looking In"

Drishti is a point of gaze or focus, yet it has little to do with our physical sight. The real "looking" is directed internally. We may fix our physical sight upon an external object or a specific point on our body, yet truly the drishti is meant to direct our attention to the subtle aspects of our practice which were discussed earlier, the breath and bandhas as well as the mind. Those of us with sight are easily distracted by our surroundings. Other students in the room, a clock on the wall, or myriad other forms may pull us away from the immediate concerns of practicing yoga with awareness. The drishti is a device designed to balance our internal and external practice. There are officially nine drishti points which I have listed below. You will find that each asana has a drishti assigned to it. It will be listed at the bottom of every asana page.

The Nine Drishtis

1) **Nasagrai** - Tip of the nose
2) **Ajna Chakra** - Between the eyebrows
3) **Nabi Chakra** - Navel
4) **Hastagrai** - Hand
5) **Padhayoragrai** - Toes
6) **Parsva Drishti** - Far to the right
7) **Parsva Drishti** - Far to the left
8) **Angustha Ma Dyai** - Thumbs
9) **Urdhva or Antara Drishti** - Up to the sky

If you find the drishtis to be too difficult, then I have a general rule of thumb which you can follow as an alternative whenever you feel the need. Let your gaze move in the direction of the stretch. As an example, if practicing a spinal twist to the right, your gaze will follow in that direction by looking over the right shoulder. When practicing a forward bend, your gaze may move toward the toes, or, if both arms are over the head, then generally the gaze will be looking up in that direction. You may think of your eyes like the eyes in a doll which will follow the movement of your head. When the head moves, the gaze will follow in the same direction.

Remember the main focus is to look inward. Create an internal checklist which you can scan in a millisecond while practicing. On this list you may have Breath, Bandhas, Flow and Equality of Opposition. Do you feel tension in particular areas of the body? Where is your awareness? Is it spread throughout the body? Are you relaxed? The list may go on but the idea is that the drishti is your microscope to examine that which may not be seen externally. The nine drishti points of Ashtanga Yoga are listed here. Utilize the prescribed one for each asana or the general rule of gazing in the direction of the stretch.

View Your Practice Through the Eyes of Drishti

Belts, Blocks and Bolsters

"To Prop Or Not To Prop"

The use of props has become increasingly popular as an aid to practicing yoga. Traditionally, the approach within the Ashtanga system has been to find methods of adjusting the asana by finding avenues of support within the body rather than through the use of any external apparatus. I have the attitude that the practitioner should utilize whatever methods or tools they find useful to enhance their practice. Whether this means using props or not, the goal is the same. Practice with awareness and create an avenue of personal progress. I look at props like training wheels on a bicycle. Eventually the reliance upon them will decrease. This may be done by using "disappearing" props. The size and quantity should lessen over time. Let's say that one is using a block for support in the triangle posture. I believe it would be beneficial to use a large book instead and upon completion of each practice session tear a page out. In this way a 300 page book would wean the practitioner away from the prop gradually and in 300 practice sessions it would disappear altogether. I have included many asana choices both with and without the utilization of props. There are an infinite number of ways to adjust an asana. I have offered a variety of possibilities. Be creative! Find new methods of your own through exploration. Work at your own capacity. Create the practice which most suits you.

Another topic I would like to address is the type of mat to use. In ancient times the yogis practiced on tiger skins and kusha grass. Due to the scarcity of these two items in modern-day yoga schools and complaints from the tigers about the difficulty of skinless existence, most practitioners in the West now use what is called a "sticky mat". This is a rubbery material that prevents the feet or hands from slipping. It is effective. I personally prefer to feel a natural substance under me such as cotton. If practicing on a wooden floor the cotton mat against it would be too slippery. If you place a sticky mat under the cotton then the problem is solved. Some people find that the cotton is slippery under the hands or feet while in **Downward Dog**. This is easily remedied by squirting a mist of water on the mat where the hands and feet are placed before practicing, then there is perfect traction. The use of cotton on top of the rubber mat is much more sanitary and environmentally sound. The cotton mat may be tossed into the washer and dryer to keep it clean. Sticky mats are problematic in this area. Rubber mats will last much longer when placing a cotton one on top. This means fewer toxic rubber mats will be clogging our bulging landfills. Cotton is biodegradable and pleasing against the skin. There are no hard-and-fast rules. Become your own teacher. Explore new methods. Play around with approaches of your own. Practice outdoors whenever possible. Feel your connection with nature. Place your cotton mat in the grass under a shade tree. Enjoy the energy of the earth. Draw fresh air deeply into your lungs. This is the greatest prop of all, **OXYGEN!**

Note - Whenever a chair is used as a prop be sure to keep the chair on a sticky mat or braced against a wall.

Yoga Chikitsa

"Yoga Therapy"

The Primary Series of Ashtanga Yoga is known in Sanskrit as "**Yoga Chikitsa**" which means yoga therapy. It is a healing process of cleansing and toning for the body, mind and senses. This therapeutic action occurs through the subtle vehicles of Ashtanga Yoga. There is an understanding in yoga that there exists within the body a complex network of energy pathways known as "**nadis**". The energy which flows in these channels is a powerful yet unseen force called "**prana**". Prana is thought to be the underlying source for all life. Along the **nadis**, obstructions can form which inhibit the free flow of prana. These hindrances are called "**granthis**" or knots. **Granthis** may arise from myriad sources. Their presence may not even be detected until their unraveling. This unraveling process is a result of a consistent and regulated practice. The clearing of **granthis** allows prana a cleaner avenue along which to travel. This is the source of the healing aspects of the Primary Series. With fewer obstacles to confront, the body, mind and senses are allowed a more fertile environment in which to function thereby operating at the utmost level of efficiency. Yoga is a self-empowering process which instills within its practitioners a confidence and a deep internal knowledge of the subtle workings of our being, both subtle and gross. The asanas are arranged in a time-tested sequence designed to specifically align the body and strengthen the nervous system. First comes the Sun Salutations and the Standing Sequence. The Primary Series begins with **Dandasana**, the first seated posture, and ends with **Setu Bandhasana** which is the final asana before the Finishing Sequence. Many practitioners of Ashtanga Yoga have found the Primary Series to be an invaluable tool to assist them in their healing process, whether it be mental or physical. As with any healing process we must be patient and determined. The greatest tool you may utilize to discover the benefits waiting for you within Yoga Chikitsa is patience. Allow time for your practice to mature and the fruits will present themselves.

The Fruits of Yoga Mature with Patience and Care

Surya Namaskara

Surya = Sun   Namaskara = Greeting or Salutation

"Sun Salutation"

Surya means the sun and Namaskara is a greeting of honor and respect to the divinity present in each of us. The entire foundation of Ashtanga Yoga is based upon the dynamic flow of **Surya Namaskara A and B**. **Surya Namaskara** is the birth of your practice. It is here that we may set the rhythm and mood for each session of yoga. The entire series, whether it be Primary, Intermediate or Advanced, is an extension and refinement of the movement learned in the sun salutations. This dynamic marriage of breath and movement into a serpentine flow is what sets this system of yoga apart from other methods. It does not mean that one system is better than the other, it is simply that there are many approaches to achieve a similar goal. Feel the relationship between movement and breath when practicing **Surya Namaskara** or the vinyasa sequence. Weaving these two actions together creates a tapestry of grace and stability both physically as well as within the subtle realms of our consciousness. Find the rhythm in your breath and allow your body to respond to it. Feel the inhales lift the body into the **Upward Dog** and the exhales propel the body into **Downward Dog**. Identify breath as the source of movement and the very core of our existence. Ride it as you would a wave in the ocean or respond to it the way your body responds to music. Use only the energy required to get you from point A to point B. Relax areas that are not required to be engaged. Feel the air move across your body as you move through space. Be free. Be light. Be joyful in the experience and expression of your personal practice.

Work Toward Practicing Five of Each Sun Salutation

If five repetitions are too many then choose a comfortable amount to begin with and increase it over time.

Discover the Essence of Ashtanga Yoga
Within the Realms of Surya Namaskara!

Surya Namaskara Options

Below you will find a variety of options to choose from when practicing Surya Namaskara. It is not the complete set of movements but rather segments that may require more attention to variety. They are numbered to correspond with the phases of **Surya Namaskara A and B** which are outlined fully on the following pages. If you find phases that are too difficult then plug in whichever option from below most suits you. Some phases are repetitive in both **Surya Namaskara A & B**. Repeat the most appropriate one. Allow your practice to mature gradually. Be patient and enjoy the journey.

Surya Namaskara A or B

Two - Take your hands to the shins or ankles instead of all of the way to the floor.

Three - Leave the hands on the shins or knees instead of the floor. Keep the spine long.

Four - You may step the feet back one at a time as in **Four A** or jump them back as in **Four B**.

Five - If necessary keep the knees on the floor. Avoid collapsing in the lower back.

Six - If you become fatigued in **Downward Dog** lower the knees to the floor and sit on the heels.

Surya Namaskara B

Seven & Eleven - If it is too much to take the foot all of the way to the hands you may step only partially forward and then raise the hands. Either way keep the front knee above the heel and the back leg working with the outer edge of the foot pressing into the floor.

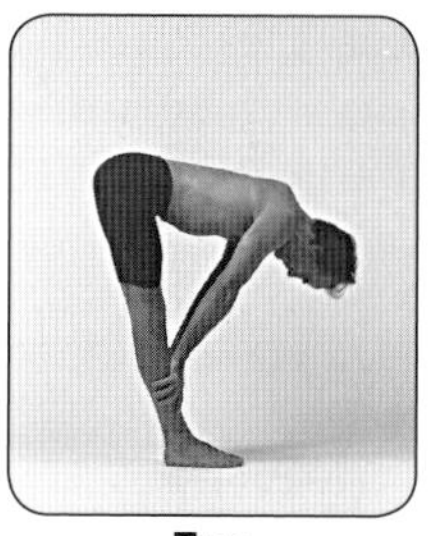

Two

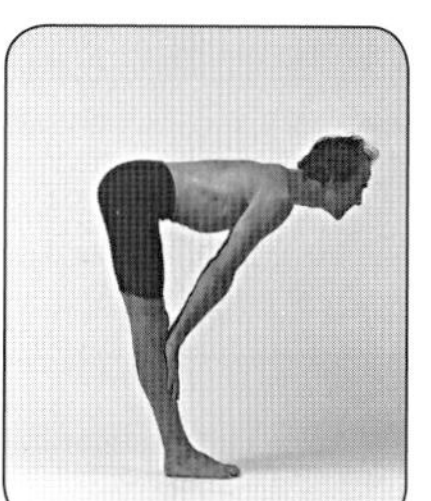

Three

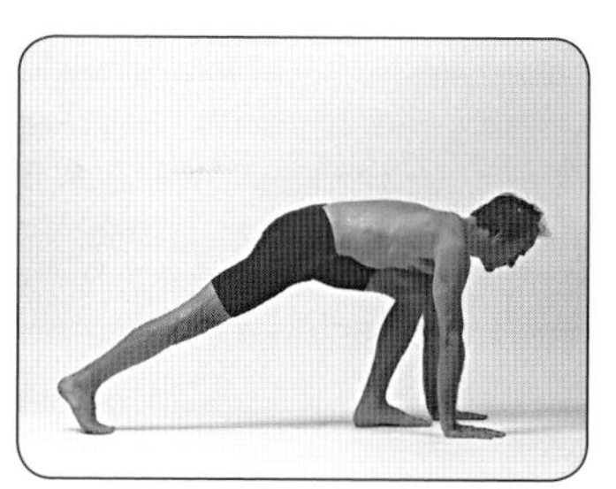

Four A

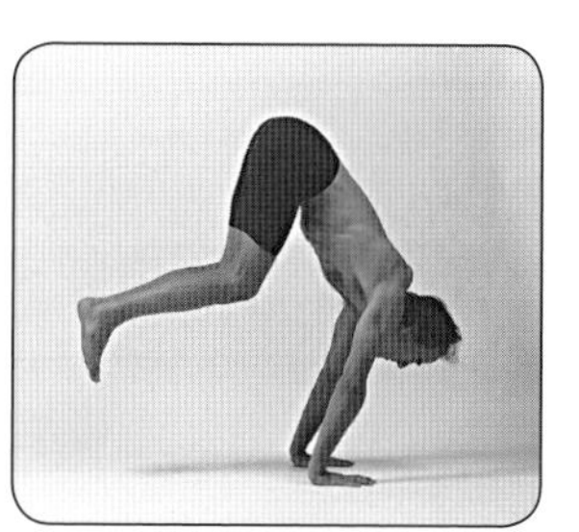

Four B

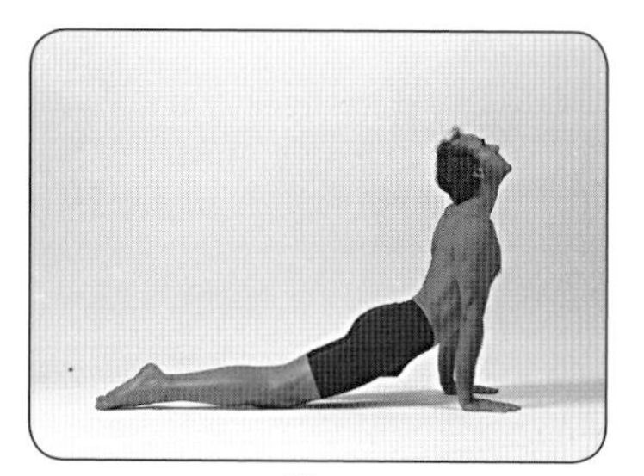

Five

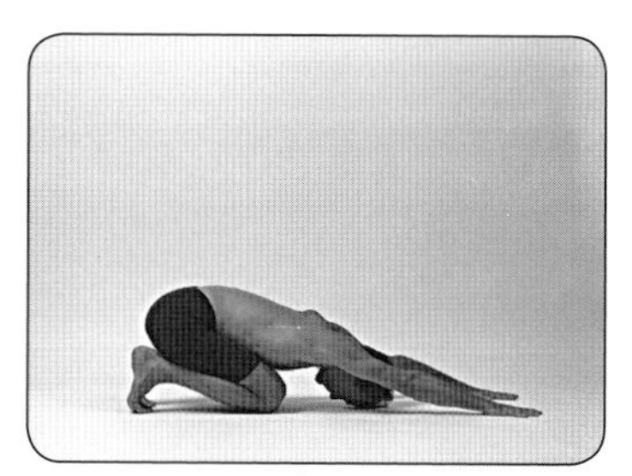

Six

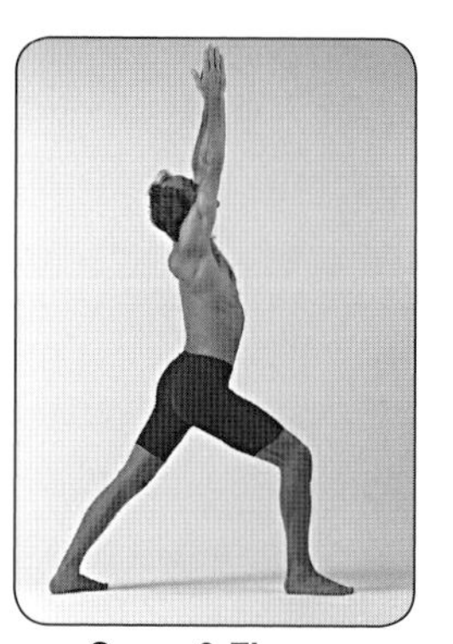

Seven & Eleven

Surya Namaskara A

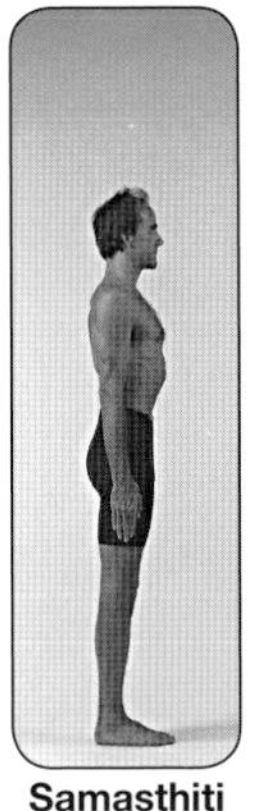
Samasthiti

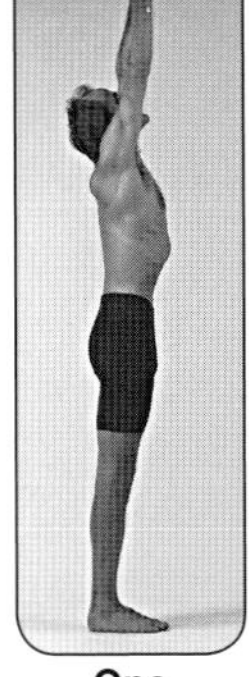
One

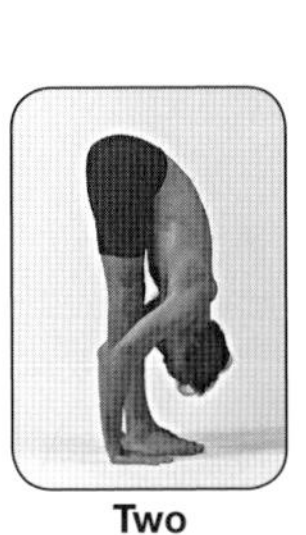
Two

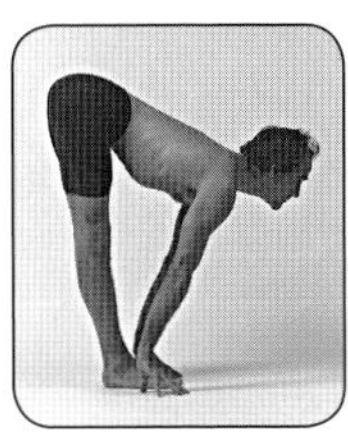
Three

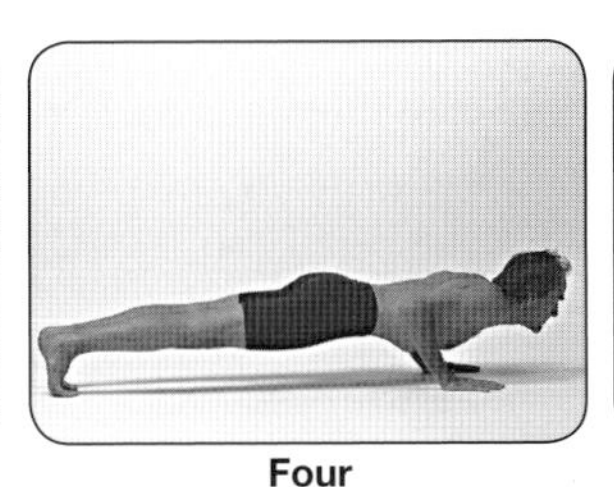
Four

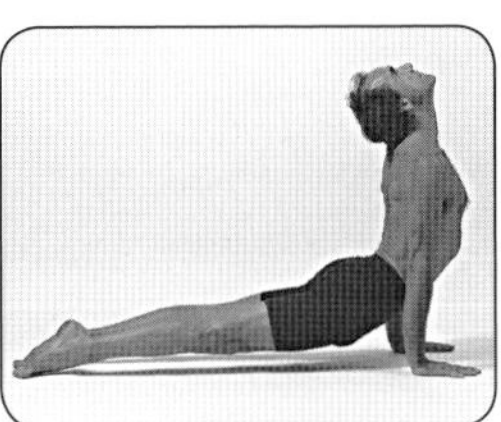
Five

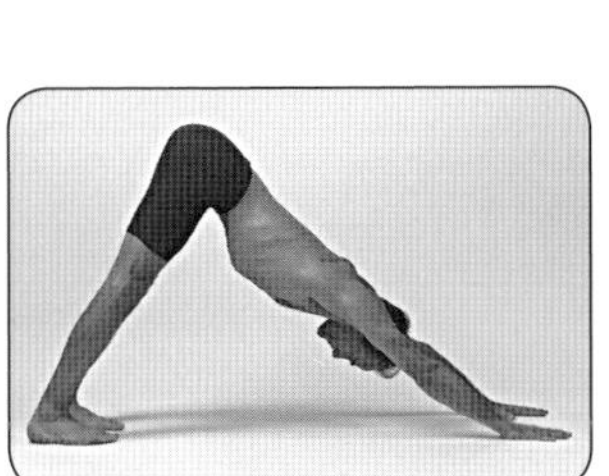
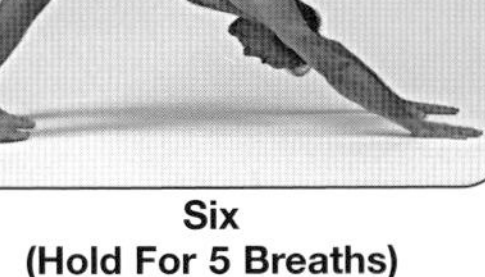
Six
(Hold For 5 Breaths)

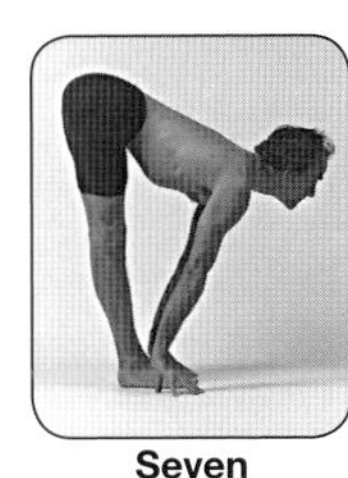
Seven

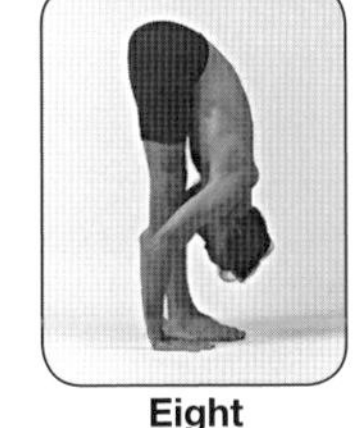
Eight

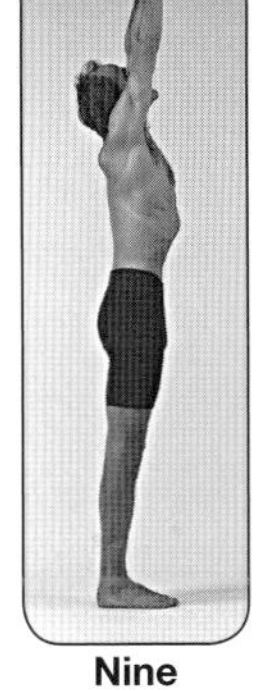
Nine

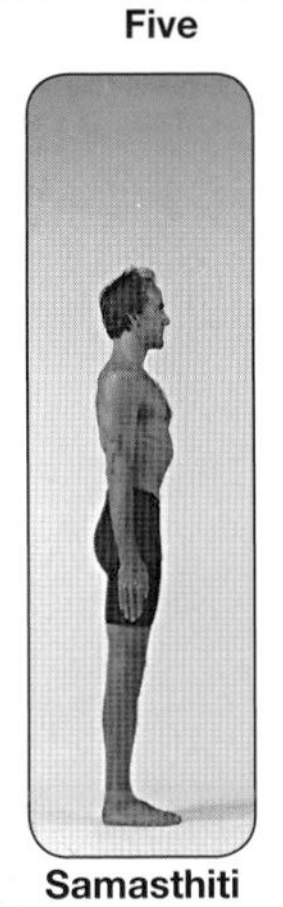
Samasthiti

Samasthiti - Stand with both feet together. Legs active. Spine long. Engage the bandhas. Breathe deep.

One - **Inhale** raising both arms. The lungs should be full just as the hands touch. Gaze at the thumbs.

Two - **Exhale** fold forward taking the chest toward the knees as you look toward the toes.

Three - **Inhale** lengthen the spine as you take your gaze to the horizon.

Four - **Exhale** step or jump back. Lower down while gazing straight ahead. You may take the knees down first or come directly toward the floor. You may either hover there or lay flat on the floor.

Five - **Inhale** straighten the arms and roll onto the tops of the feet. Knees lifted. Toes pointed.

Six - **Exhale** as you push the hips up. Lengthen the spine from your sacrum through the top of your head. Press the heels toward the floor and lift the kneecaps. Gaze at your navel. Engage the bandhas.

Remain Here for 5 Deep Breaths

Seven - **Inhale** as you either jump or walk the feet forward. Lengthen the spine and take your gaze to the horizon.

Eight - **Exhale** fold forward taking the chest toward the knees and your gaze toward the toes.

Nine - **Inhale** raising both arms high over the head until the palms touch. Gaze at the thumbs.

Samasthiti - **Exhale** lower your arms in preparation for the next Surya Namaskara or Vinyasa.

Surya Namaskara B

Samasthiti - Stand with both feet together. Legs active. Spine long. Engage the bandhas. Breathe deep.

One - **Inhale** as you bend your knees and raise both arms. Fill the lungs fully. Gaze at the thumbs.

Two - **Exhale** fold forward. Take the chest toward the knees as you straighten the legs.

Three - **Inhale** lengthen the spine as you take your gaze to the horizon.

Four - **Exhale** and either step or jump back. Lower down while keeping your gaze straight ahead. You may either hover one inch from the floor or take your torso fully down to the earth, whichever is most appropriate.

Five - **Inhale** straighten the arms and roll onto the tops of the feet. Engage the legs. Lift the chest high.

Six - **Exhale** as you push the hips up. Lengthen the spine from your sacrum through the top of your head.

Seven - **Begin** inhaling as you pivot the left heel in and press the outer edge of the foot down. Step forward with your right foot. Place it between or near your hands. Raise your hands over your head with the arms straight until the palms touch. Gaze at the thumbs.This entire sequence should comprise one **inhale**. If it is too much of a strain, then take an extra breath but work toward making it in one.

Eight - **Exhale** as you place your hands on the floor and lower your body down to the plank position. Either hover one inch from the floor or come all of the way down.

Nine - **Inhale** roll onto the tops of the feet. Straighten the arms with the legs engaged and the chest lifted.

Ten - **Exhale** as you push the hips up. Lengthen the spine from your sacrum through the top of your head.

Eleven - **Inhale** as you pivot the right heel and press the outer edge of the foot down. Step forward with the left foot placing it between or near your hands. Continue inhaling as you take your hands up over your head, arms straight. The breath should be complete when your palms touch. Control your breathing. Keep it connected with the movement. Gaze at the thumbs. This movement should comprise one **inhale**.

Twelve - **Exhale** as you place your hands on the floor and lower your body down to the plank position. Remember your option of either hovering or lowering all of the way down.

Thirteen - **Inhale** roll onto the tops of your feet and straighten the arms. Keep the legs engaged and the chest lifted high with the heart open. Stay with your breath as you ride from one phase to the next.

Fourteen - **Exhale** as you push the hips up. Lengthen the spine from your sacrum through the top of your head. Engage the muscles above the knees while pushing the heels toward the floor. Gaze at you navel.

Remain Here for 5 Deep Breaths

Fifteen - **Inhale** as you either jump or walk the feet toward the hands. Lengthen the spine as you gaze to the horizon.

Sixteen - **Exhale** fold forward lowering the chest toward the knees and your gaze toward the toes.

Seventeen - **Inhale** bend the knees and raise both arms over the head. Gaze at the thumbs.

Samasthiti - **Exhale** lower your arms and straighten the legs in preparation for the next Surya Namaskara or Vinyasa. Gaze straight ahead.

Surya Namaskara B

Samasthiti

One

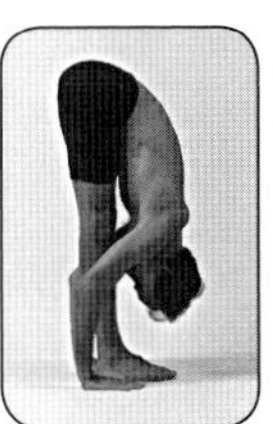

Two

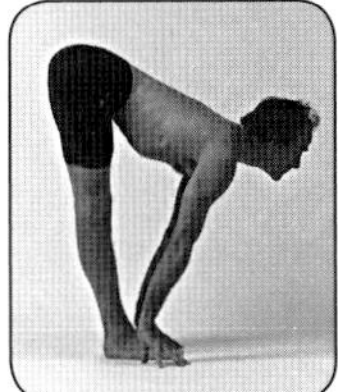

Three

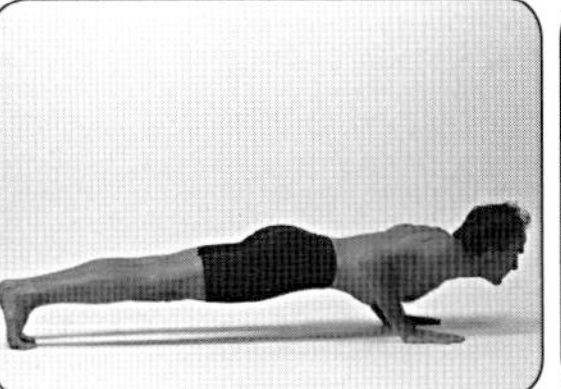

Four

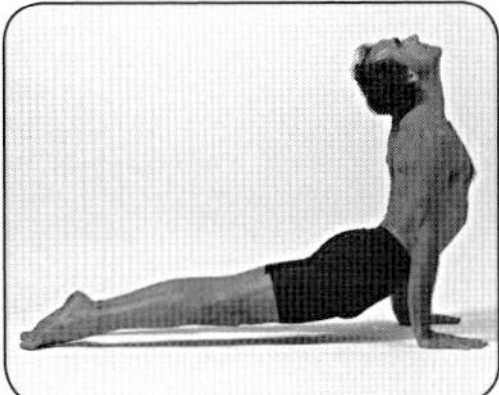

Five

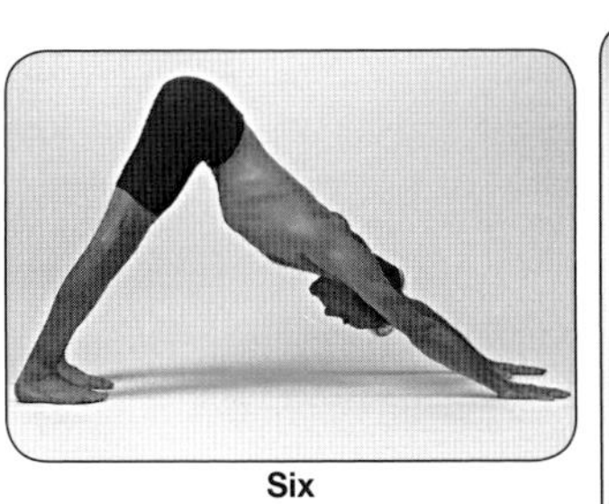

Six

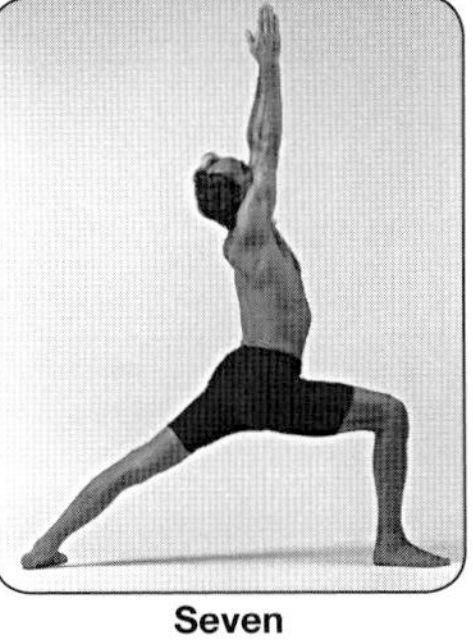

Seven

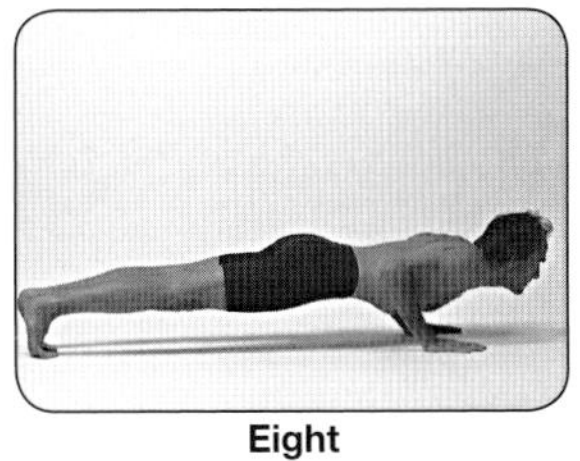

Eight

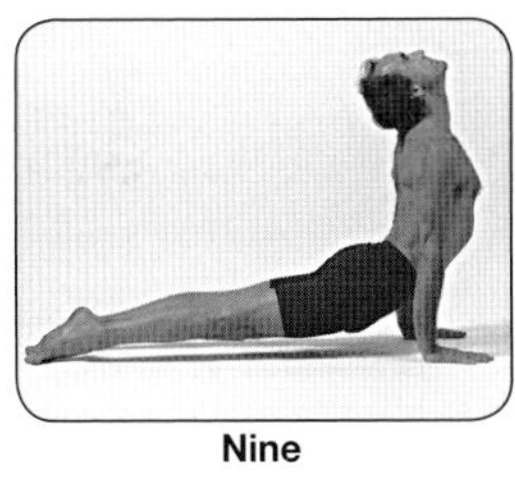

Nine

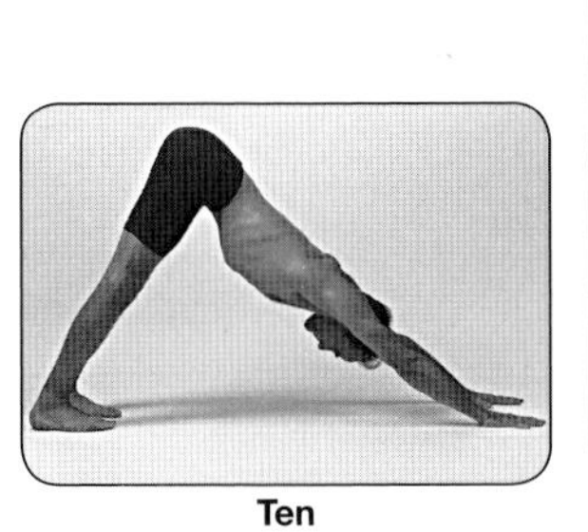

Ten

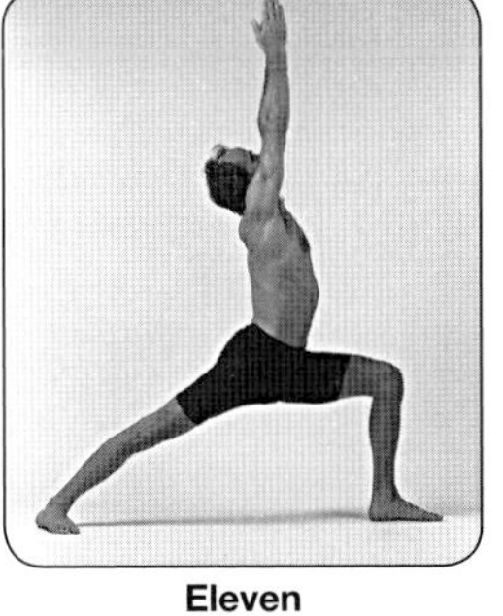

Eleven

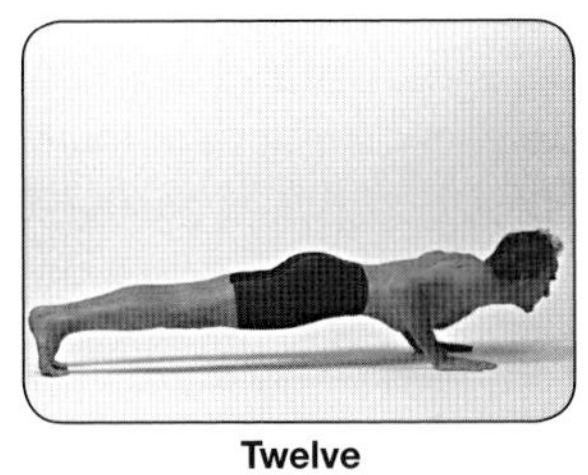

Twelve

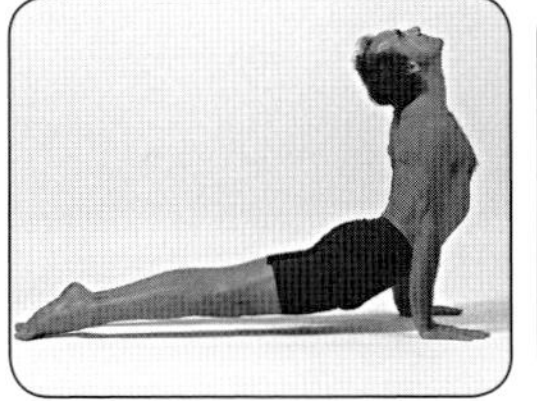

Thirteen

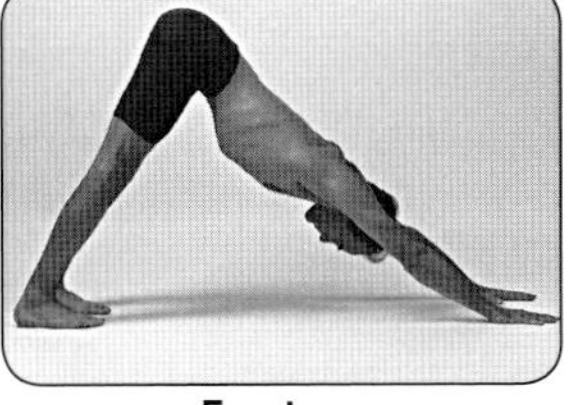

Fourteen
(Hold For 5 Breaths)

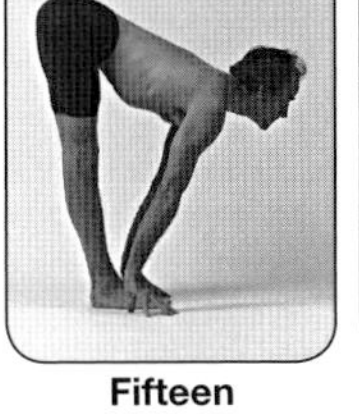

Fifteen

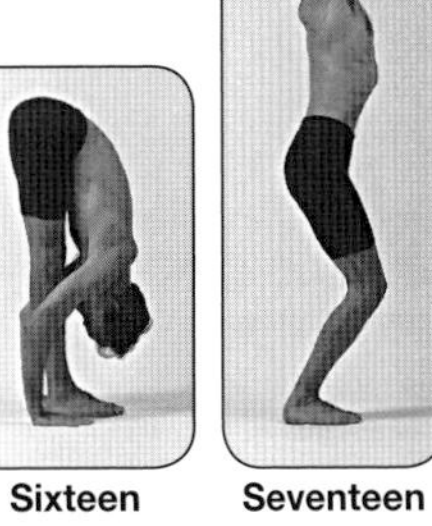

Sixteen

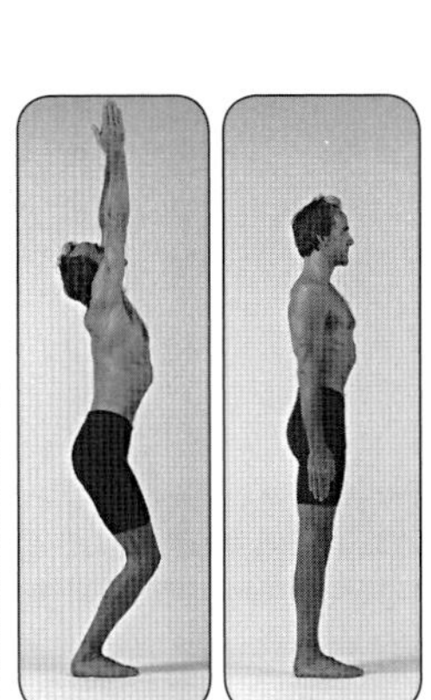

Seventeen

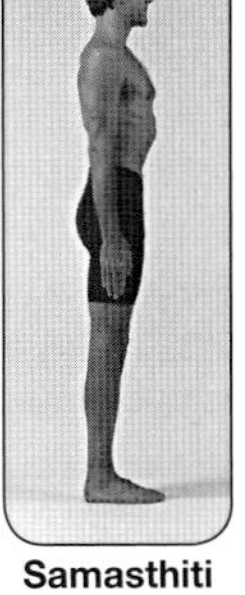

Samasthiti

Balance

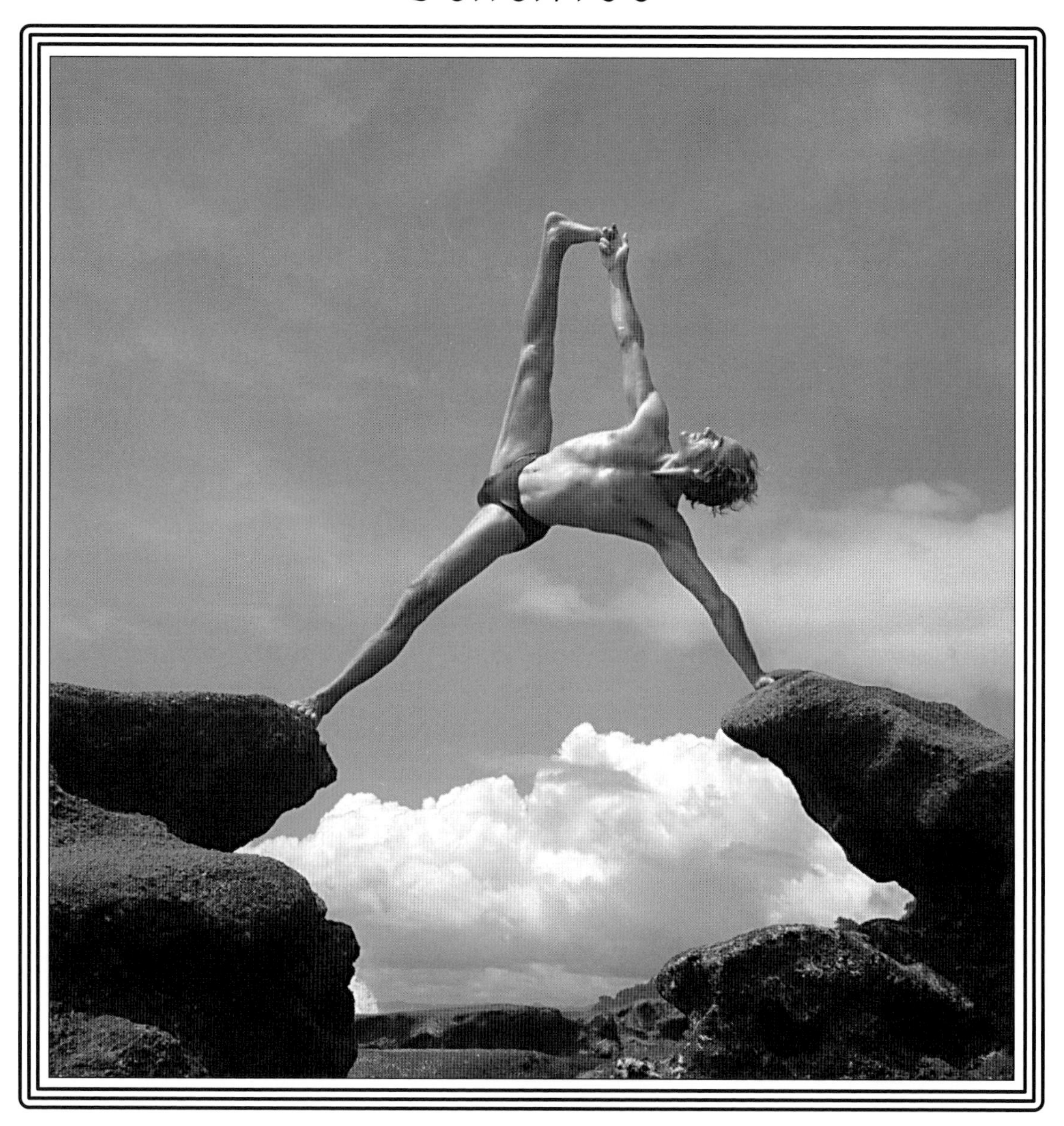

Vasishtasana
Advanced A Series
David Swenson ~ Costa Rica

The Standing Sequence

"Seeking the Balance"

The rhythm and the foundation for practice has been set through the flowing nature of **Surya Namaskara A and B**. The standing sequence initiates the weaving of one asana to the next to form, what K. Pattabhi Jois calls a garland of asanas. The sun salutations combined with the standing sequence act as one slice of bread. The second piece of bread is the finishing sequence which will be discussed later on.

In the standing sequence our balance is challenged and the understanding of how to work with the forces of gravity is developed. In all asanas there is a point of equality of opposition in which we may find the greatest sense of stability and comfort. This point may be discovered in the simultaneous rooting and rising energies within the body. In the standing sequence the feet are the roots of our body which reach far down into the earth in order to gain a stable foundation. From this base we may then grow and expand, lifting and lengthening into each asana. The soles of the feet become our connection with the earth. We must learn to feel that contact point. The triangle formed between the balls of the feet and the center of the heel is the region which we will draw upon for stability. From here the energy may rise up the legs and spread throughout the body. Be aware that over emphasis upon the lifting qualities of an asana will weaken the foundation and stability will become diminished. With an over-compensation of the rooting quality we will find it increasingly difficult to keep the body erect and lightness will be hindered.

Ideally we must **seek a balance** between these two forces in order to feel free in our expression of yoga. The practice of yoga is a perfect arena to explore the dynamics of balance in all things. Balance is more than just not falling over. It is the learning of an internal composure which translates into self-awareness. This internalization of understanding is an invaluable tool. It is not the external appearance of an asana that matters, but rather the internal level of balance achieved on both a physical and mental plane. The standing sequence is a laboratory to explore the physics of balance as understood on both the gross and subtle realms.

Balance Exists in the Equality of Oppositon

Padangusthasana

Pada = Foot   Angustha = Big Toe

"Foot Big Toe Posture"

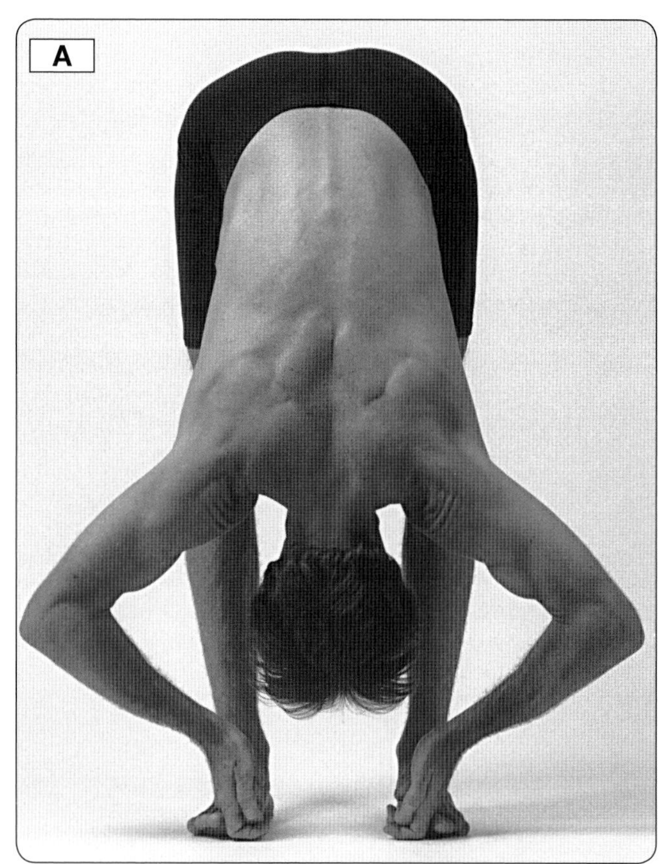

1) Inhale as you hop or step your feet to a hip-width distance apart.

2) Exhale place your hands on your waist.

3) **Inhale** as you lift your gaze to the sky and open your heart while keeping the shoulders back. ***(Do not collapse in the lower back)***

4) Exhale fold forward and clasp the big toes with two fingers of each hand **(A)** or take the hands behind the legs as in **(B)**. Another option is to rest the hands on the ankles with the knees bent and the ribs touching the thighs **(C)**.

5) Inhale look to the horizon and lengthen the spine.

6) Exhale while moving into whichever phase is most appropriate for you. Avoid rounding the back. Keep the neck long.

Remain Here For 5 Deep Breaths

7) Inhale lengthen the spine as you gaze to the horizon.

Enter the Next Asana from Here

Drishti ~ **Nose**

If you feel discomfort in an asana come out and return to your breath.
Never sacrifice the breath to achieve an asana.

If You Can't Breathe Fully You Shouldn't Be There!

Padangusthasana

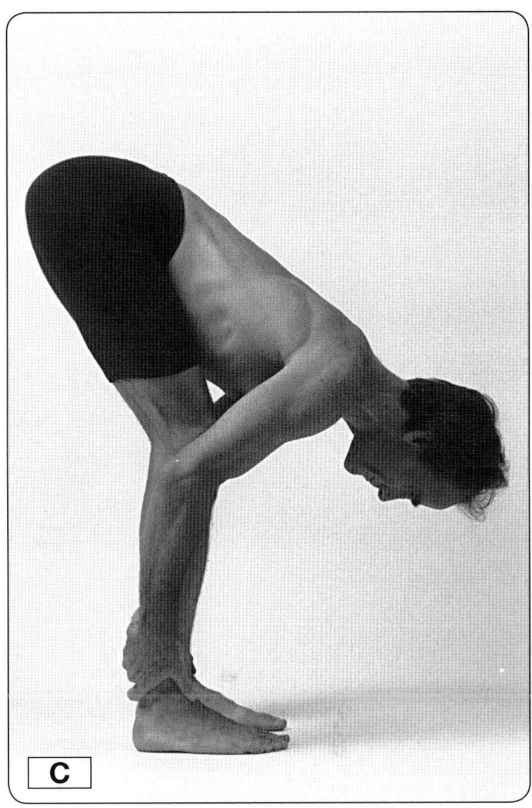

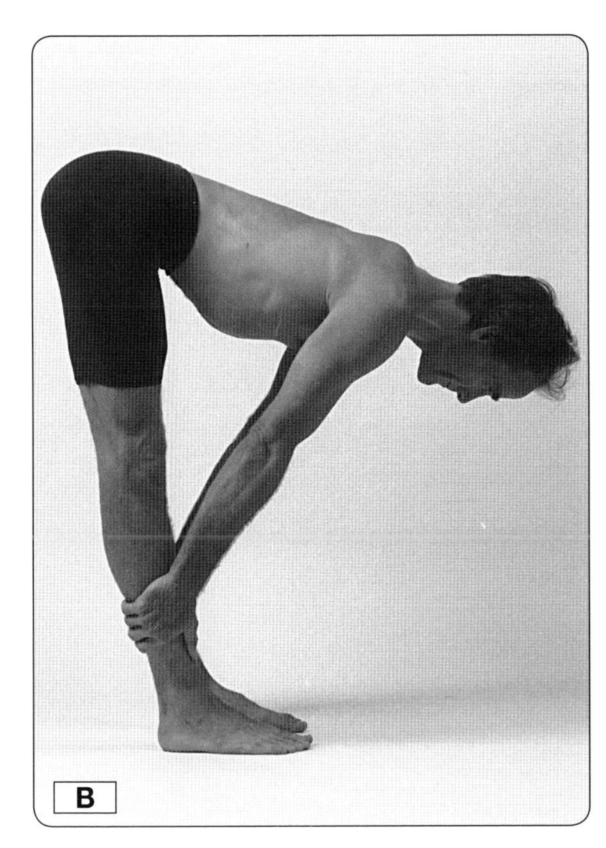

Comments - It is important in all forward-bending asanas to keep length in the spine. Tilt the upper pelvis forward slightly to avoid rounding in the lower back. The bandhas are a great aid in achieving this. Imagine that you have an eye in the middle of your chest at the sternum. Extend forward from that point. Position the "eye" in your chest so that it has a view of the toes. It is also beneficial to engage the quadriceps, above the knees, in order to release the hamstrings. In this way you may strengthen the front of the legs while lengthening the back side. If holding the toes, you may gently pull with the hands to deepen the asana but be aware of the potential of over-stretching. Keep your shoulders moving away from the ears as you point the elbows out to the sides. Lengthen the neck.

Padahastasana

Pada = Foot   Hasta = Hand

"Foot to Hand Posture"

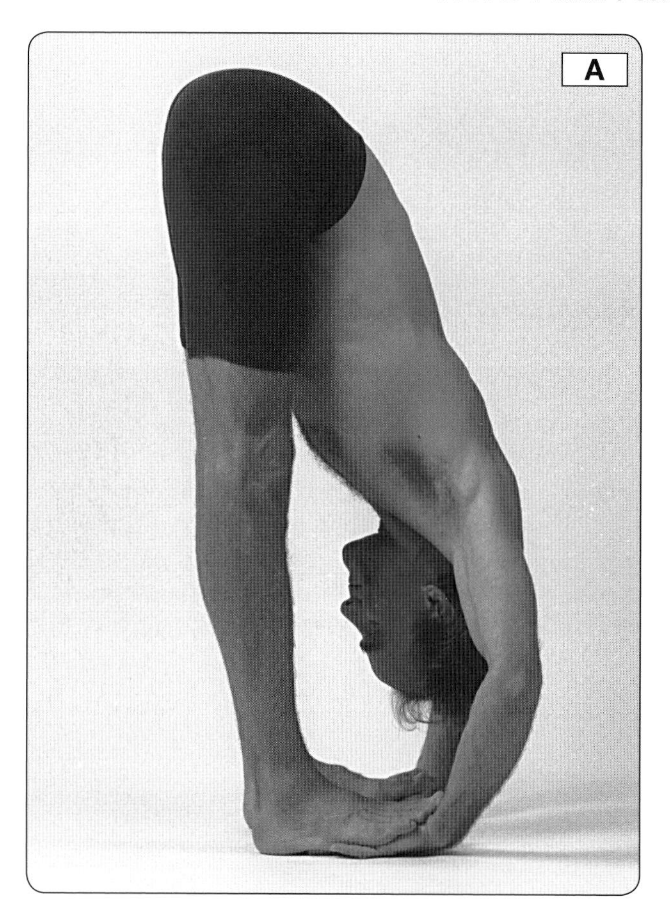

1) **Exhale** place the hands under the feet with the palms facing up and the toes touching the wrist crease **(A)**. If this is too extreme then take only the fingers under the feet **(B)** or bend your knees bringing the ribs onto the thighs **(C)**. You may also repeat one of the options from the previous posture.

2) **Inhale** look up and lengthen the spine.

3) **Exhale** fold forward.

Remain Here For 5 Deep Breaths

4) **Inhale** lengthen the spine as you gaze to the horizon.

5) **Exhale** bring your hands to your waist with a flat back and legs straight. If that is too intense then bend your knees slightly.

6) **Inhale** up to a standing position.

7) **Exhale** hop or step your feet together facing the front again.

Drishti ~ **Nose**

Feel the effect of the breath upon the asanas. Exhales tend to move us deeper and inhales encourage length and lightness.

Allow the Breath to be Your Guide

Padahastasana

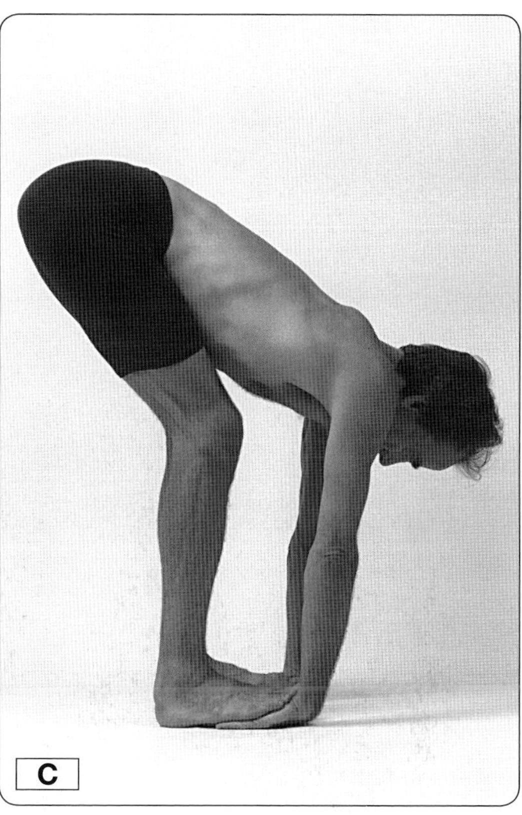

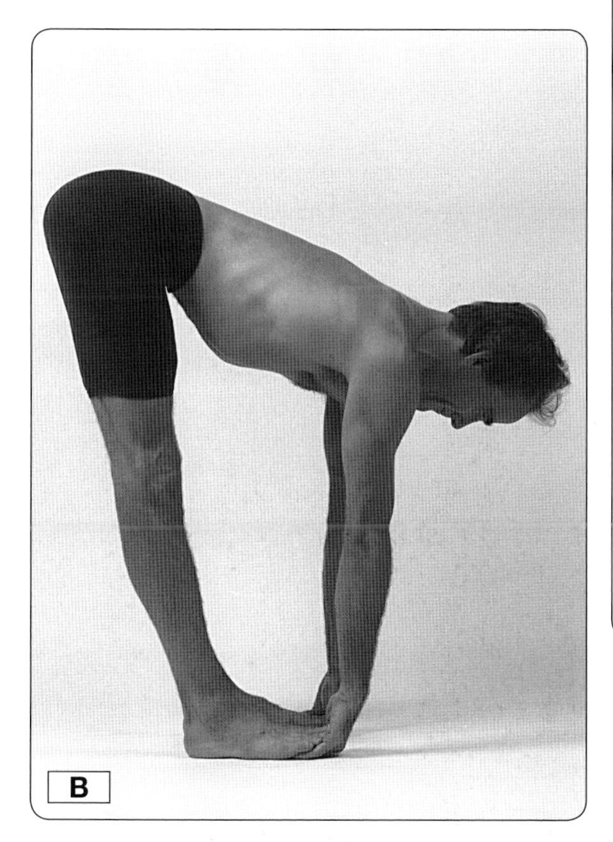

Comments - If you are choosing the **(A)** option for **Padahastasana** you may play a bit with the weight distribution of the feet. Transfer some of the weight from your heels toward the balls of your feet which are resting on the palms of your hands. You will feel an increase in the stretch on the hamstrings. **Do Not** push forward too much, however, due to the risk of falling over or putting undue pressure on your hands. Move only slightly and feel the difference in the dynamic of the asana. **Breathe Deep!**

Utthita Trikonasana

Utthita = Extended Tri = Three Kona = Angle

"Extended Triangle Posture"

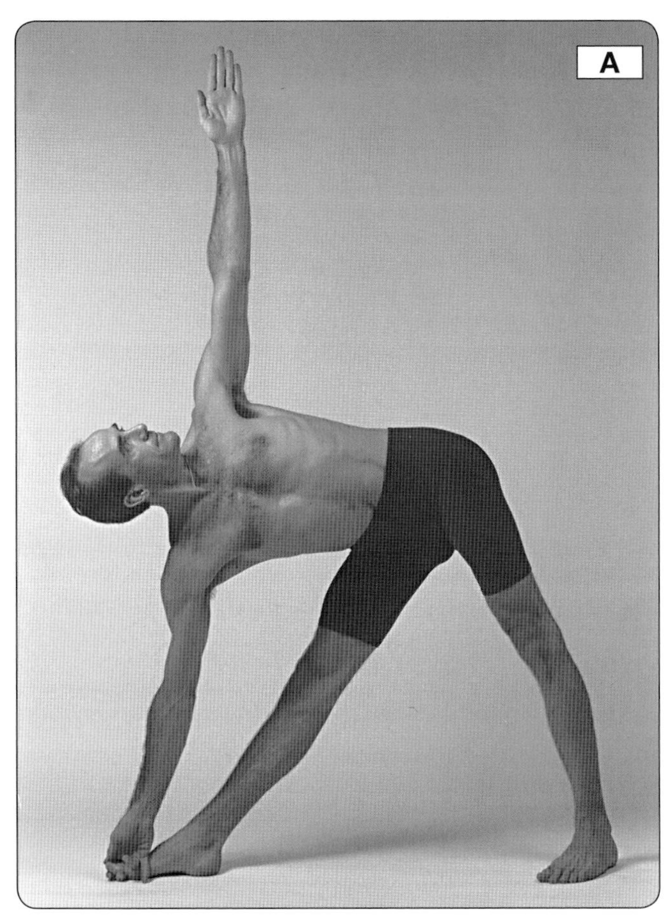

1) **Inhale** jump or step your feet a quarter turn to your right with arms outstretched. The feet should be positioned one leg-length apart.

2) **Exhale** as you turn your right foot out. Point it in the same direction as the right hand. Turn the left toes in slightly. Extend the right hand toward the right foot. Clasp the big toe with two fingers **(A)** or rest the right hand on your shin **(B)**. You may also use a block for support **(C)**. Keep the upper body aligned with the right leg. Rotate the torso while keeping the shoulders broad and the neck long.

Remain Here for 5 Deep Breaths

3) **Inhale** come up slowly. Turn the feet parallel.

4) **Exhale** lower into the other side as in **#2**.

Remain Here for Five Deep Breaths

5) **Inhale** come up slowly. Turn the feet parallel.

Enter the Next Asana from Here

Drishti ~ **Hand**

If the mind wanders bring it back to the sound, quality and texture of your breath.
Remain relaxed and present.

Each Asana and Each Breath is a Complete Journey

Utthita Trikonasana

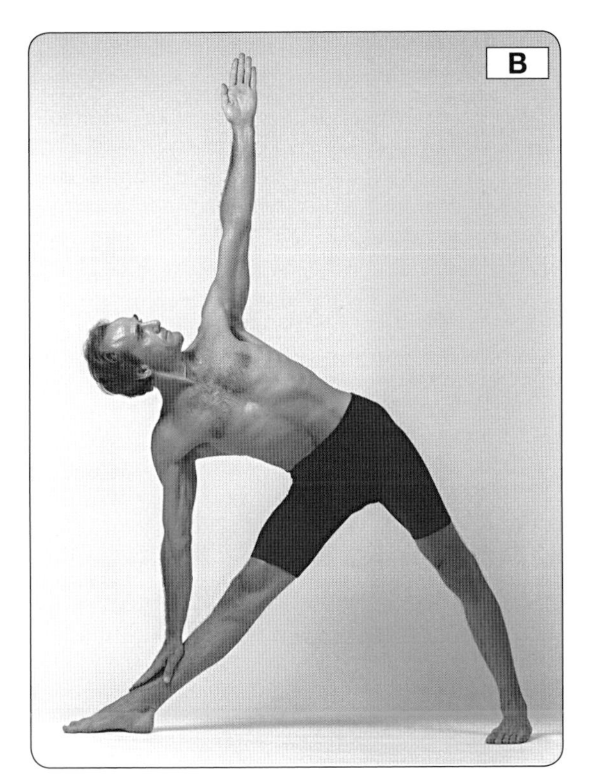

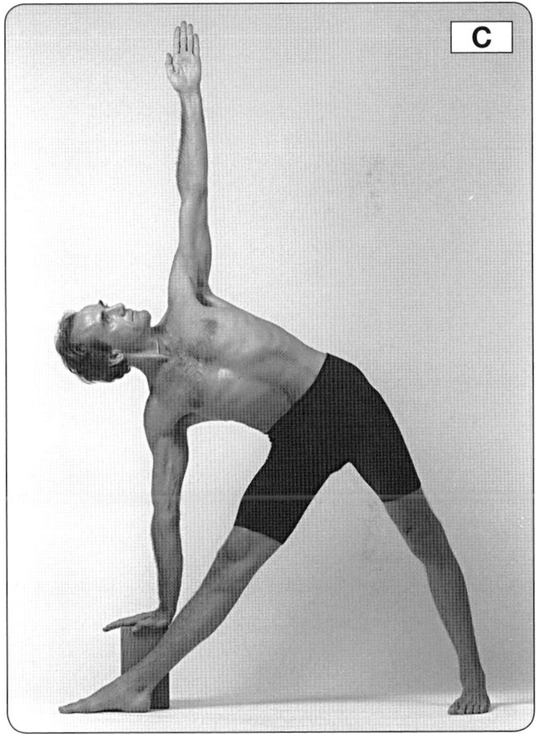

Comments - One of the challenges of this asana is to avoid collapsing in the lower back. Keep the torso rolling open so that it remains in line with the extended leg. This may mean that you will have to back off from clasping the toe until you are able to align the shoulders with the front leg. Be aware of the upper and lower ribs. Extend through both sides of the torso evenly to achieve balance. If you feel discomfort in the neck then gaze at the front foot instead of upward. Lengthen the spine from the base of the sacrum all of the way through the top of your head. Broaden the shoulders by sending energy through the arms and out the fingertips. Feel an equal weight distribution on both feet and press the balls of the feet into the floor. Keep the back foot grounded.

Parivritta Trikonasana

Parivritta = Revolved Tri = Three Kona = Angle

"Revolved Triangle Posture"

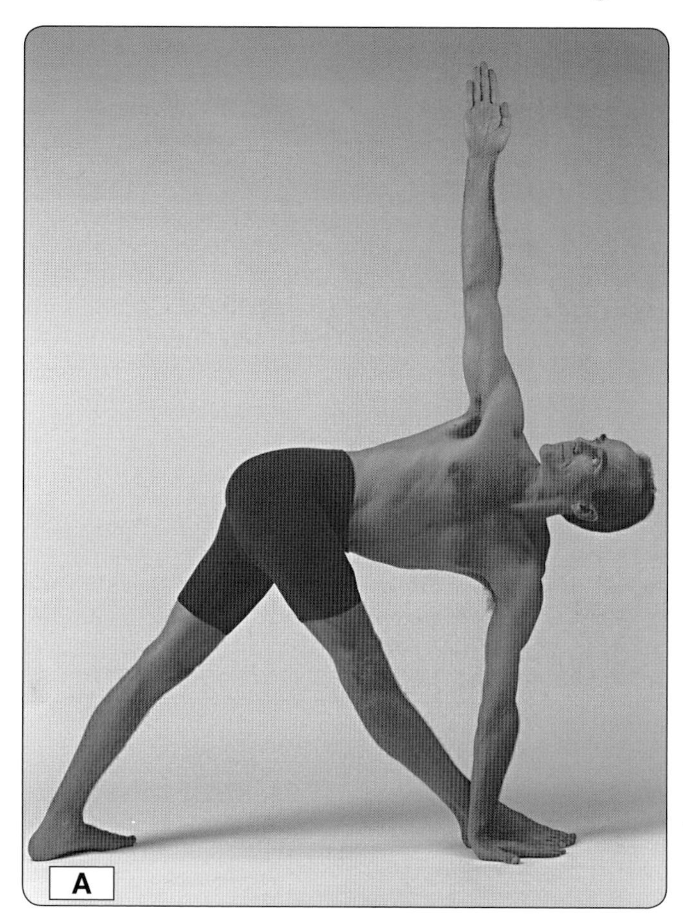

1) **Exhale** as you turn your right foot out pointing it in the same direction as the right hand. Turn the left toes in until the foot is at a forty-five degree angle. Square your hips to the right and take the arms around like a windmill. Place the left hand on the floor outside the right foot and press it into the floor **(A)**. If you are unable to reach the floor with the left hand then rest it on your shin **(B)** or take both hands to the right shin **(C)**. Broaden the shoulders. Move the right hip back and the left hip forward so that they are aligned. Keep both legs active. Keep the spine long as you rotate the torso. Gaze at the right thumb.

Remain Here for Five Deep Breaths

2) **Inhale** come up slowly. Turn the feet parallel.

3) **Exhale** lower into the other side as you did in **#1**.

Remain Here for Five Deep Breaths

4) **Inhale** come up slowly. Turn the feet parallel.

5) **Exhale** jump or step the feet together facing the front again.

Drishti ~ **Hand in A & B or Toes in C**

Can you feel the locks working? What is their effect on each asana?
Find and create avenues of length from the sacrum to the top of the head.

Feel the Internal Flow of Prana and Expand With It

Parivritta Trikonasana

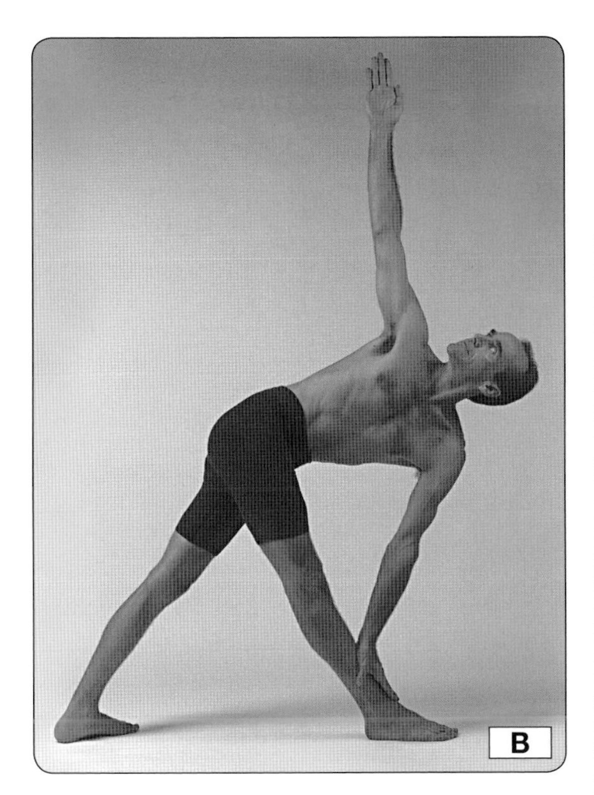

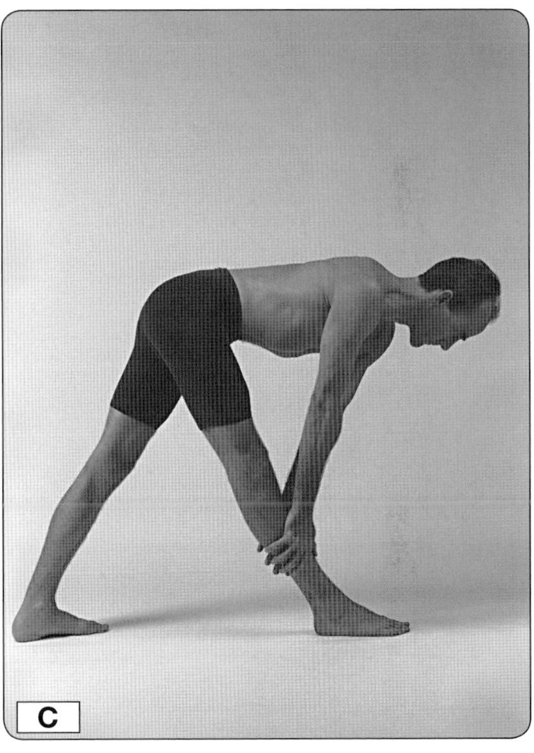

Comments - For this revolving version of the triangle posture it is important to lengthen the spine in a **spiraling** motion from the sacrum through the top of the head. This may be achieved by squaring the hips and then extending through both sides of the torso evenly. Distribute the weight equally across the base of both feet. Broaden the shoulders by pressing the hand firmly into the floor. Take that energy across the shoulders and shoot it out the fingertips of the upward extended hand. Move the right hip back as you pull the left hip forward until they come into balance. Work the base of the big toes.

Utthita Parsvakonasana

Utthita = Extended   Parsva = Side   Kona = Angle

"Extended Side Angle Posture"

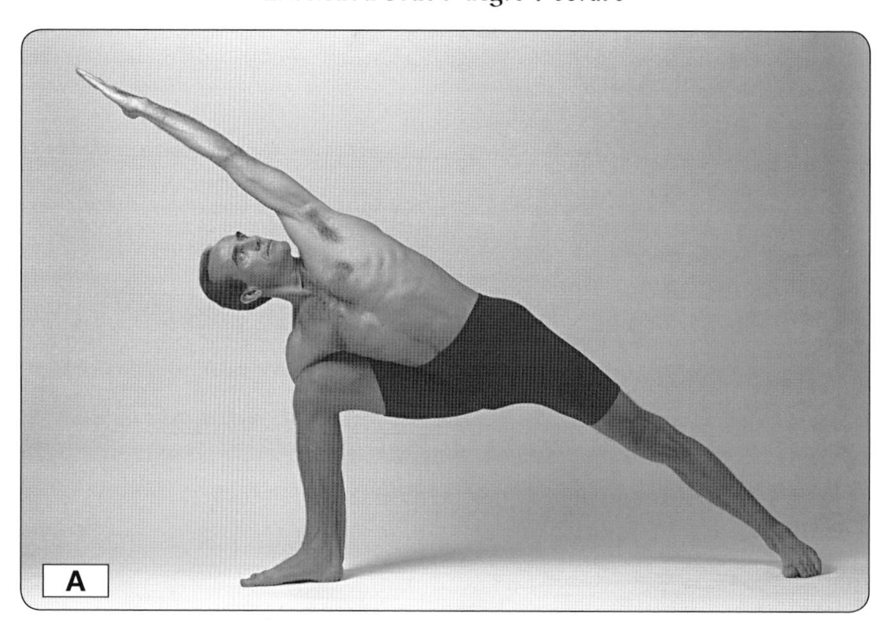
A

1) **Inhale** jump or step your feet a quarter turn to the right with the arms outstretched. Position the feet wider than the previous posture. Eventually the feet should be aligned under the wrists with the distance between them being greater than the length of one of your legs.

2) **Exhale** as you turn your right foot out. Point it in the same direction as the right hand. Turn the left foot in slightly. Bend the right leg until the knee is directly above the heel. Lower the right hand to the floor outside the right foot **(A)** or place the right forearm on top of the knee **(B)**. You may also use a block to support the right hand **(C)**. Lengthen and rotate the torso. Left arm beside the head. Back foot flat.

Remain Here for Five Deep Breaths

3) **Inhale** come up slowly. Turn the feet parallel.

4) **Exhale** lower into the other side as in **#2**.

Remain Here for Five Deep Breaths

5) **Inhale** come up slowly. Feet parallel.

Enter the Next Asana from Here

Drishti ~ **Hand**

Utthita Parsvakonasana

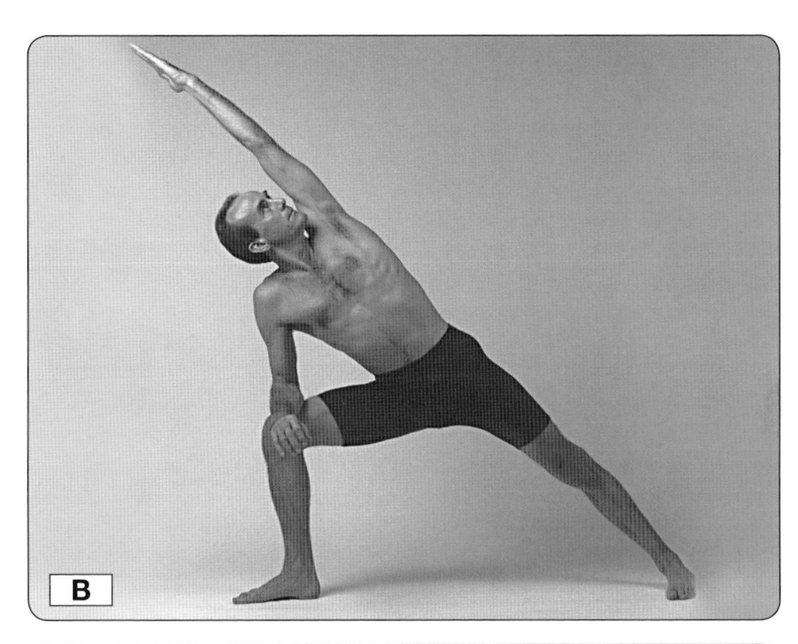

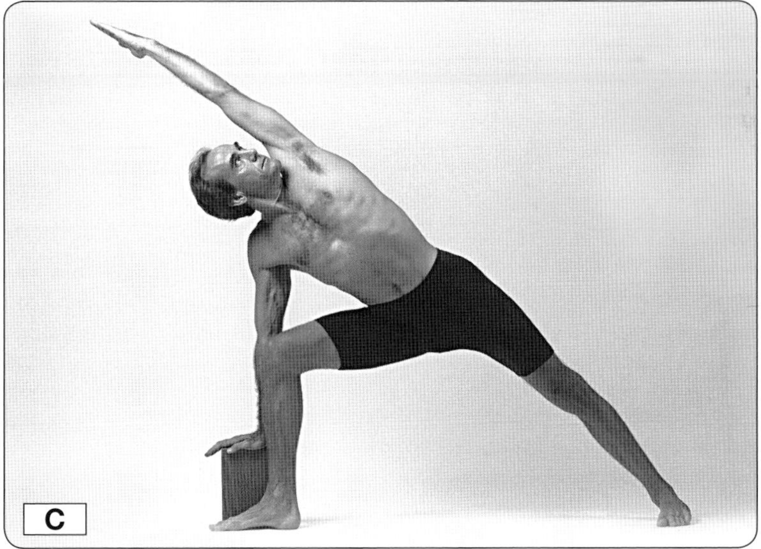

Comments - For the **(A)** version press the front knee against the arm to increase the rotation of the torso. In all variations create length from the outer edge of the back foot to the fingertips of the upper arm. Keep the neck long.

Parivritta Parsvakonasana

Parivritta = Revolved Parsva = Side Kona = Angle

"Revolved Side Angle Posture"

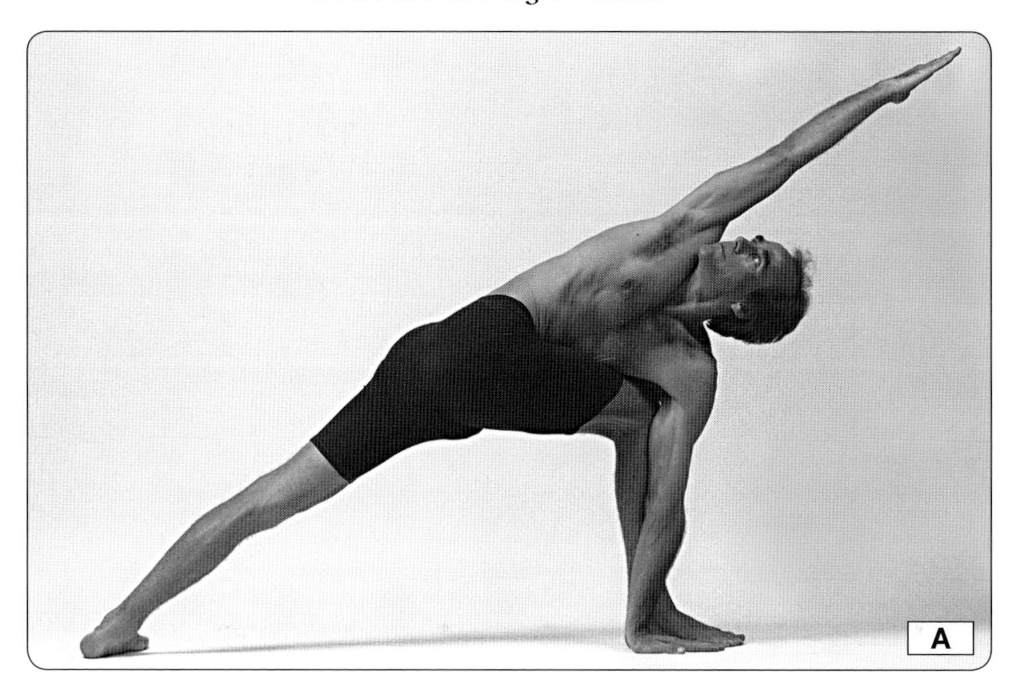

1) **Exhale** turn your right foot out. Point it in the same direction as the right hand. Turn the left foot in slightly. Bend the right leg. Keep the knee directly above the heel. Bring your left elbow to the outside of the right knee. Keep the back foot flat on the floor by pressing the outer edge down. Either place the left hand on the floor outside the right foot **(A)** or place the palms together and point the right elbow to the sky **(B)**. Gaze at the fingertips in **(A)** or in the direction that the right elbow is pointing in **(B)**. If necessary you may lower the left knee to the floor for additional support as in **(C)**.

Remain Here for Five Deep Breaths

2) **Inhale** come up slowly. Turn the feet parallel.

3) **Exhale** lower into the other side as in **#1**.

Remain Here for Five Deep Breaths

4) **Inhale** release and come up slowly. Feet parallel.

5) **Exhale** jump or step the feet together. Face the front of your mat in preparation for the next asana.

Drishti ~ **Hand in A & C or Upward in B**

Parivritta Parsvakonasana

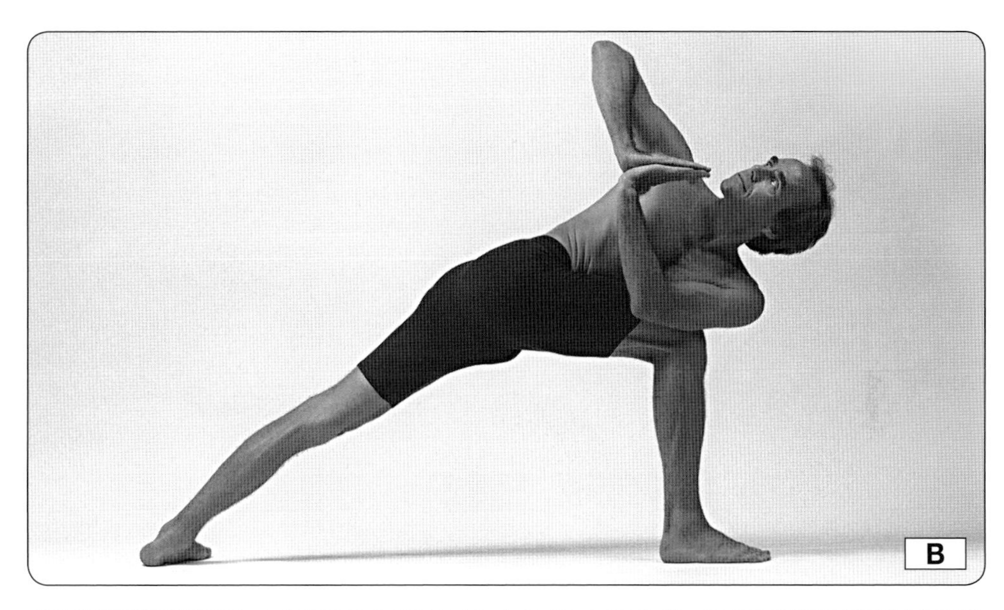
B

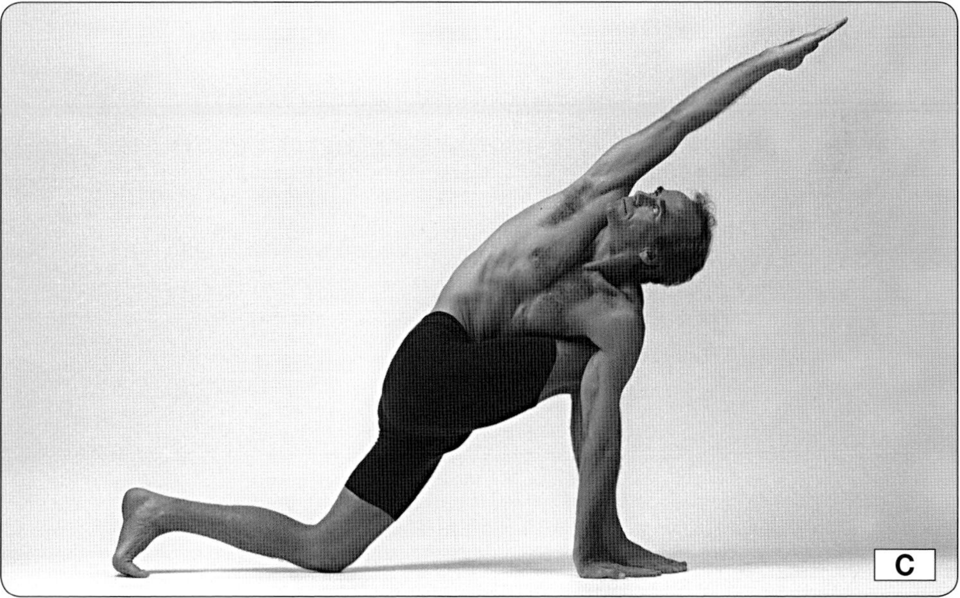
C

Comments - Use opposing forces between the arm and the knee to create a more stable rotation of the torso. Lengthen the spine from the sacrum through the top of the head to create a spiraling motion.

Prasarita Padottanasana A

Prasarita = Spread Out   Pada = Foot   Uttana = Intense Stretch

"Feet Spread Intense Stretch Posture"

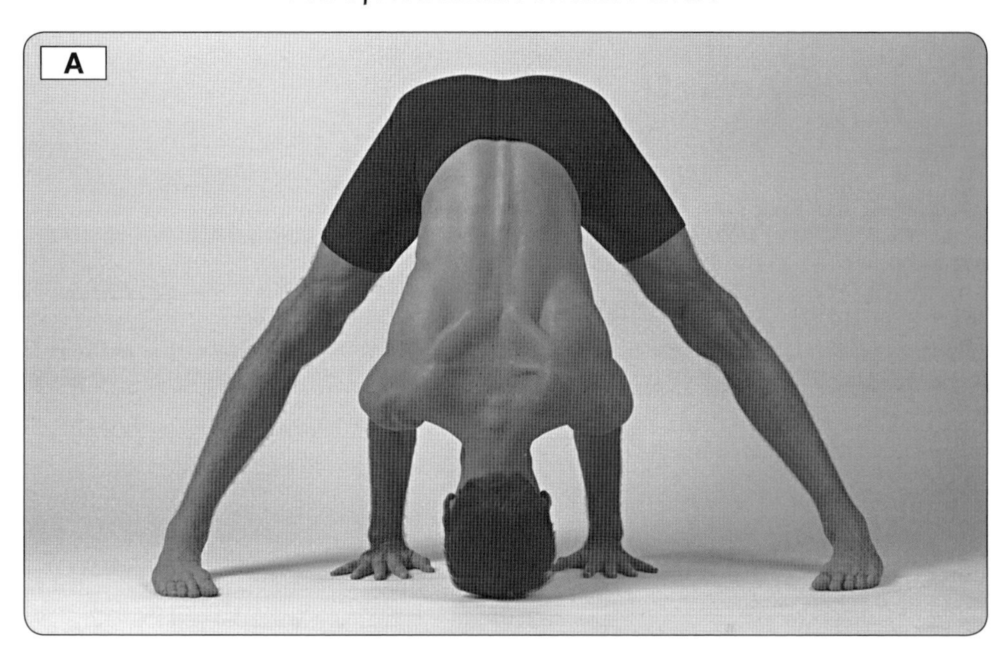

1) **Inhale** jump or step a quarter turn to your right. The feet should be the same distance apart as the previous posture with the outer edges of the feet parallel. Arms outstretched, parallel to the floor.

2) **Exhale** lower your hands to your waist.

3) **Inhale** lift your chest. Open the heart and gaze upward. **Do not collapse in the lower back**.

4) **Exhale** fold forward, hands to the floor between the feet with the legs active **(A)** or rest your hands on the shins **(B)**. You may also bend the knees and take the hands to the floor **(C)**.

5) **Inhale** as you lengthen the spine and gaze to the horizon.

6) **Exhale** fold into the posture at the appropriate level for you as shown in **(A)**, **(B)**, or **(C)**.

Remain Here For 5 Deep Breaths

7) **Inhale** lengthen the spine and gaze to the horizon.

8) **Exhale** bring your hands to your waist with a flat back.

9) **Inhale** come all of the way up to standing.

Enter Prasarita Padottanasana 'B' from Here

Drishti ~ **Nose**

Prasarita Padottanasana A

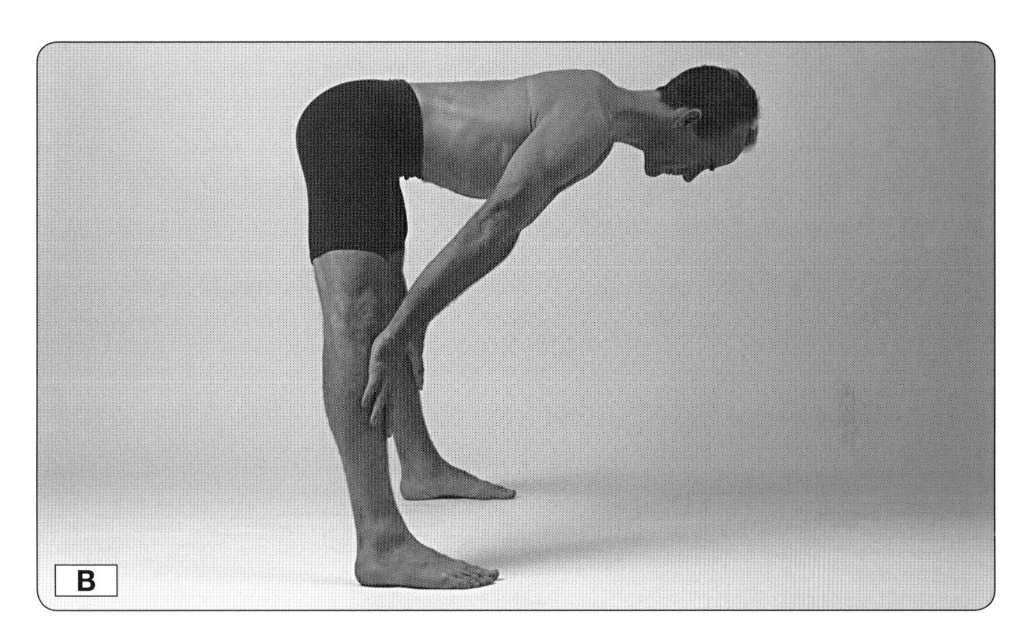

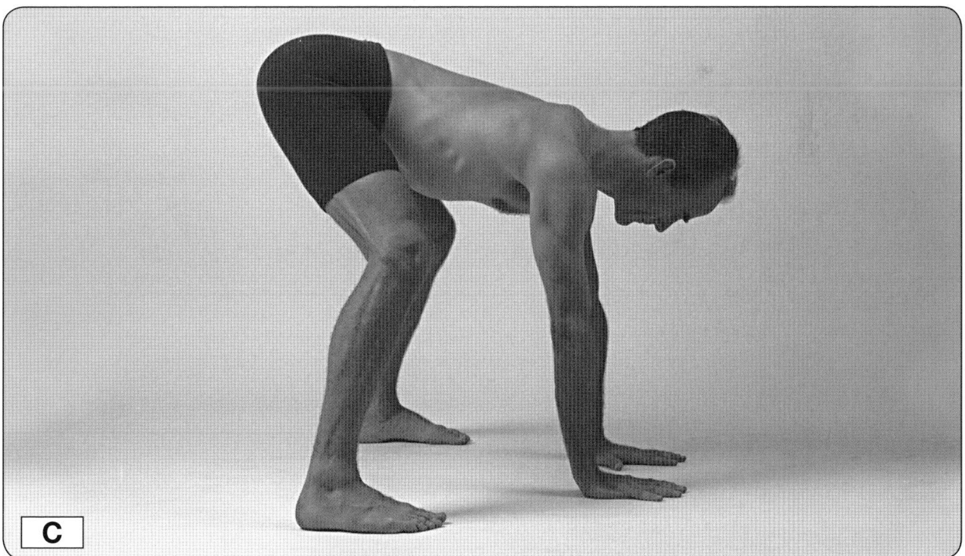

Comments - Avoid rounding the back. Use the hands against the floor or against the legs to assist in creating greater length in the spine. This will support the lower back. This support is enhanced by the engagement of your bandhas. Keep both legs active. **Breathe!**

Prasarita Padottanasana B

Prasarita = Spread Out   Pada = Foot   Uttana = Intense Stretch

"Feet Spread Intense Stretch Posture"

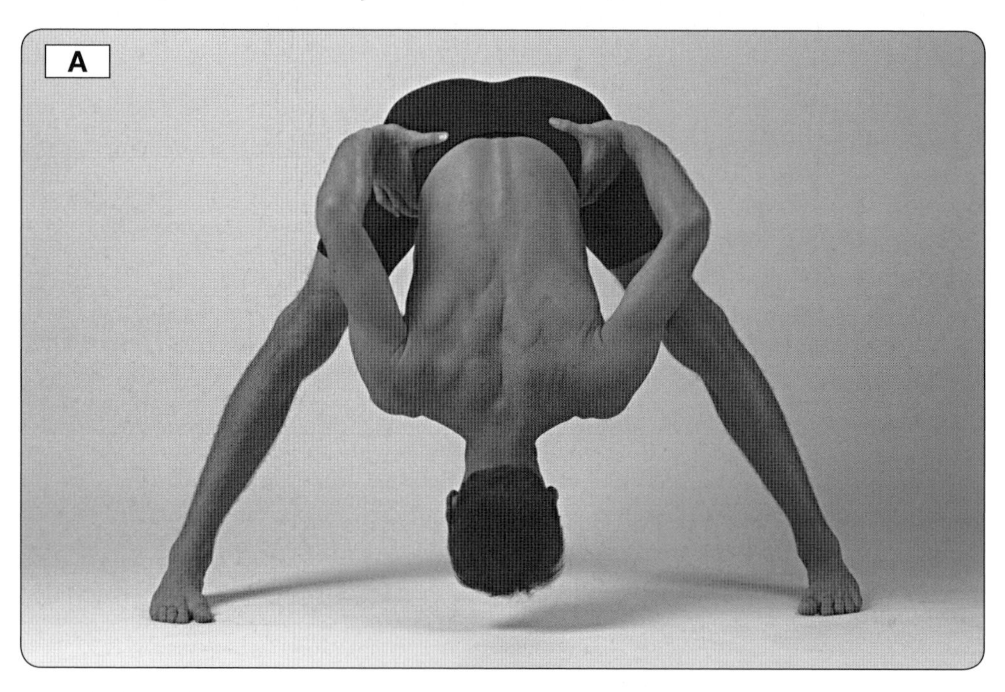

1) **Exhale** fold forward keeping the hands on your waist and the legs straight as the upper body pulls through the legs **(A)** or fold only halfway down **(B)**. A third option is to bend the knees and take the elbows to the thighs for support as in **(C)**.

Remain Here For 5 Deep Breaths

2) **Inhale** come all of the way up to standing. Move slowly so as not to become dizzy.

Enter Prasarita Padottanasana 'C' from Here

Drishti ~ **Nose**

Prasarita Padottanasana B

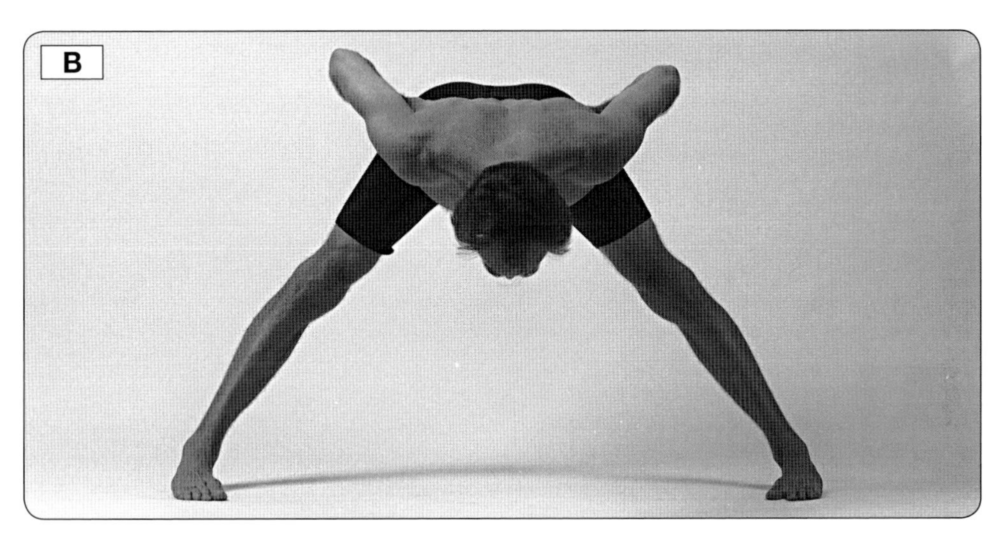

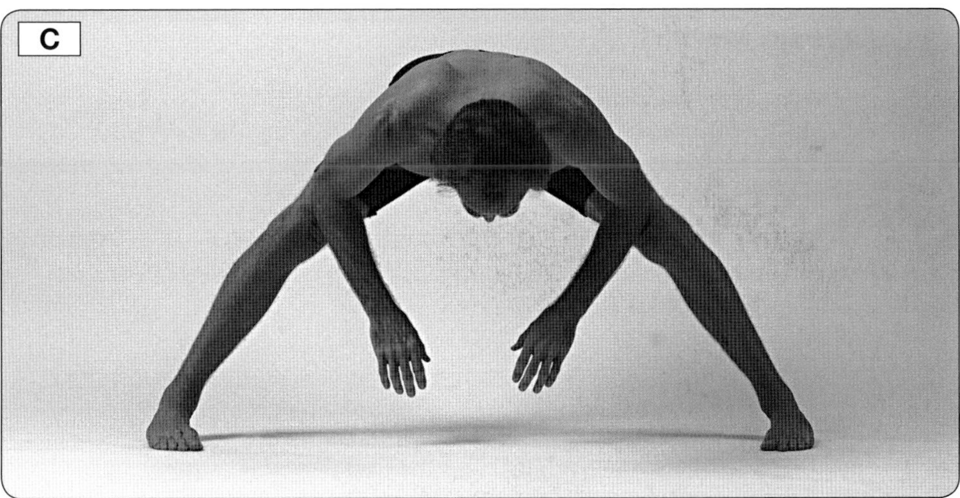

Comments - Use your bandhas and the quadriceps to assist in finding greater depth and stability in this asana. Feel the feet fully grounded so that the weight is evenly distributed across the balls of the feet and heels. Maintain firm contact at the base of the big toes. Keep your eyes open and the neck long with the shoulders broad. Avoid the tendency for the shoulders to raise toward the ears. Use your breath to find your way further into the asana. With each **exhale** you may travel a bit deeper and with each **inhale** the spine may lengthen slightly more. In this way there is a sensation of settling into the asana by riding upon each breath.

Prasarita Padottanasana C

Prasarita = Spread Out   Pada = Foot   Uttana = Intense Stretch

"Feet Spread Intense Stretch Posture"

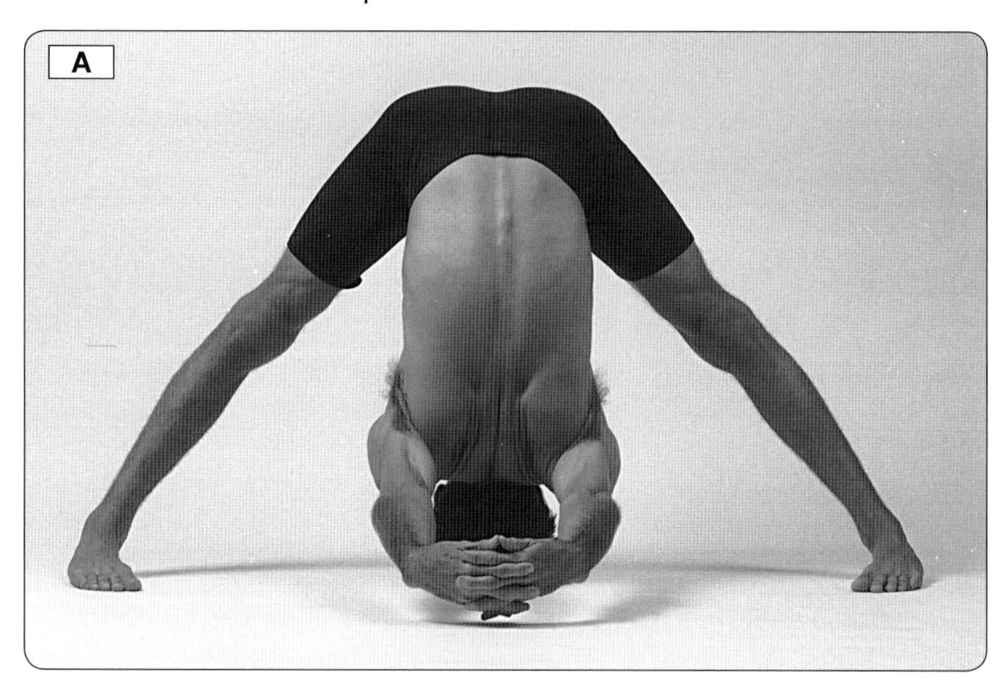
A

1) **Exhale** clasp the hands behind the back by interlacing the fingers and straightening the arms. If this is too much just hold your elbows.

2) **Inhale** lift the chest. Open the heart and raise your gaze.

3) **Exhale** fold forward pulling the hands to the floor with the legs straight **(A)** or part of the way down with the knees slightly bent **(B)** or you may choose to hold the elbows instead of clasping the hands **(C)**.

Remain Here For 5 Deep Breaths

4) **Inhale** come all of the way up to standing. Rise slowly with control and breathe fully to avoid dizziness.

5) **Exhale** take your hands to your waist in preparation to enter the next asana.

Enter Prasarita Padottanasana 'D' from Here

Drishti - **Nose**

Prasarita Padottanasana C

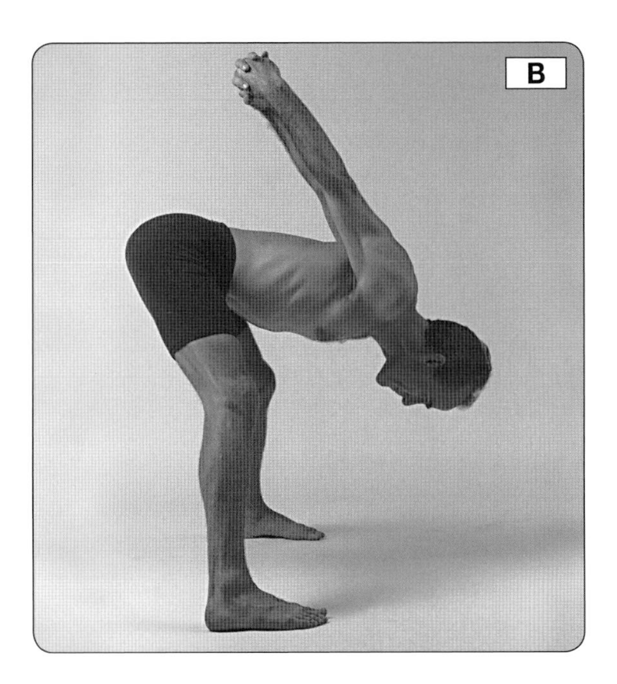

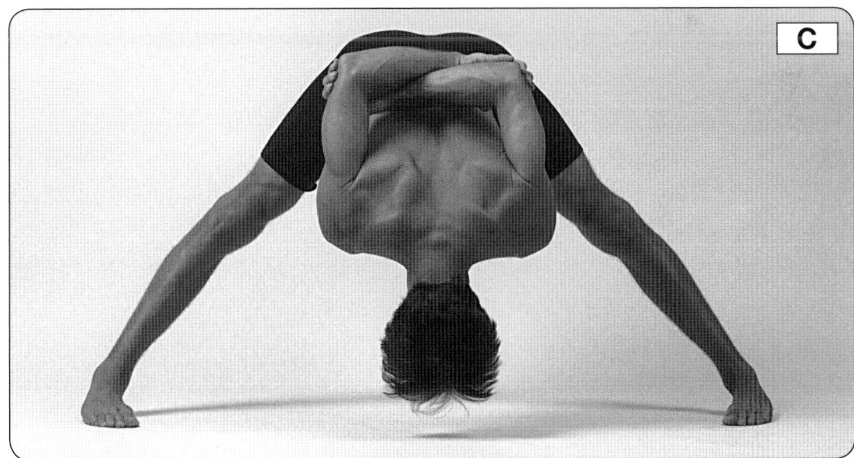

Comments - Use the force of gravity to assist you. Allow your body to follow the natural downward pull as the hands move closer to the floor. Keep the legs active to create a balanced foundation. Just as in the previous variations of **Prasarita Padottanasana** it is important to engage the bandhas fully in order to find the maximum level of stability. Distribute the weight evenly across the bottom of each foot. Do not grip with the toes. If you feel discomfort on the back of your knees you may bend them slightly.

Prasarita Padottanasana D

Prasarita = Spread Out   Pada = Foot   Uttana = Intense Stretch

"Feet Spread Intense Stretch Posture"

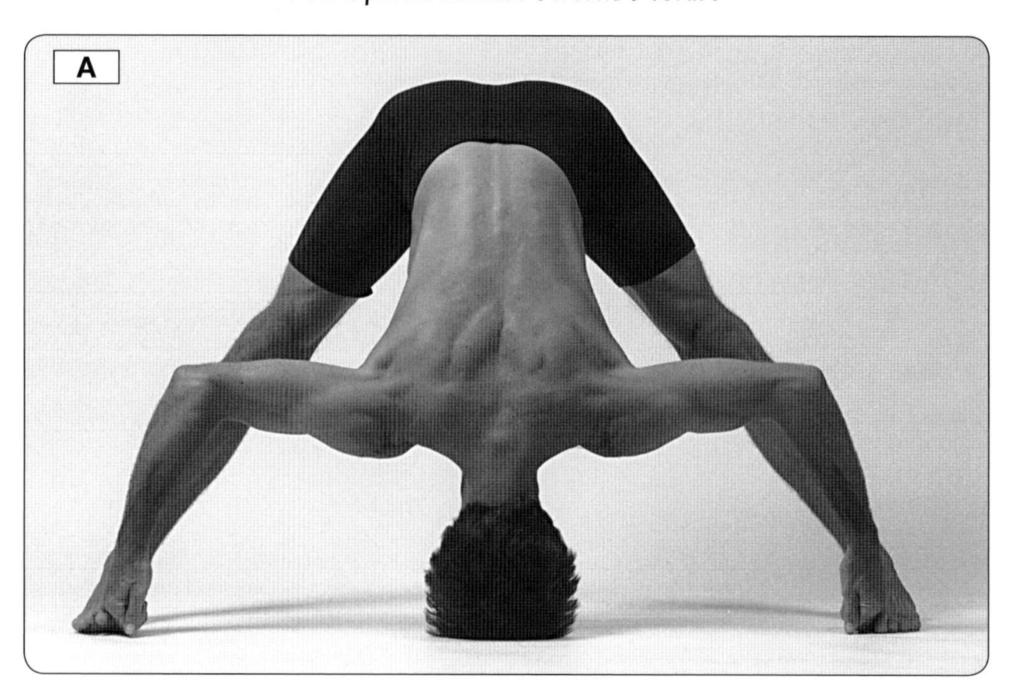

1) **Inhale** lift your chest. Open the heart and gaze upward. Use your bandhas to support the lower back.

2) **Exhale** fold forward and clasp the big toes with two fingers of each hand **(A)** or rest your hands on the shins or above the knees **(B)**. You may also take the hands to the floor **(C)**.

3) **Inhale** as you lengthen the spine and gaze to the horizon.

4) **Exhale** fold into the posture at the appropriate level for you by choosing either **(A)**, **(B)**, or **(C)**.

Remain Here For 5 Deep Breaths

5) **Inhale** lengthen the spine and gaze to the horizon.

6) **Exhale** bring your hands to your waist with a flat back.

7) **Inhale** come all of the way up to standing.

8) **Exhale** jump or step your feet together again facing the front in preparation for the next asana.

Drishti ~ **Nose**

Prasarita Padottanasana D

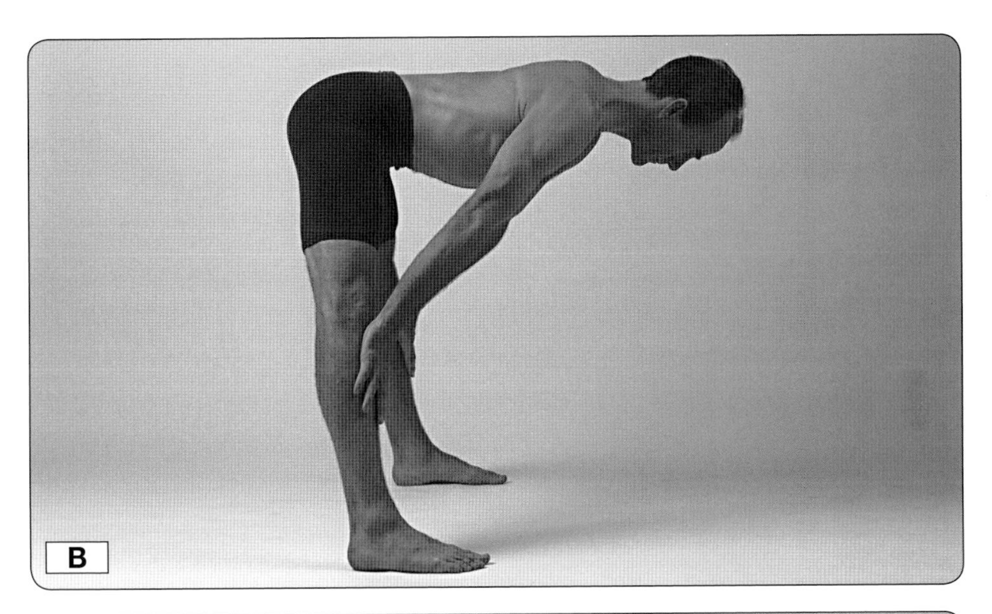

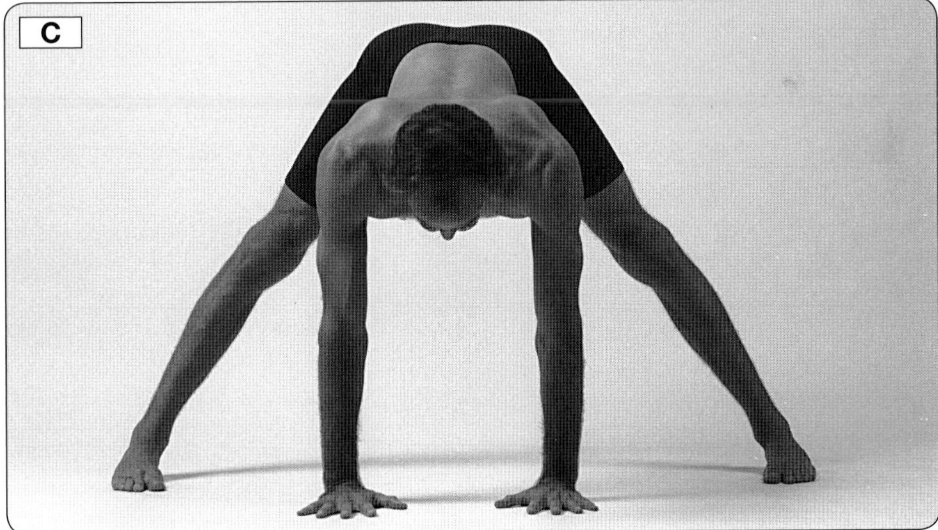

Comments - For option **(A)** use the fingers to pull against the toes to broaden the shoulders and pull the chest through the legs. In all options maintain length in the spine, strong bandhas and deep breathing. If you feel too much strain on the outer ankles you may bring the feet a bit closer together. Engage the adductor muscles on the inner legs to avoid rolling out onto the outer edges of the feet. Keep the balls of the feet firmly planted on the floor. The neck is an extention of the spine so keep it lengthening as you seek depth.

Parsvottanasana

Parsva = Side   Uttana = Intense Stretch

"Intense Side Stretch Posture"

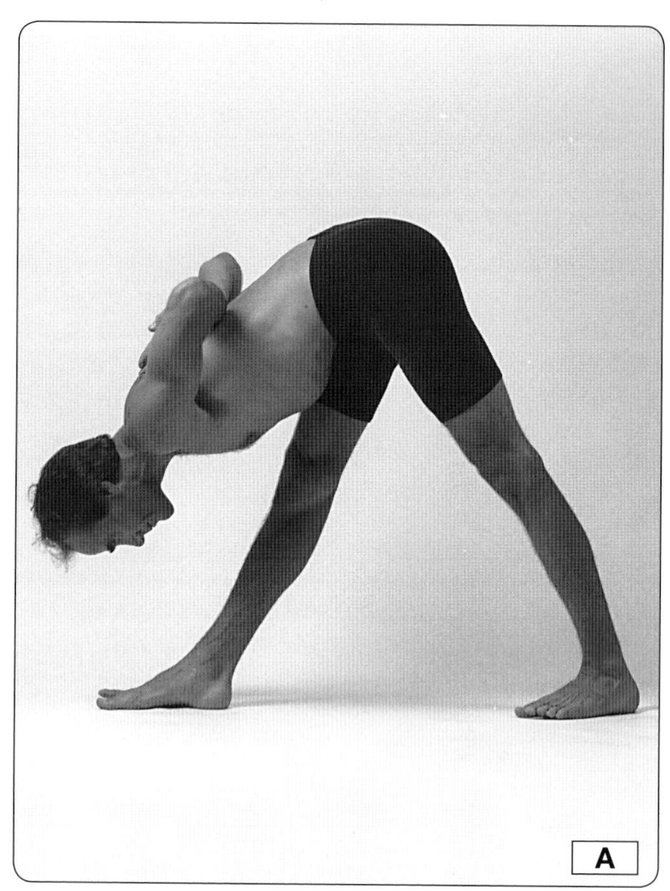

1) **Inhale** and hop or step a quarter turn to your right with one leg-length distance between the feet. Arms up.

2) **Exhale** pivot the feet. Turn the right foot out ninety degrees and turn the left foot into a forty-five degree angle. Square the hips. Arms behind the back in prayer-fashion or clasp the elbows.

3) **Inhale** open the heart. Look up.

4) **Exhale** fold out over the right leg leading with your chest. Keep both legs straight and take the ribs toward the thigh **(A)**. Otherwise come only halfway down **(B)** or bend the front leg slightly **(C)**. If it is too much to place the hands in prayer-fashion then you may hold the elbows instead **(D)**.

Remain Here For 5 Deep Breaths

5) **Inhale** up. Turn the feet parallel.

6) **Exhale** turn the left foot out ninety degrees and the right foot in to forty-five degrees. Square the hips.

7) **Inhale** and lift your chest.

8) **Exhale** and fold out over the left leg. Choose an option from **#4**.

Remain Here For 5 Deep Breaths

9) **Inhale** come up.

10) **Exhale** take the hands to your waist. Turn the feet parallel.

11) **Inhale** arms outstretched.

12) **Exhale** jump or step your feet together facing the front. Lower the arms to your sides in preparation to enter the next asana.

Drishti ~ **Nose**

Parsvottanasana

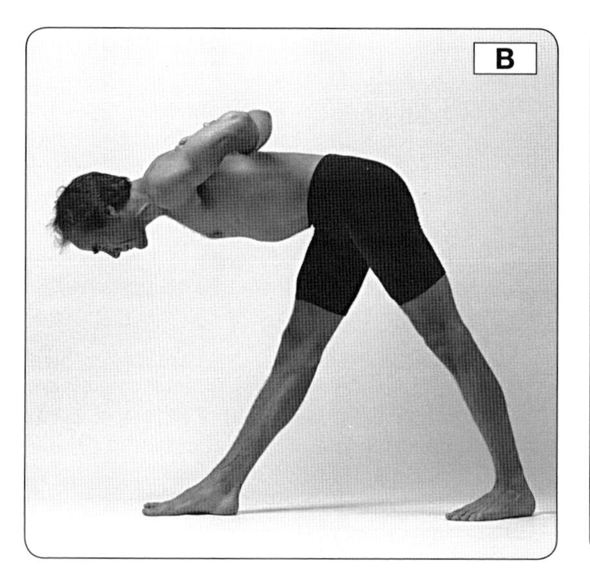

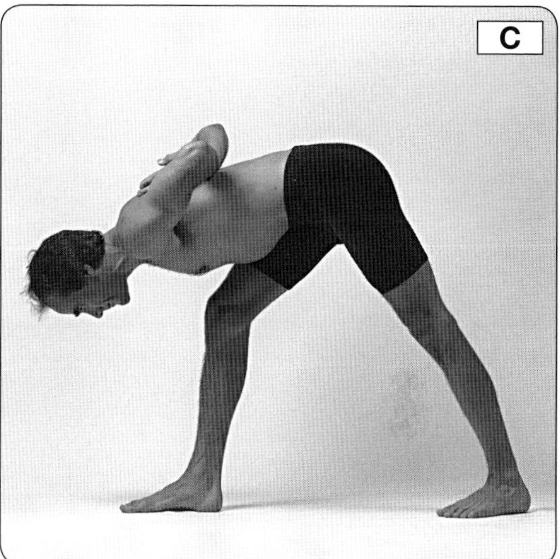

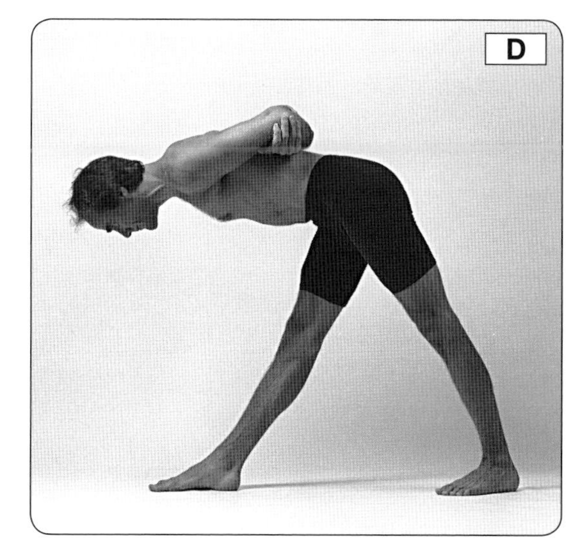

Comments - Lead with your sternum. If you had a flashlight in the middle of your chest it should be shining on the toes of the front foot. Roll the shoulders back to keep the heart area open. Lengthen the neck. Keep the hips squared with both legs active. Press the base of the big toe of the front foot into the floor while keeping the back foot fully grounded. Let the exhales draw you deeper and feel the inhales creating greater length.

Utthita Hasta Padangusthasana A

Utthita = Extended   Hasta = Hand   Padangustha = Big Toe

"Extended Hand Big Toe Posture"

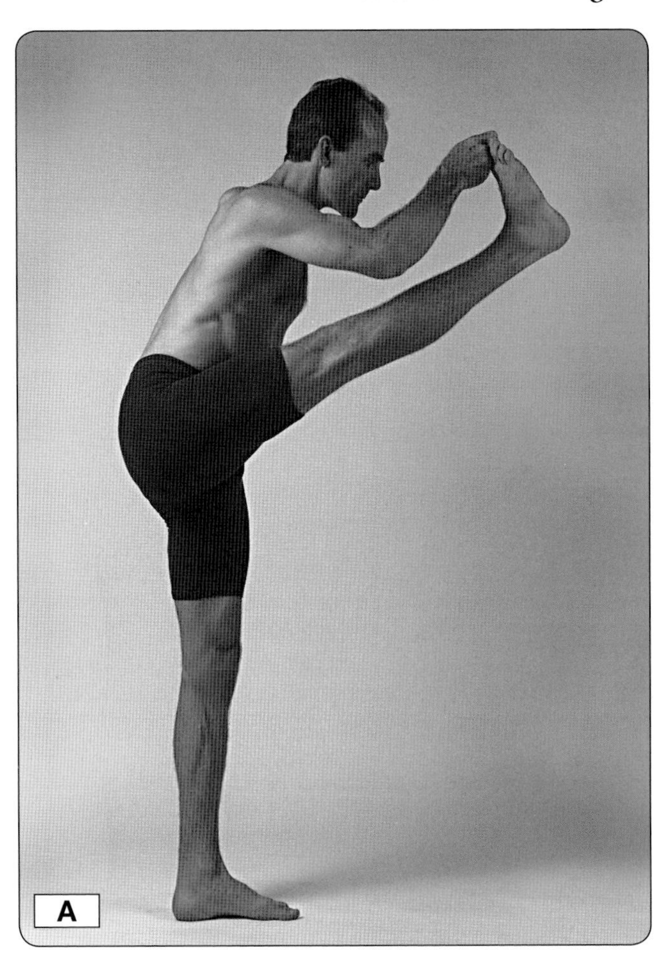
A

1) **Inhale** raise your right foot. Grab the big toe with two fingers of the right hand. Straighten the leg or hold the knee with two hands. Place the left hand on the left side of your waist unless you are holding the knee in which case you would take both hands to the knee as described in option **(D)**.

2) **Exhale** lift the right leg toward the chest and also extend the chest out over the leg simultaneously **(A)** or remain standing up straight with the leg extended **(B)**. If it is too extreme to straighten the right leg then keep it bent slightly **(C)** or hold the right knee with two hands **(D)**.

Remain Here For 5 Deep Breaths

3) **Inhale** lift your chest. Gaze to the horizon.

Enter
Utthita Hasta Padangusthasana B
from Here

Drishti ~ **Toes in A & B**
Straight Ahead C & D

Utthita Hasta Padangusthasana A

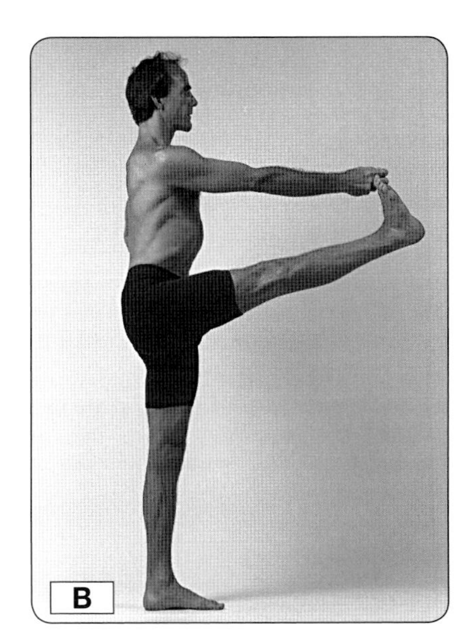

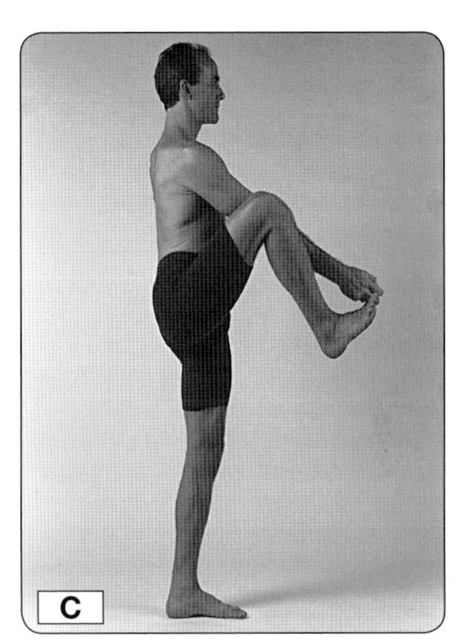

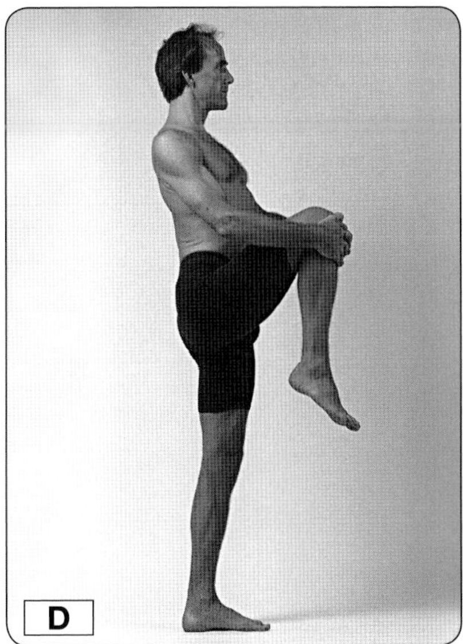

Comments - Keep the supporting leg working by lifting the muscles above the knee. It should be straight but ***not*** locked back. The supporting foot is rooted to the earth while the leg grows tall and extends upward throughout the body. Keep the spine long and the shoulders rolled back and down away from the ears.

Utthita Hasta Padangusthasana B

Utthita = Extended Hasta = Hand Padangustha = Big Toe

"Extended Hand Big Toe Posture"

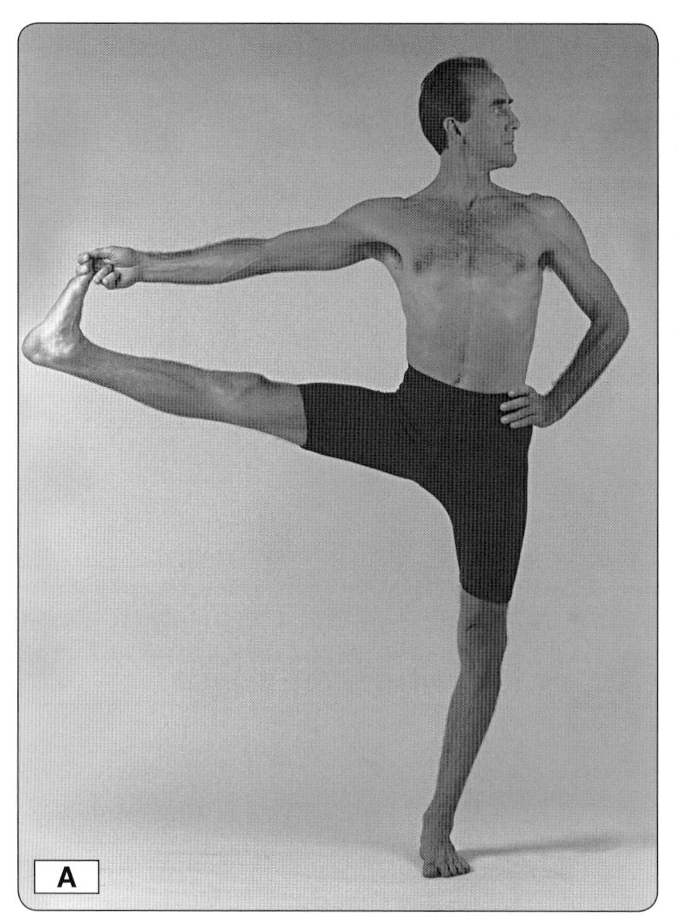
A

1) **Exhale** open the right hip. Take the right foot to the side. Turn your gaze to the left. Extend fully through the heel of the right foot and pull the toes back **(A)**. If this is too extreme then you may bend the right leg slightly **(B)** or hold the knee with your right hand as in **(C)**. Keep the left hand on the left hip in all of the above options.

Remain Here For 5 Deep Breaths

2) **Inhale** bring the right leg back to the front.

Enter
Utthita Hasta Padangusthasana C
from Here

Drishti ~ **Side**

Utthita Hasta Padangusthasana B

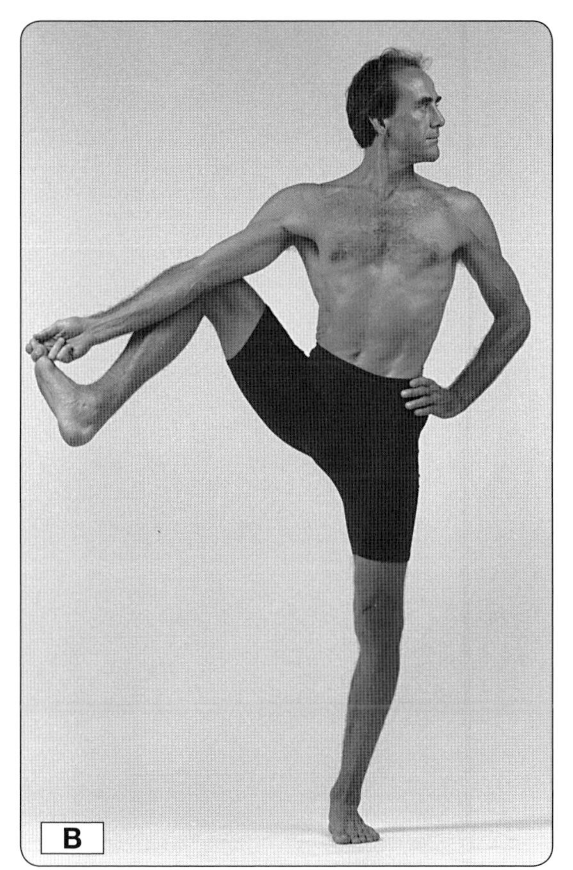

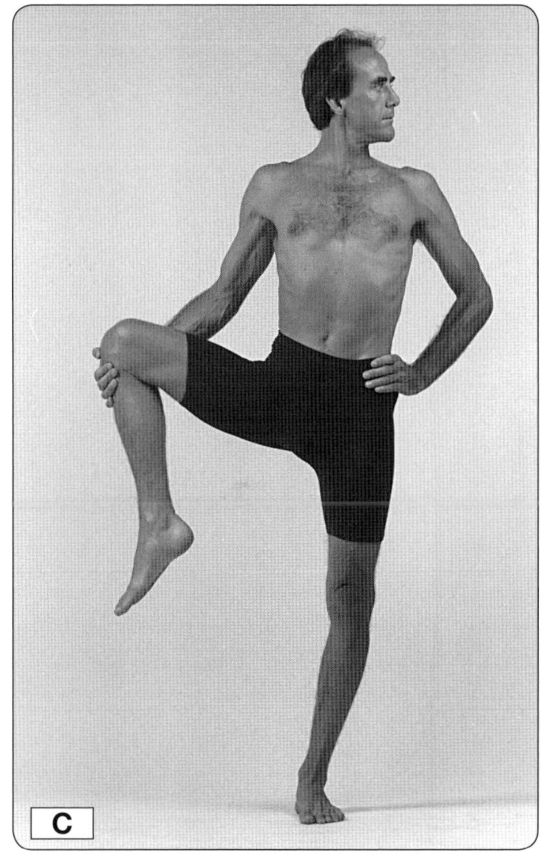

Comments - Balance will be challenged in this asana. Use your drishti and the breath as stabilizers. Breathe fully. That will relax the mind. Less effort is the key. If it is too difficult to gaze to the side then look straight ahead. Focus on a fixed point near you. Hold on to that object with the power of your drishti. Feel the weight distribution across the bottom of your supporting foot. Distribute it evenly from the mid-point of the heel to the balls of the foot. Root into the earth from the foot while you simultaneously extend upward.

Utthita Hasta Padangusthasana C

Utthita = Extended   Hasta = Hand   Padangustha = Big Toe

"Extended Hand Big Toe Posture"

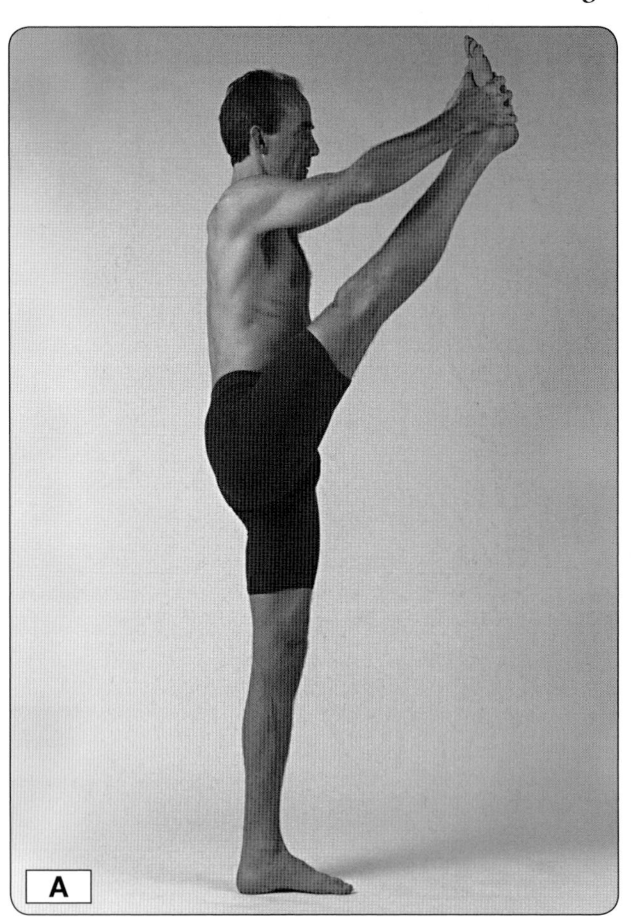
A

1) **Exhale** as you take the foot with both hands and raise it. Keep the upper body erect and bring the leg toward your chest **(A)**. Or you may keep the right leg bent while holding the foot with two hands **(B)** or bend the right leg and hold the knee with both hands and lift as in **(C)**.

Remain Here For 5 Deep Breaths

2) **Inhale** lower the leg slightly while maintaining your grip.

Enter
Utthita Hasta Padangusthasana D
from Here

Drishti ~ **Toes in A & B**
Straight Ahead in C

Utthita Hasta Padangusthasana C

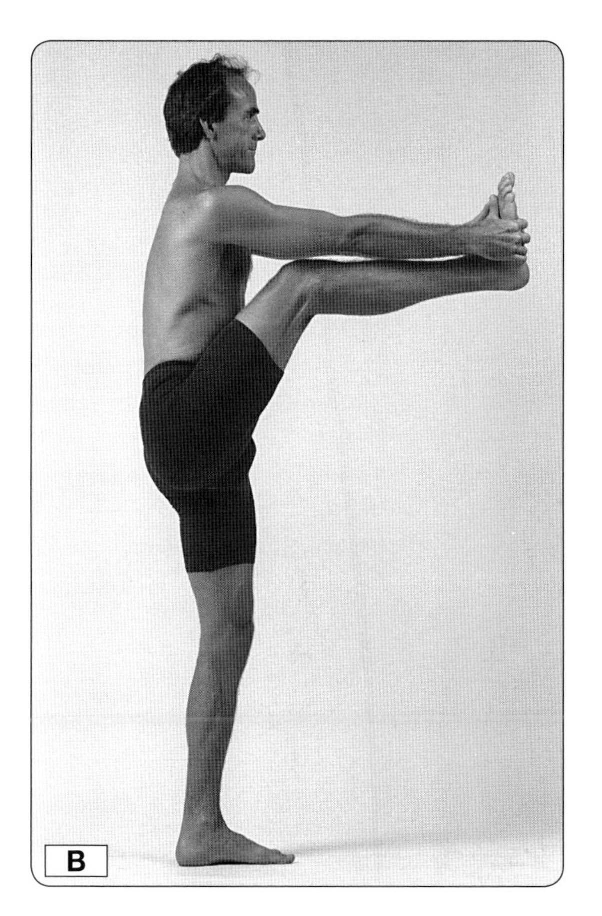

B

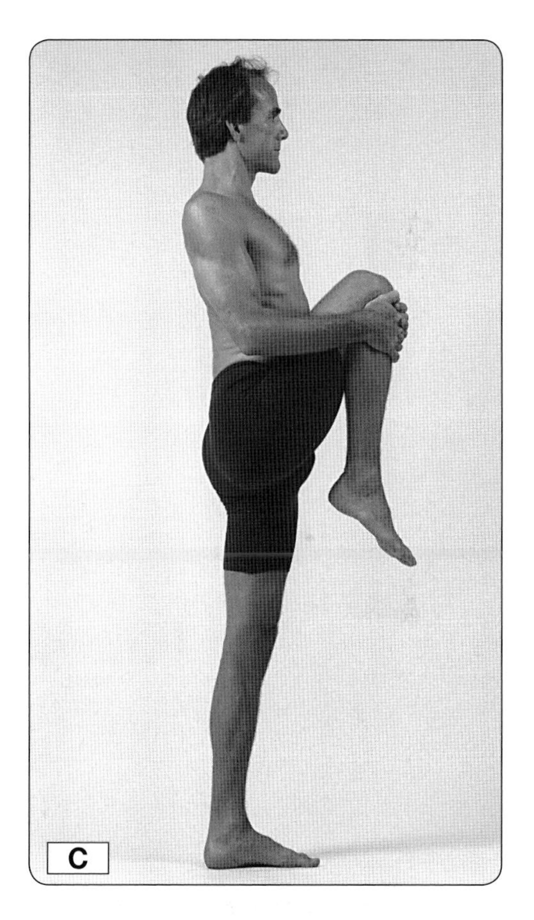

C

Comments - Avoid being pulled forward by the force of the right leg. If you find yourself leaning too far forward then back off and choose one of the other options until you find the appropriate one for you. Send energy down into the earth from the core of the supporting leg and simultaneously lift upward internally to create an equality of opposition from which balance will manifest.

Note - This asana is sometimes omitted from the Primary Series or instead of holding it for a full five breaths the nose is touched to the knee upon an exhale and then the foot released to proceed into **Utthita Hasta Padangusthasana D**. It is also called **Trivikramasana** in the Advanced Series.

Utthita Hasta Padangusthasana D

Utthita = Extended Hasta = Hand Padangustha = Big Toe

"Extended Hand Big Toe Posture"

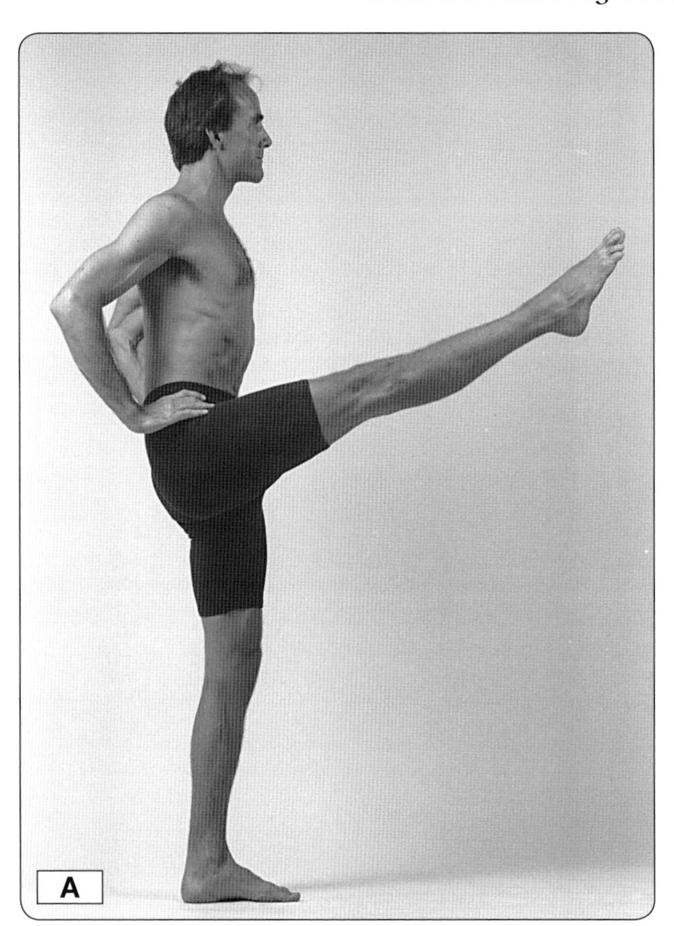
A

1) **Exhale** release the foot without lowering it. Keep the leg straight and lifted high with the toes pointed **(A)** or you may keep the leg straight and let it hover closer to the floor **(B)**. A third option is to keep the right leg bent with the knee lifting and the toes pointing toward the floor **(C)**. In all of the above options keep both hands pressing into the waist.

Remain Here For 5 Deep Breaths

2) **Inhale** lift the foot or knee slightly higher.

3) **Exhale** lower the right foot to the floor.

Repeat Utthita Hasta Padangusthasana A,B,C,D on the Left Side

Drishti ~ **Toes in A**
Straight Ahead B & C

Utthita Hasta Padangusthasana D

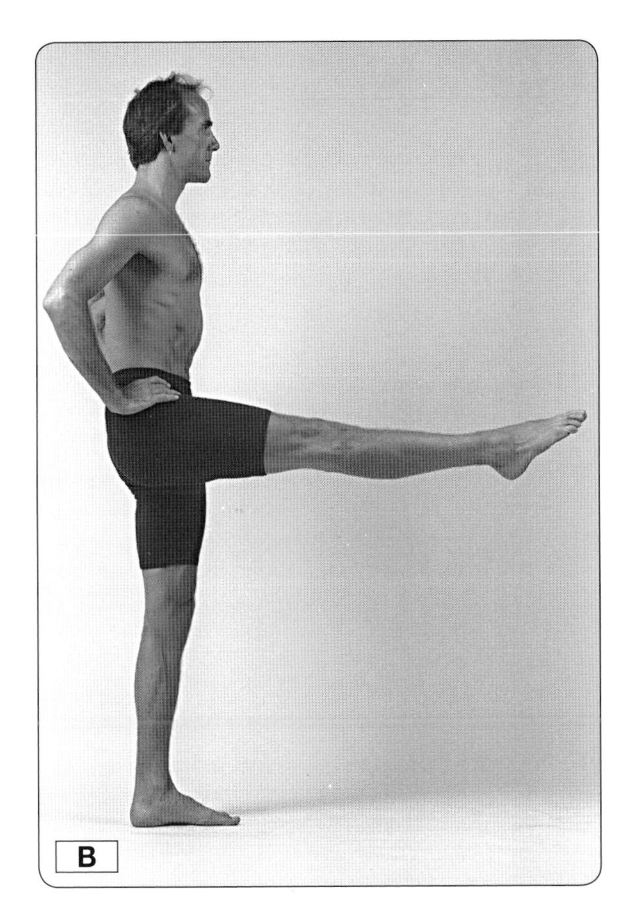

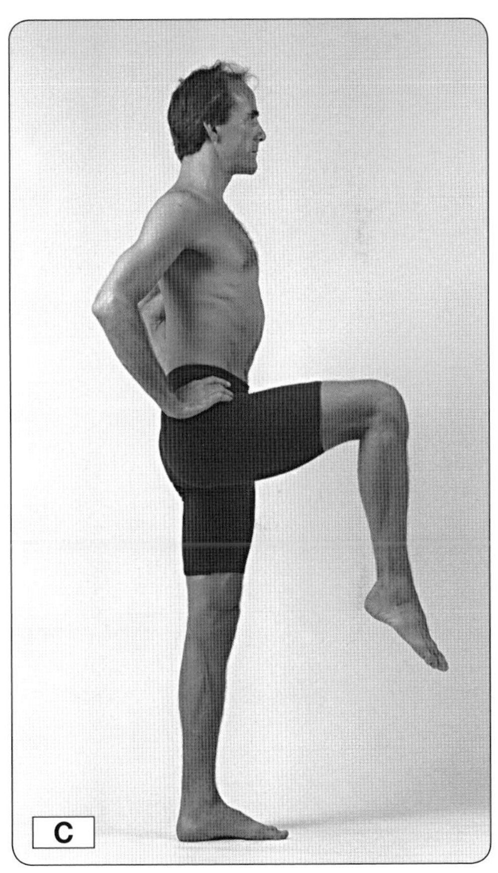

Comments - Avoid leaning back when you release the foot or knee to enter this asana. Press your hands firmly into the waist. You may use the fingertips to feel that **uddiyana bandha** is engaged. Use the bandhas to find stability. Keep the supporting leg active with the kneecap lifting. Relax the face and mind.

Ardha Baddha Padmottanasana

Ardha = Half   Baddha = Bound   Padma = Lotus   Uttana = Intense Stretch

"Half Bound Lotus Intense Stretch Posture"

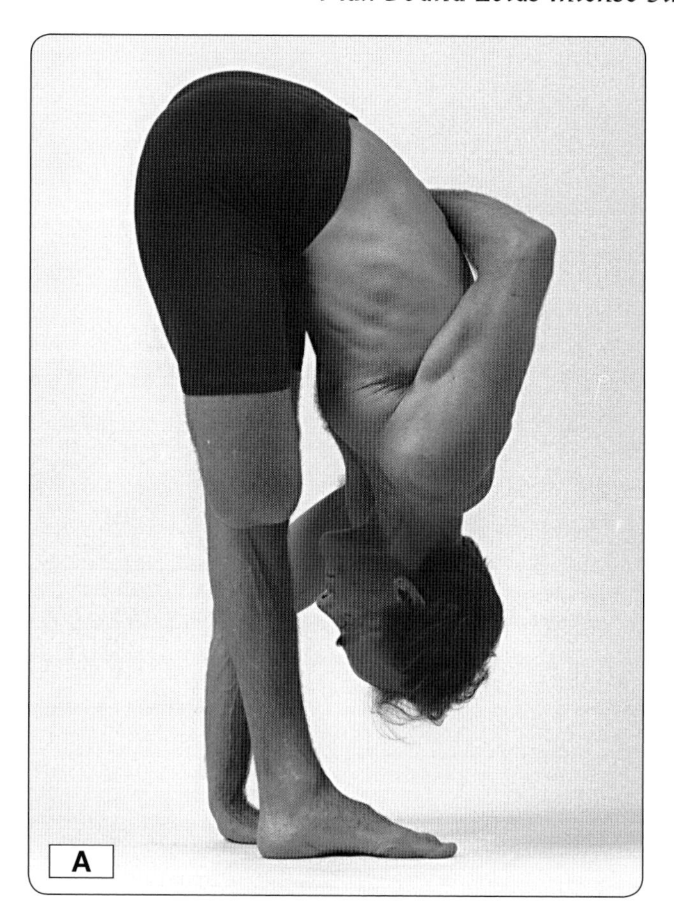
A

1) **Inhale** lift the right foot with both hands.

2) **Exhale** place the foot on the upper left thigh. Reach behind the back with the right hand and clasp the foot. If this is too extreme then move on to **# 6 B** or **# 6 C**.

3) **Inhale** raise the left arm.

4) **Exhale** fold forward and place the left hand on the floor outside the left foot.

5) **Inhale** lengthen the spine as you gaze to the horizon.

6) **Exhale** lower the chest toward your thigh **(A)**. If it is too extreme to clasp the right foot with the right hand then hold it with the left hand. Reach around the back with the right hand and grab the left elbow. Remain standing as in **(B)**. Or place the right foot on the inner left thigh and remain standing with the palms in prayer fashion **(C)**.

Remain Here For 5 Deep Breaths

(If practicing option **A** in which you are bending all of the way forward with the left hand on the floor then follow **#7**, **#8**, **#9** and **#10**. Otherwise move ahead to **#10** only)

7) **Inhale** lengthen the spine and look up.

8) **Exhale** bend the left leg slightly to engage the quadriceps muscles above the knee.

9) **Inhale** stand up and raise the left arm.

10) **Exhale** release the asana. Extend the right leg and lower the foot to the floor.

Repeat Steps 1-10 on the Left Side

Drishti ~ **Nose in A**
Straight Ahead in B & C

Ardha Baddha Padmottanasana

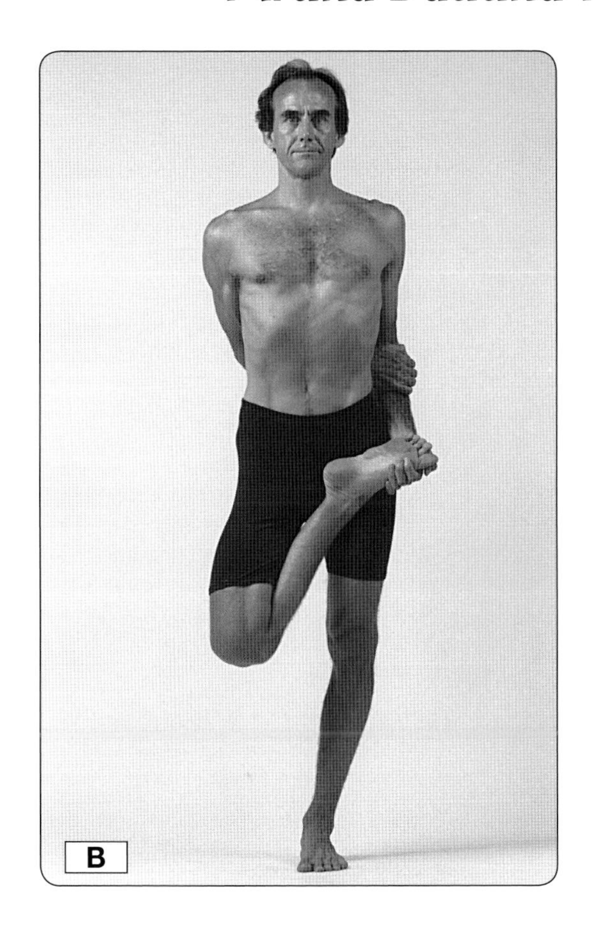

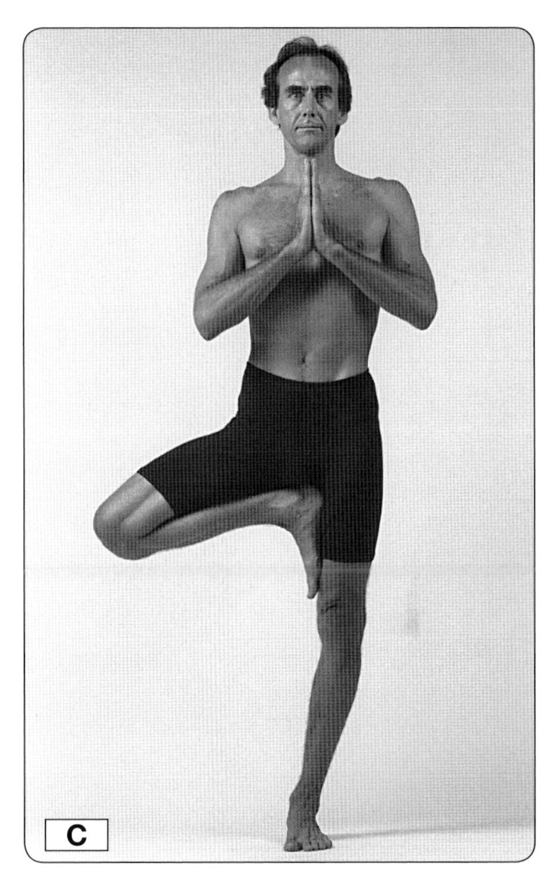

Comments - Listen to your knees! If any section of this asana feels too extreme for your joints then back off. Find the option that is most suitable for you. If all options feel too intense then leave this asana out for now. Work toward it over time. Listen to the inner wisdom of your body. No one knows it better than you.

Utkatasana

Utka = Fierce or Powerful

"Fierce Posture"

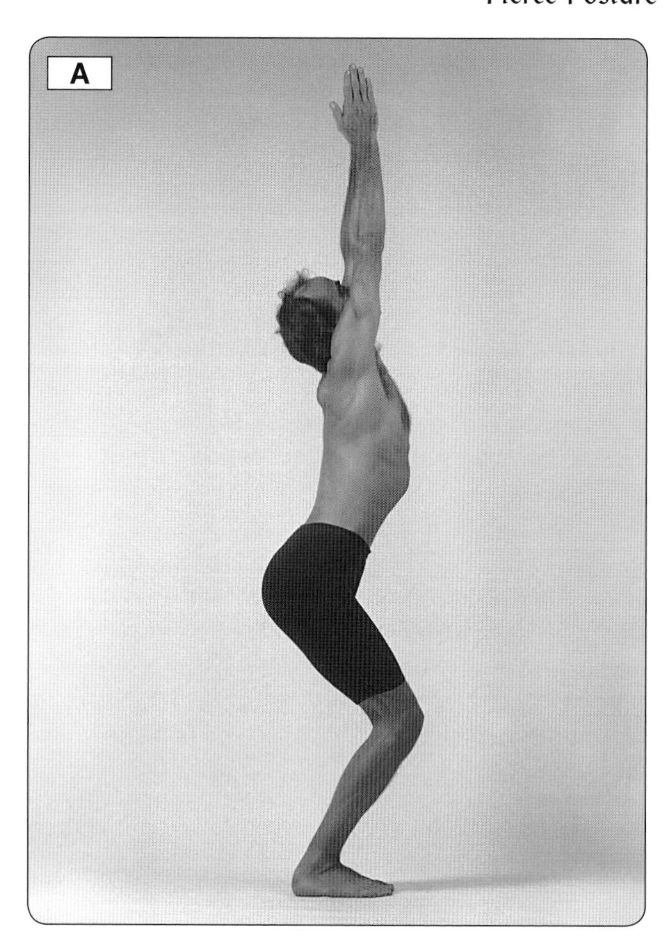

To Enter **Utkatasana** move through **Suryanamaskara A** but do not stay in the **Downward-Facing Dog** position for five breaths. Instead follow the steps below from **Downward Dog**.

1) **Inhale** jump or step both feet forward so that they are positioned between the hands. Drop the hips as though you are sitting in a chair and raise the arms overhead pointing the fingers toward the sky with the palms pressing together **(A)**.You may find it difficult to get a full extension in the shoulders with the palms in this position. If this is the case then interlace all but the index fingers which remain pointing straight up toward the sky. Use that extra support to gain greater length in the arms **(B)** or hold the elbows as shown in **(C)**.

Remain Here For 5 Deep Breaths

2) **Exhale** fold forward lowering the hands toward the floor or to your shins.

3) **Inhale** lengthen the spine and look up.

4) **Exhale** jump or step back and lower to the floor.

5) **Inhale** into **Upward-Facing Dog**.

6) **Exhale** into the **Downward-Facing Dog** in preparation to enter the next asana.

Drishti ~ **Thumbs in A & B**
Straight Ahead in C

Utkatasana

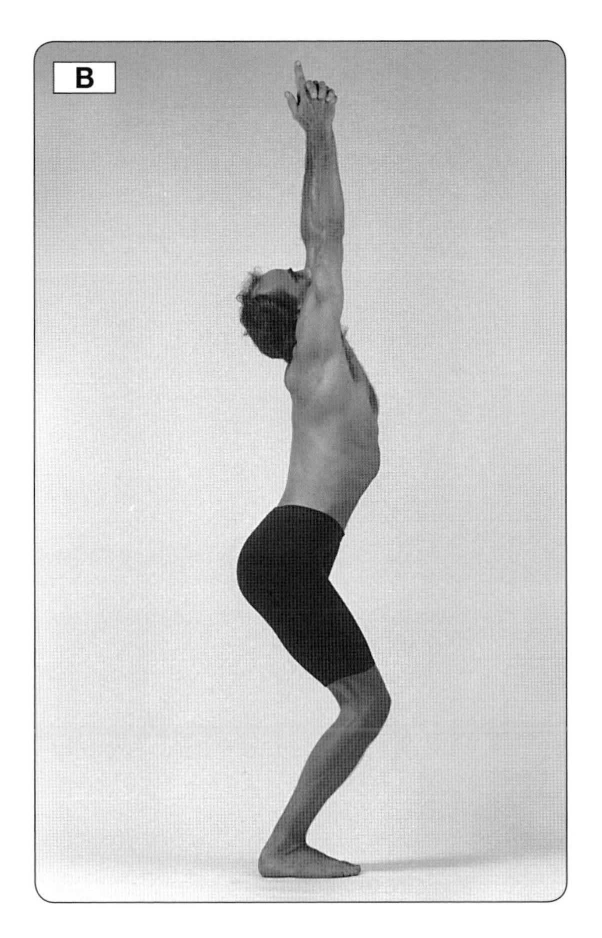

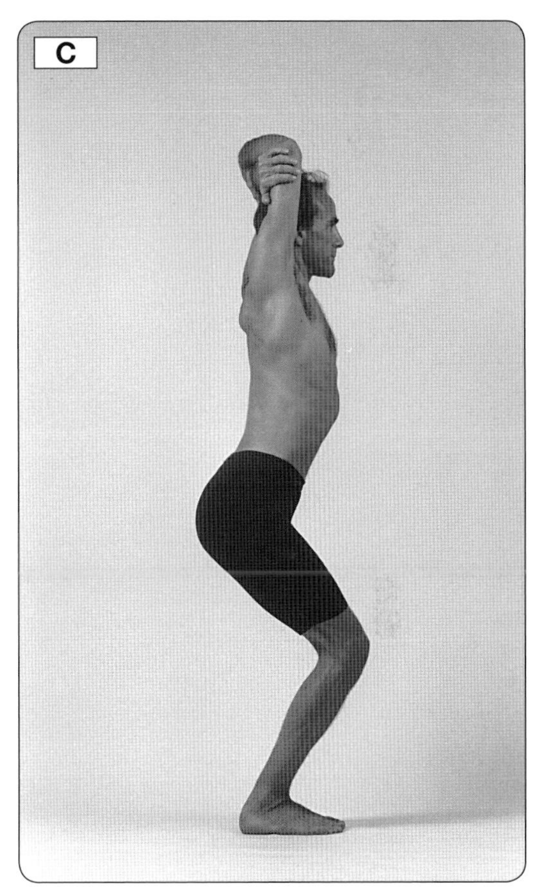

Comments - Keep your knees touching, ankles touching and the toes touching. The heels should remain grounded with the sit-bones dropped. Feel gravity pulling you into the earth from the waist down and an opposing force lifting you from the sacrum up the spine through the top of your head and out the fingertips. Find your equality of opposition within the point of stillness between effort and effortlessness.

Virabhadrasana A

Virabhadra = Hero or Warrior

"Warrior Posture"

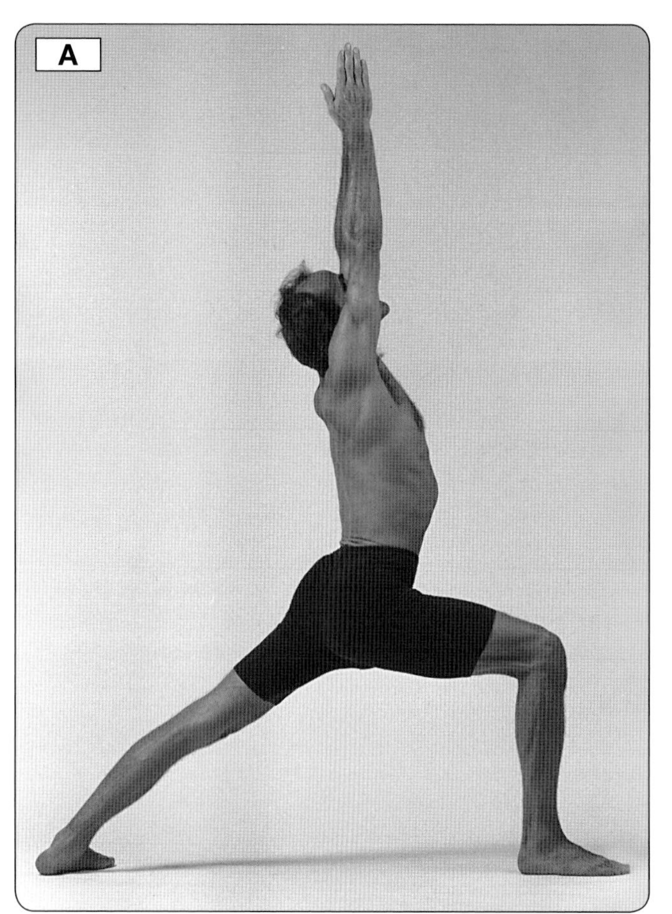

1) **Inhale** step the right foot in between the hands from the **Downward Dog** position. Raise both arms overhead. Keep the front leg at a ninety degree angle with the knee directly above the heel and the spine long with the outer edge of the back foot turned in slightly and pressed firmly into the floor **(A)**. If it is too much to step the foot all of the way to the hands then bring it only partially forward and come up from there. The front knee still needs to remain above the heel **(B)**. If it is too much to bend the front leg then keep it straight **(C)**.

Remain Here For 5 Deep Breaths

2) **Inhale** and straighten the right leg and then pivot the feet by turning the right foot in and the left foot out. Bend the left leg and repeat one of the options above for the left side.

Remain Here For 5 Deep Breaths

Enter the Next Asana from Here

Drishti ~ **Thumbs**

Virabhadrasana A

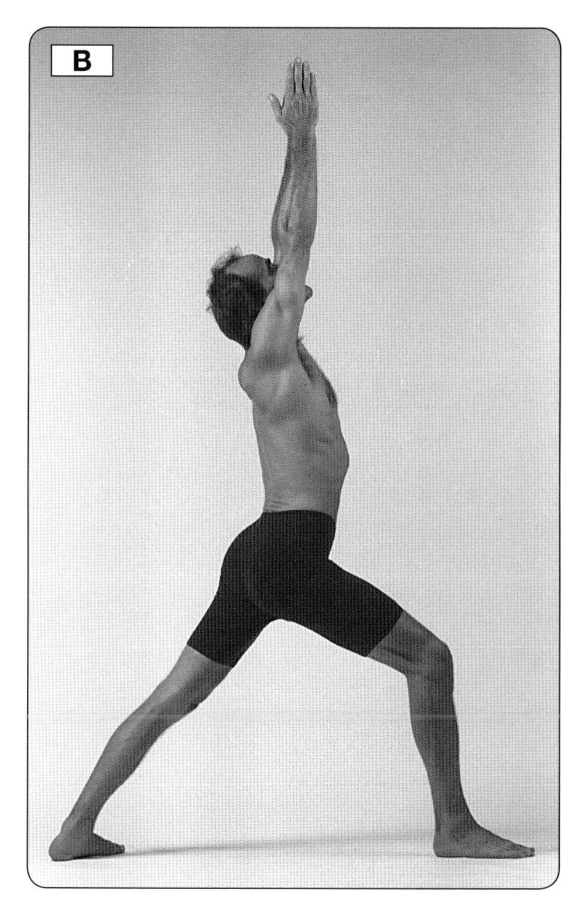

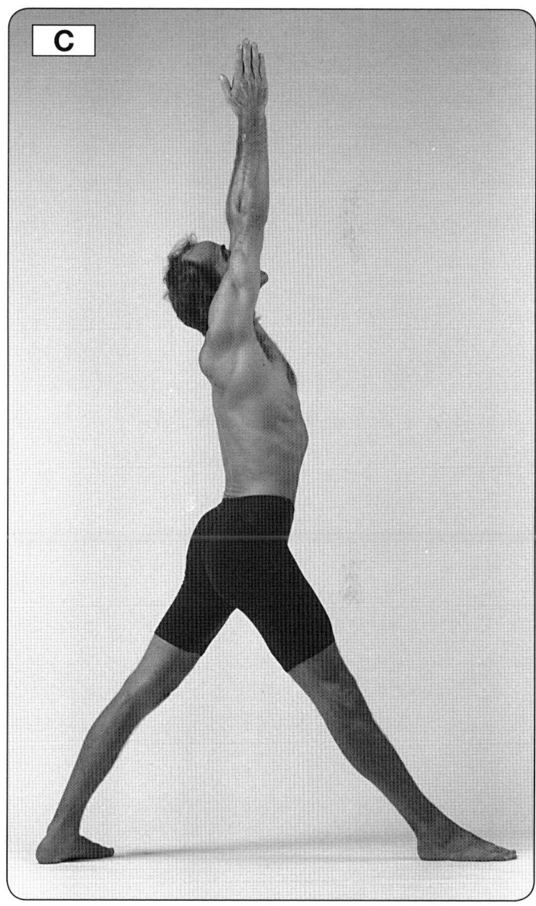

Comments - Keep the knee directly above the heel of the front foot in options **A** and **B**. The back leg should be fully active with the outer edge of the foot pressing into the floor. Create an equality of opposition with the sit-bones falling toward the earth and an upward expanding extension growing from the sacrum up through the spine and flowing out the fingertips. Draw the ribs in to avoid collapsing in the lower back. Move the hips and pelvis so that your torso is facing forward as much as possible. Drop the head back only as far as is necessary to see the thumbs.

Virabhadrasana B

Virabhadra = Hero or Warrior

"Warrior Posture"

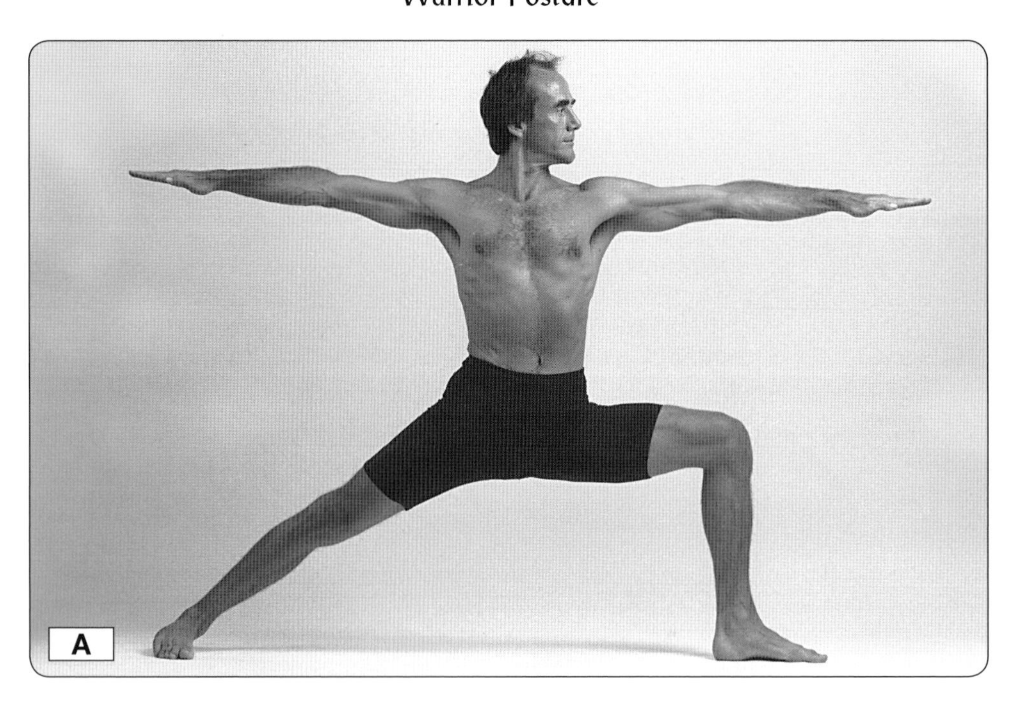

1) **Exhale** from **Virabhadrasana A**. Open your arms parallel to the floor and in line with the legs. Move the upper **right** pelvis back and the inner **left** knee forward. The left leg should remain at a ninety-degree angle as in **(A)**. If it is too extreme to have the left leg at a ninety-degree angle then back off a bit as in **(B)**. You may also practice it with both legs straight **(C)**.

Remain Here For 5 Deep Breaths

2) **Inhale** straighten the left leg and pivot the left foot in.

3) **Exhale** turn the right foot out. Bend the right leg and repeat one of the options above for the right side.

Remain Here For 5 Deep Breaths

4) **Exhale** and take both hands to the floor on each side of the right foot. Step back and lower to the floor.

5) **Inhale** into the Upward Dog.

6) **Exhale** into **Downward Dog** in preparation for entry into the ***Primary Series on page 60** or the ***Intermediate Series on page 129**.

Drishti ~ **Hand**

***If you are practicing Primary Series proceed to page 60.**

***If you are entering Intermediate Series go to page 129.**

Virabhadrasana B

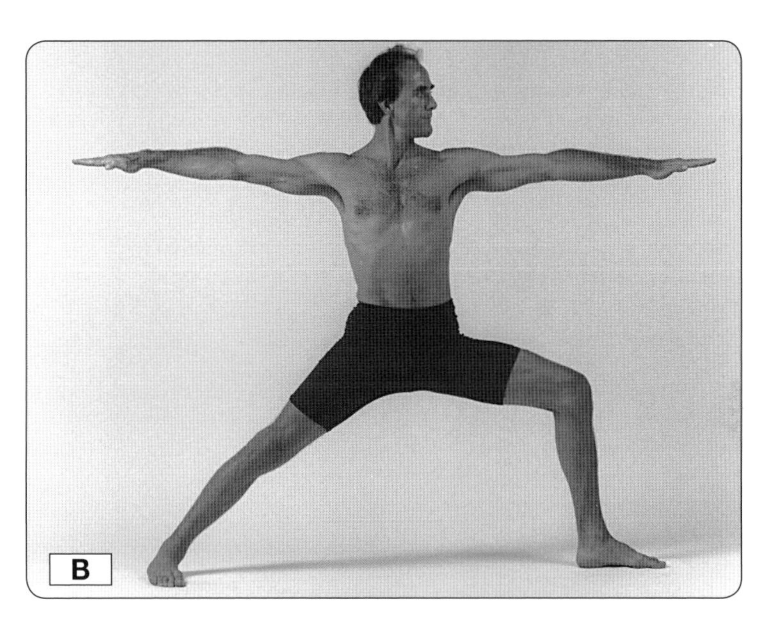

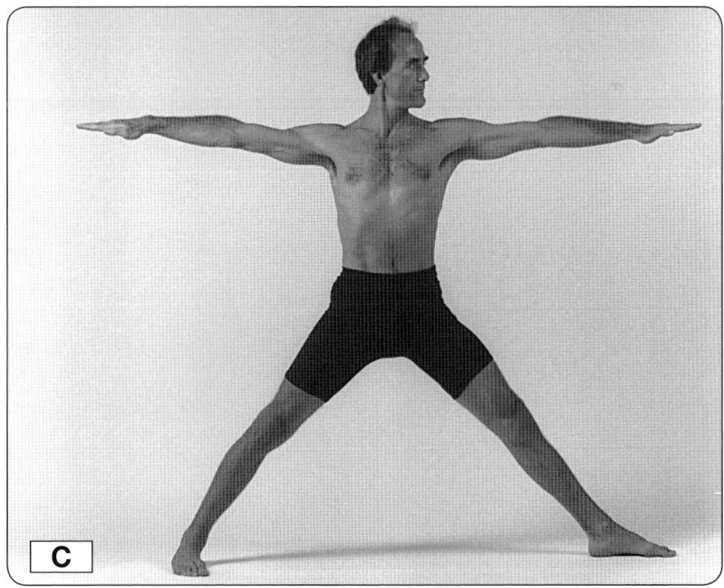

Comments - The spine and arms should form a cross with the spine being perpendicular to the floor and the arms being parallel to the floor. Extend across the shoulders and out the fingertips. Use your bandhas.

Entering the Primary Series

"Applying the Physics of Flight"

The pathway from the standing sequence into **Dandasana** requires the application of the first jumping Vinyasa of Ashtanga Yoga. To maneuver from the **Downward-Facing-Dog** into a seated position requires an understanding of the "Physics of Flight". In order to explore this action more fully, I've created a set of rules which apply to the aerodynamics of flight accompanied by photos.

Rule One - "Engage Your Bandhas"

Truly this rule is the essence of all flying capabilities. Within the bandhas you will find lightness and control throughout the practice. Move into the **Downward Dog** position and pause there. Create a lifting effect from the inner knees all of the way up into the groin. Feel the locks engaged fully **(Photo 1)**.

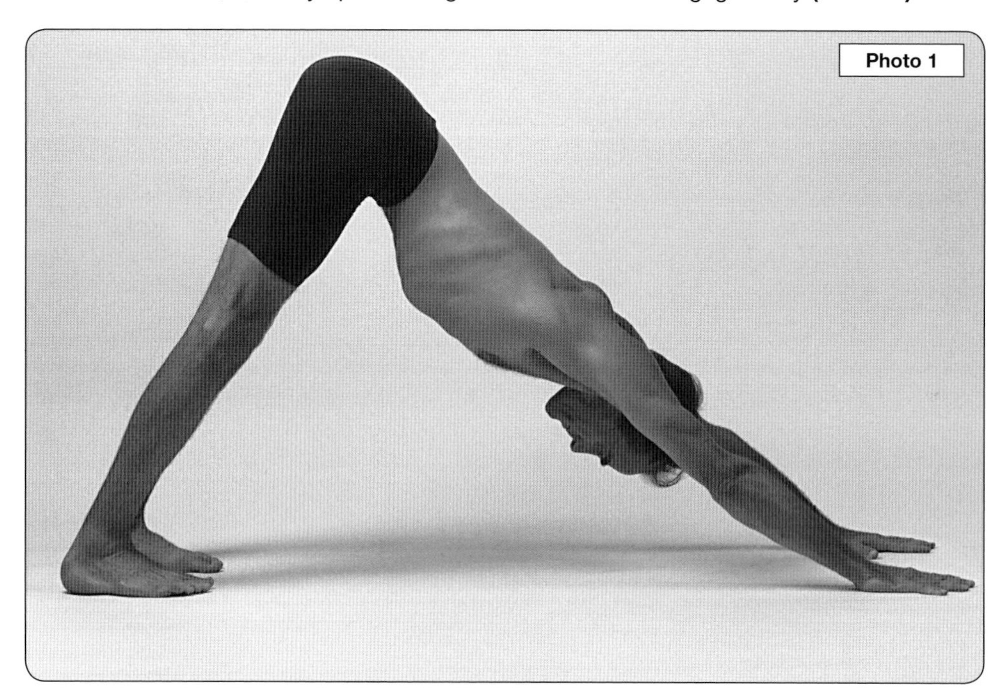

Photo 1

Entering the Primary Series

"Applying the Physics of Flight"

Rule Two - "Lift Your Landing Gear During Flight"

Many people do not even know that we have landing gear. It is located in the region comprised of the sit-bones, sacrum and pelvis. In order to fly, the landing gear must be lifted. This is achieved by raising the sit-bones toward the sky and tilting the upper front portion of the pelvis toward the toes **(Photo 2)**. When this dynamic is engaged then it is possible to propel the hips upward with less effort and greater control. There is a tendency however to drop the sit-bones as soon as the legs are bent to initiate a jump as in **(Photo 3)**. That is wrong and will hinder the flight potential. This dropping action places the hips in a landing mode which is ***not*** conducive to flight. Rather, it will draw the feet back to earth prematurely causing an abbreviated flight pattern. When you bend your knees in preparation to jump keep the landing gear lifted as shown already in **(Photo 2)**.

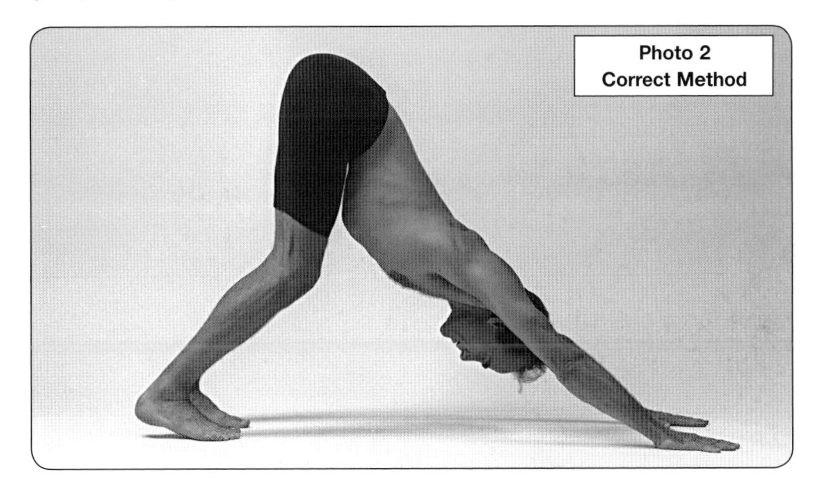

Photo 2
Correct Method

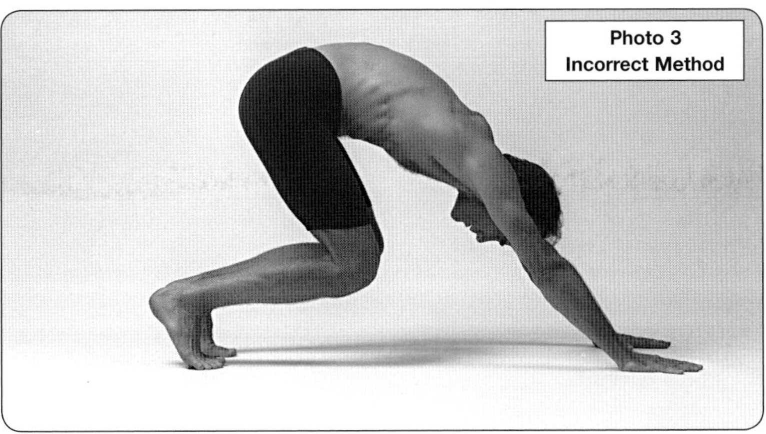

Photo 3
Incorrect Method

Entering the Primary Series

"Applying the Physics of Flight"

Rule Three - "Lead With Your Hips"

Your legs are connected to your hips. This is an anatomical truth which at first appearance seems to be very obvious yet can be elusive. While jumping forward there is a tendency to lead with the feet instead of the hips. When this happens the feet fly up like a kicking mule **(Photo 4)** and the hips either move only slightly or remain in the same position. This causes the center of weight to remain behind the hands which will bring the feet crashing down to the floor due to the lack of sufficient forward projection. Conversely, when the hips are the leading force of the jump then the legs will naturally follow with less effort and greater control bringing the center of weight over the hands **(Photo 5)**. You may experiment a few times. Feel the weight transfer to your hands each time that you jump, then let the feet return to the **Downward-Facing-Dog** position.

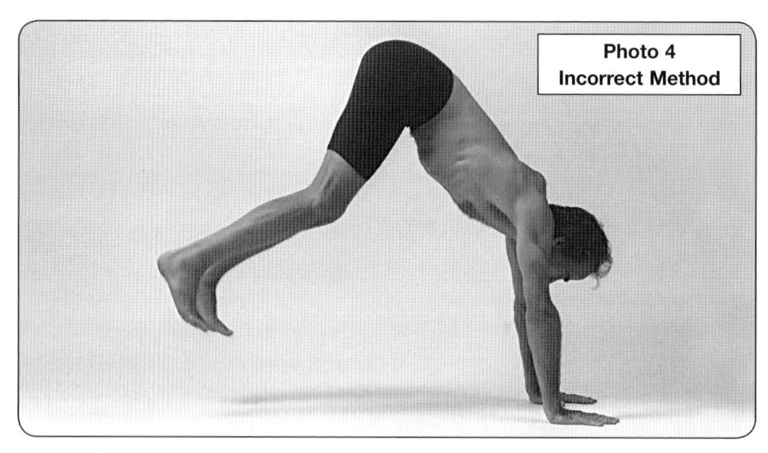

Photo 4
Incorrect Method

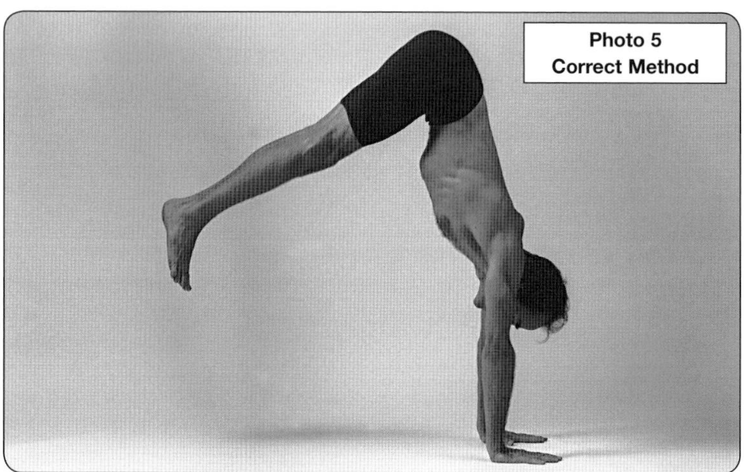

Photo 5
Correct Method

Entering the Primary Series

"Applying the Physics of Flight"

Rule Four - "Raise Your Ceiling"

To explore the dynamics of this rule I am going to give you an image to assist in clarification. Imagine that you are in a room that is thirty feet long, seven feet wide with a ceiling height of only four feet. You are seated at the far end of the room and there is a window at the opposite end thirty feet away. You are holding a mango in your hand which you would like to throw out of the window without moving from where you are. How would you need to throw it so that it can reach the window without touching the ceiling or floor first? You would need to propel it with great velocity. Now lets say that you are in the same room but now the ceiling has been raised up to a height of forty feet. How could you throw it differently now? With such a great expanse overhead it would be possible to toss the mango in a grand arch using little effort to achieve the same goal. This principle may be applied to the dynamics required to jump forward with control. If the imaginary ceiling above your hips, while in the **Downward-Facing-Dog**, is too low as in **(Photo 6)** then when it comes time to jump forward there is no room to rise and it will be necessary to shoot ahead like an arrow in order to initiate the Vinyasa. If on the other hand you raise your imaginary ceiling high into the sky **(Photo 7)** then with such an expanse above you may project the hips in a graceful arch with less effort to achieve the same results as shown earlier in (**Photo 5**). The bandhas play a crucial role here. The hips must be the leading force.

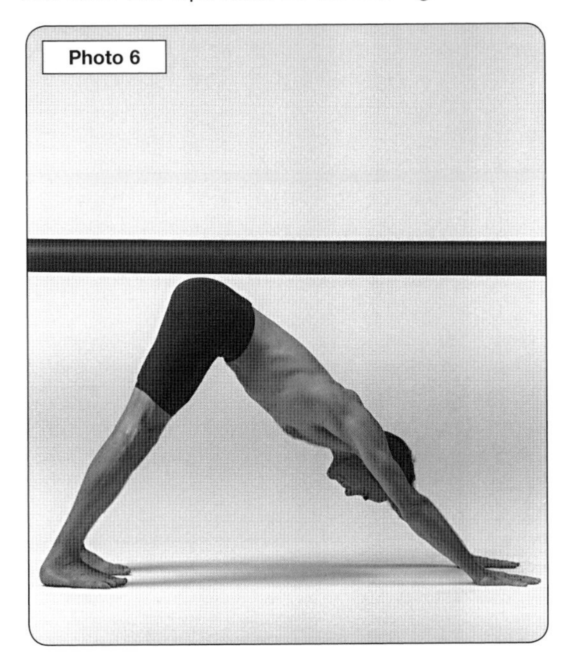

Photo 6

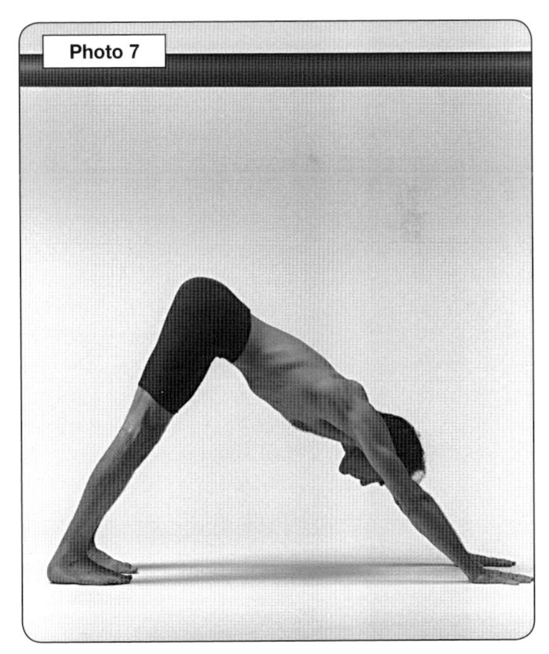

Photo 7

Entering the Primary Series

"Applying the Physics of Flight"

Rule Five - "Drop Your Landing Gear When Landing"

Just as it is necessary for the landing gear to be lifted during flight, it must be dropped when it is time to land. I will share with you two methods of "flying" which I call **"Jumping"** and **"Floating"**. They are both achieved by curling the sit-bones under after you have reached the top of your arch. It is necessary to wait for the moment that your weight is fully over your hands before engaging the landing gear. There is a point of weightlessness when you are neither rising nor falling. At that precise moment you may tuck the sit-bones under and place your bandhas on full alert. For the **"Jumping"** method, as soon as you begin to drop the landing gear draw your knees in toward your chest **(Photo 8)** and land the feet on the floor near your hands before coming through to a seated position. You may work toward bringing the feet through without touching the floor. If you have particularly flexible hamstrings then you may apply the **"Floating"** method. For this approach you must keep the legs straight. At the peak of the arch you may pull the thighs close in to the chest as you drop your sit-bones **(Photo 9)**. In addition to flexibility you must maintain control of your bandhas as you float through to a seated position in order to assist in a smooth landing. When dropping your landing gear you may find further assistance in the drishti. The drishti is intimately connected with the movement of the pelvis in this maneuver. When in the **Downward-Facing-Dog** position, preparing to jump through, the gaze should be between the hands. It should remain there through all phases of the jump until you reach the stage that you are going to drop your landing gear. At that point, as soon as you begin to drop the sit-bones you should then lift your gaze to the horizon. It is as though the gaze is connected to the pelvis. When you lift your gaze it assists in the lifting of the frontal portion of the pelvis and pubic bone. That rising action in the mid-section is crucial to bringing the feet through the hands in the "flying" methods above. These "flying" approaches to vinyasa are quite advanced and may require years of practice before proficiency is realized. For this reason I have developed other methods of vinyasa. They are called, **"Ground Transportation"**. The first is **"Walking"**. From **Downward Dog** you may step the feet one-at-a-time forward toward the hands **(Photo 10)** and then drop the hips, sit down and walk the feet through to sitting. The other **"Ground Transportation"** option is known as **"Jogging"**. You may simply "jog" the feet forward in a series of small steps toward the hands **(Photo 11)** in order to transfer the feet from the **Downward Dog** and then drop the hips and come through into a seated position. There is no one method that is correct for everybody! You may utilize a variety of approaches in any one given practice session. **The main thing is to enjoy your yoga practice so that it is something to look forward to and not something to loathe.** My hope is to give a variety of options for the asanas and other aspects of this practice so that anyone who chooses may enjoy its fruits. Have fun with these variations of vinyasa and choose the one that most suits you. You may even wish to switch off from time to time to experience the different approaches.

Entering the Primary Series

"Applying the Physics of Flight"

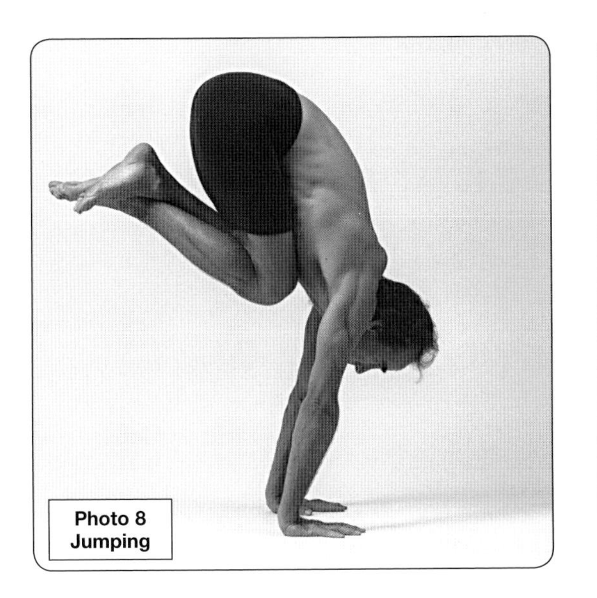

Photo 8
Jumping

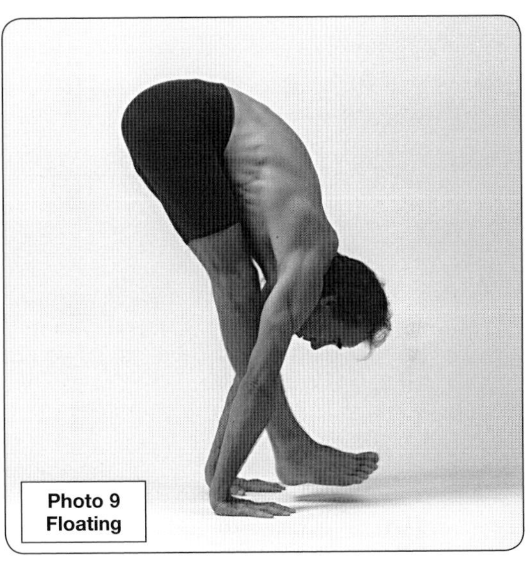

Photo 9
Floating

"Ground Transportation"

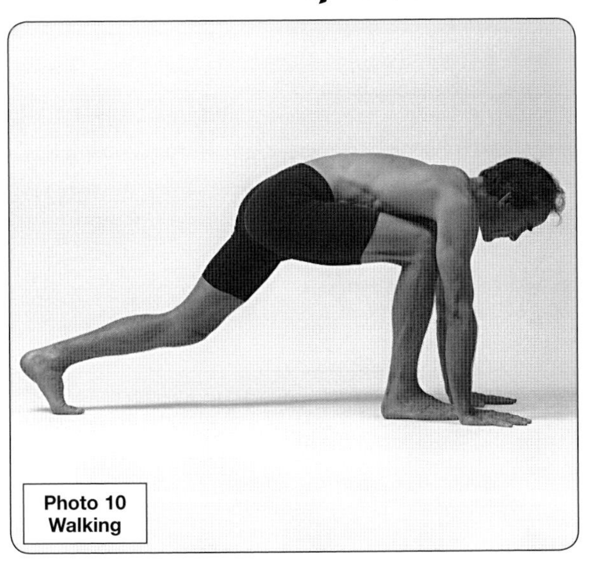

Photo 10
Walking

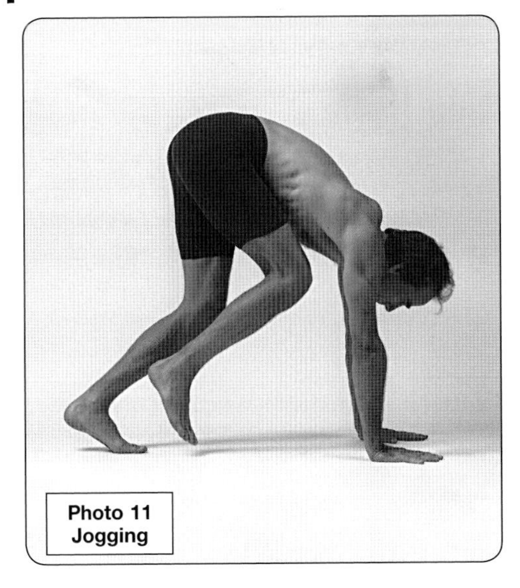

Photo 11
Jogging

Dandasana

Danda = Stick or Staff

"Staff Posture"

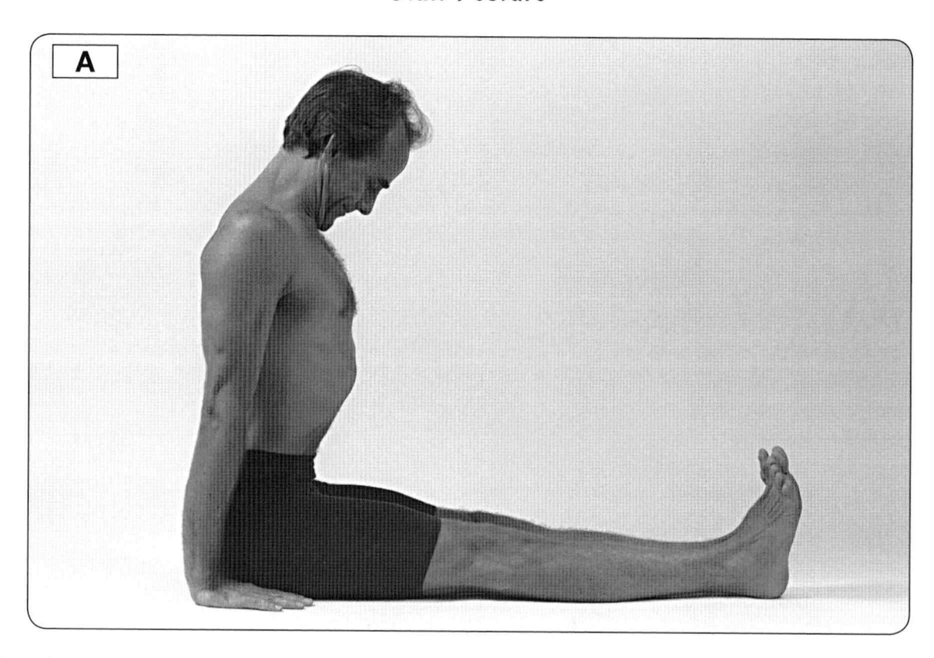

1) **Inhale** using either **"flight"** or **"ground transportation"** to enter a seated position from **down dog**.

2) **Exhale** drop your chin to your chest. Legs active. Spine long. Arms straight. Hands pressing down with the palms flat **(A)**. If it is too extreme to straighten the legs then you may bend them slightly **(B)**. Another option is to place the hands slightly behind the hips instead of directly beside them while slightly leaning back. This will create slack in the hamstrings to allow the legs to straighten more easily **(C)**.

Remain Here For 5 Deep Breaths

3) **Inhale** raise your arms straight up over the head.

Enter Paschimottanasana A From Here

Drishti ~ **Nose**

Comments - This asana is called the stick posture because of the straight lines formed in the legs, arms, feet, and spine. From external appearances it seems to be a passive posture yet **Dandasana** is quite dramatic when practiced with full awareness within the inner workings of it. There are numerous opposing forces. The heels and sit-bones move away from each other, the sacrum sinks down and the spine lengthens, the shoulders move down the back as the hands press into the floor and the chest opens and lifts. To keep all of this energy moving the bandhas must be engaged fully including **jalandhara bandha**, the chin lock. Keep the back of the knees pressing down but do not lift the heels from the floor. Instead of lifting the heels push them forward in order to create length in the legs. Remain focused yet relaxed.

Dandasana

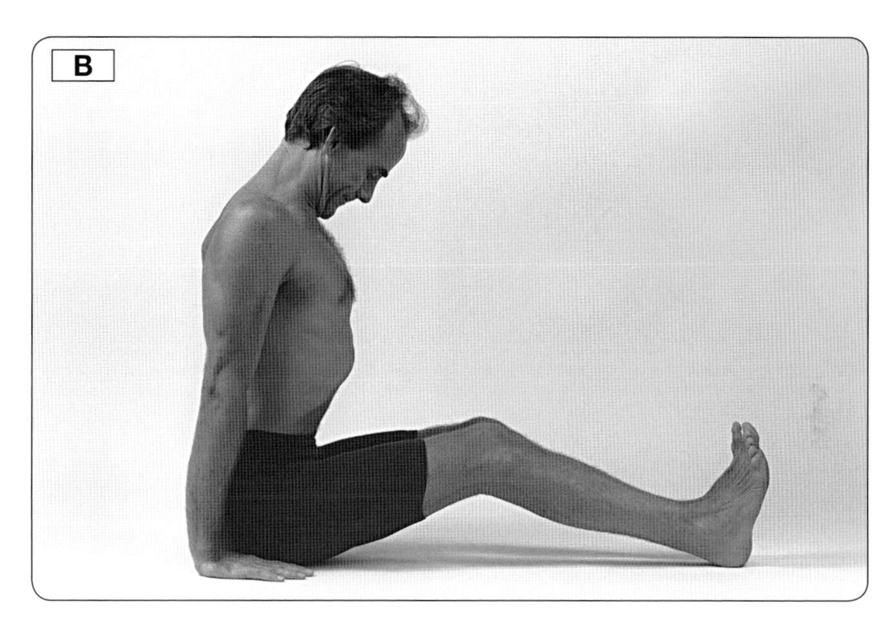

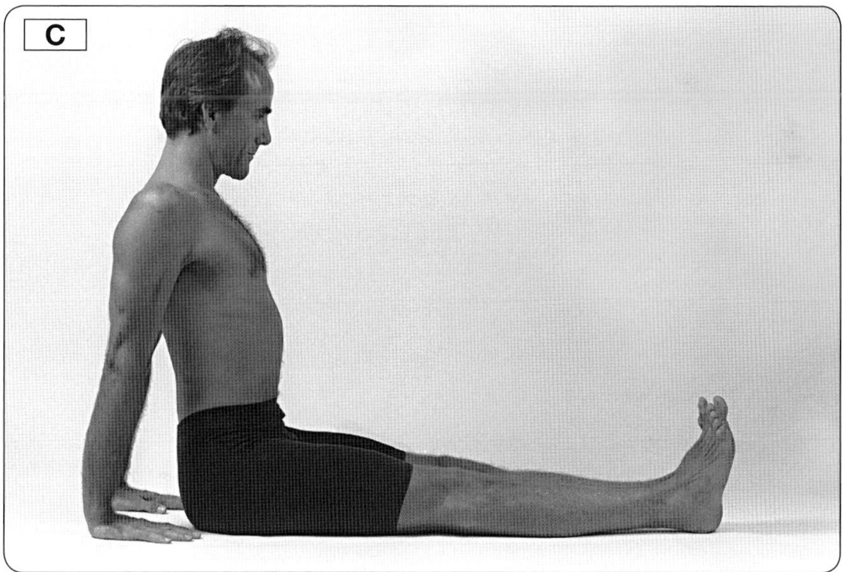

Paschimottanasana A

Paschima = Western Uttana = Intense Stretch

"Western Intense Stretch Posture"

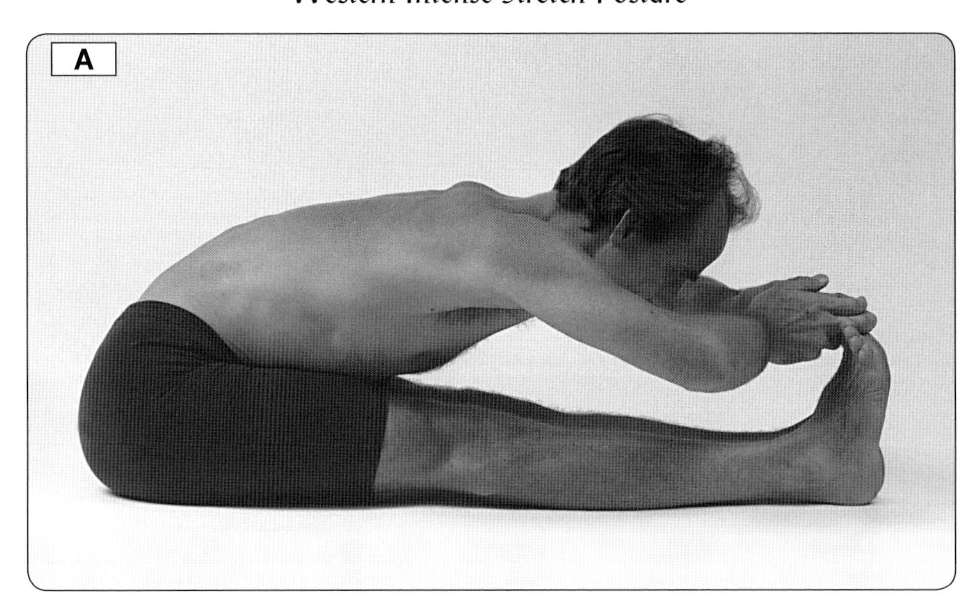

1) **Exhale** fold forward. Clasp the big toes with two fingers of each hand **(A)**. If that is too much then hold the ankles or shins with the legs straight and spine long **(B)** or you may bend the knees and either hold the toes or ankles **(C)**. (If you enjoy using a strap see **Paschimottanasana B**, pg. 71).
2) **Inhale** lengthen the spine and lift the chest. Gaze to the horizon. Open the heart.
3) **Exhale** fold forward into whichever option is most appropriate for you.

Remain Here For 5 Deep Breaths

4) **Inhale** lengthen the spine and look to the horizon.

Enter Paschimottanasana B From Here

Drishti ~ **Toes**

Comments - If you feel discomfort in the lower back, bend your knees or come out of the asana. Lead with your sternum. If you had a flashlight in the middle of your chest it should be shining on the toes. Keep both legs active with the heels moving ahead and the toes pulling back. Be aware of the outer edges of your feet. There is a tendency for them to roll in. If you push through from the base of the big toes it will help to alleviate this and also keep the ankles active. Keep the neck long and shoulders broad with the elbows lifted.

Paschimottanasana A

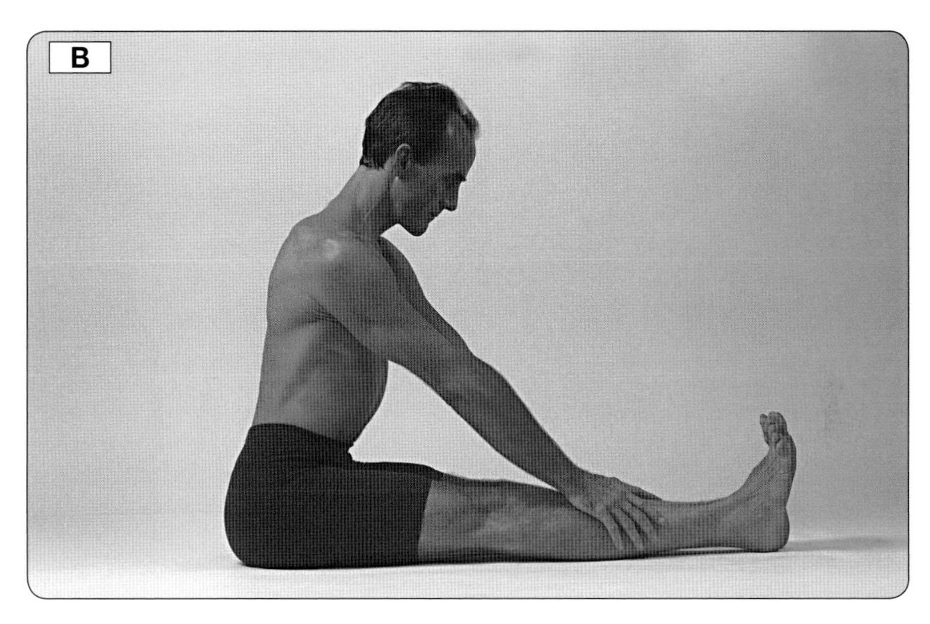

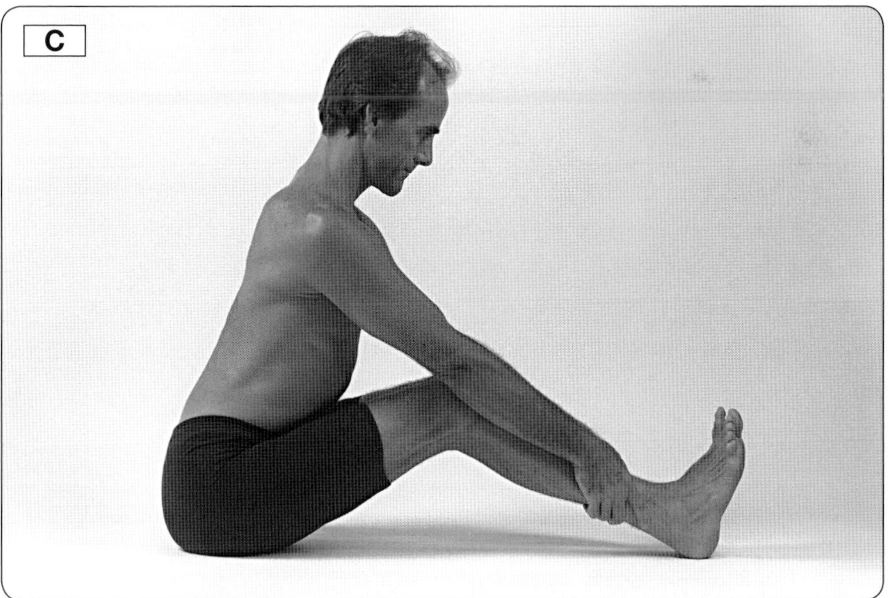

Paschimottanasana B

Paschima = Western Uttana = Intense Stretch

"Western Intense Stretch Posture"

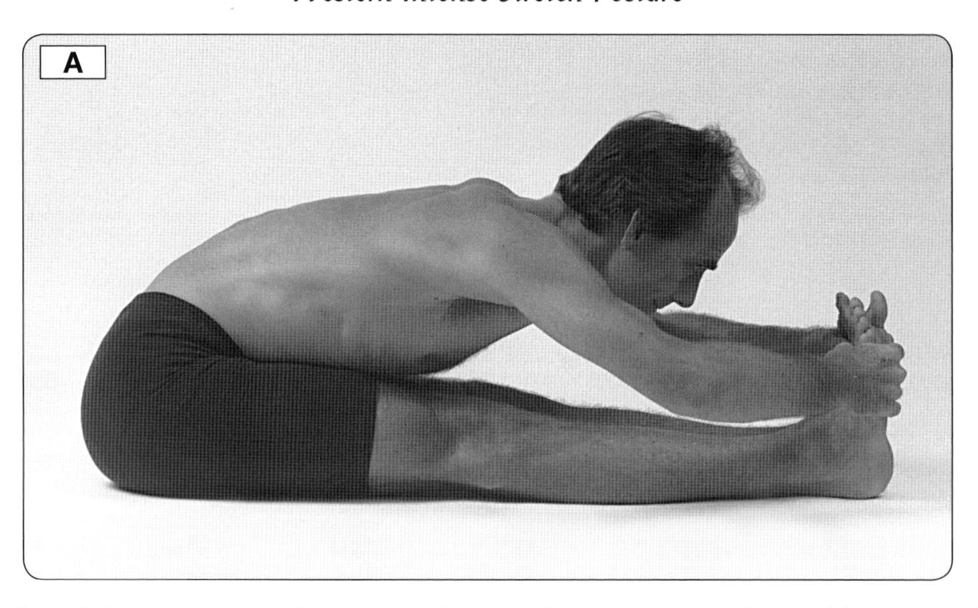

1) **Exhale** and change your grip unless you are already working at your capacity in which case you should remain in an option from **Paschimottanasana A**. If you are continuing then clasp the feet with the fingers on the soles and the thumbs on top **(A)**. If you enjoy using props you may utilize a strap around the feet with legs straight as in **(B)** or bend the legs **(C)**. **Listen to your body**.

2) **Inhale** with the new grip. Lengthen the spine and lift your gaze to the horizon.

3) **Exhale** fold into whichever level is appropriate for you.

Remain Here For 5 Deep Breaths

4) **Inhale** lengthen the spine and look to the horizon.

Enter Paschimottanasana C From Here

Drishti ~ **Toes**

Comments - The same lengthening aspects should apply here as in **Paschimottanasana A**. In all of the **Paschimottanasana** postures the legs should remain active so that in addition to lengthening the back side you are also strengthening the front by engaging the quadriceps. The grip on the feet in this version of **Paschimottanasana** is designed to assist in pulling the outer edges of the feet back. This action keeps the stretch focused directly in the hamstring area and keeps the ankles from collapsing or rolling out. It is best to keep the elbows away from the floor to keep them awake and fully engaged rather than sleeping.

Paschimottanasana B

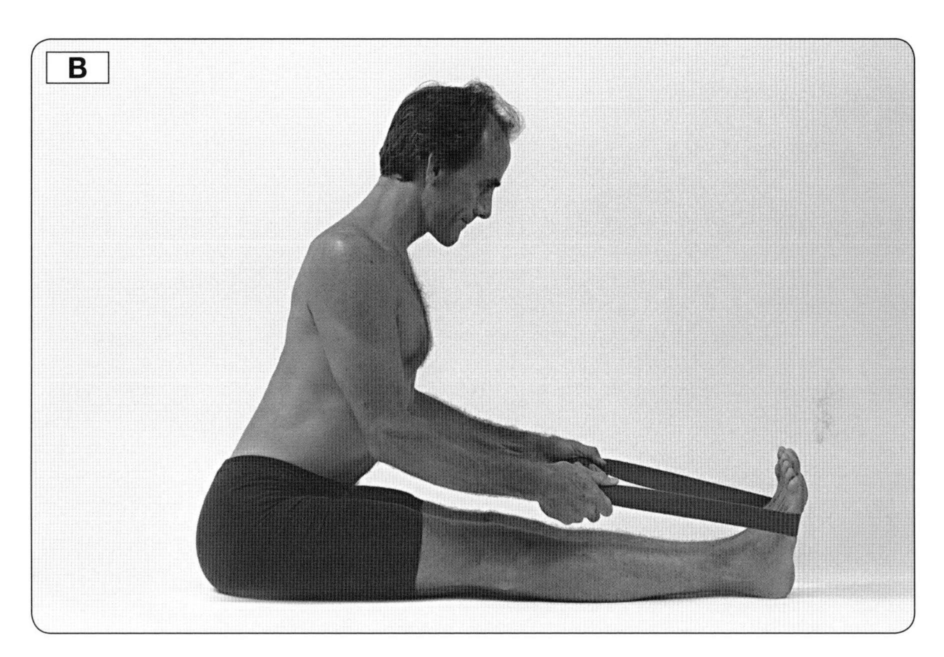

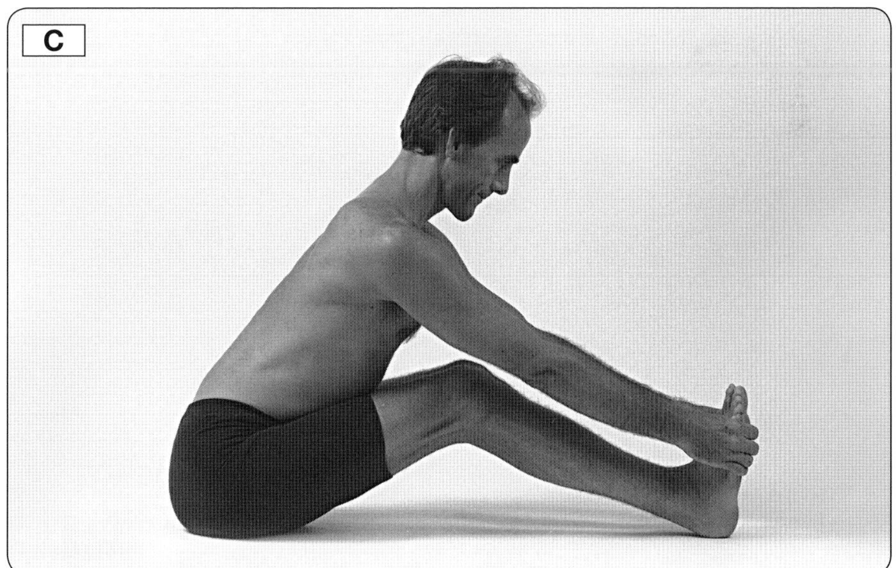

Paschimottanasana C

Paschima = Western Uttana = Intense Stretch

"Western Intense Stretch Posture"

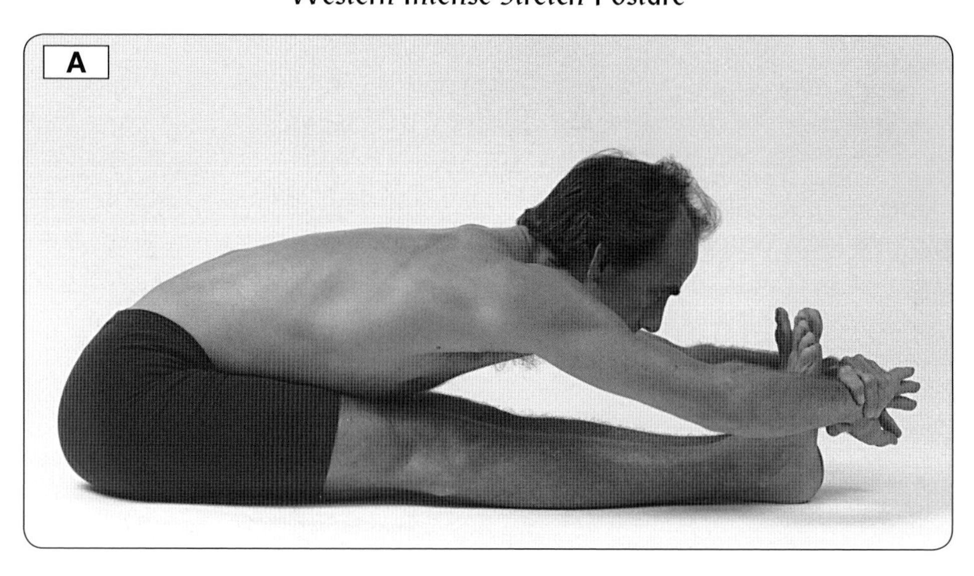

1) **Exhale** change your grip again unless you are now working at your capacity in which case you should remain in one of the previous levels. If you are continuing then reach around the feet and clasp your wrists **(A)**. You may also use one of the previous alternatives with a strap **(B)** or bend the legs **(C)**.
2) **Inhale** with the new grip. Lengthen the spine and lift your gaze to the horizon.
3) **Exhale** fold into whichever level is appropriate for you.

Remain Here For 5 Deep Breaths

4) **Inhale** lengthen the spine and look to the horizon.
5) **Exhale** release the feet and take the hands to the floor beside your hips in preparation for the first jumping vinyasa from a seated position. **See pages 74-77 for details**.

~VINYASA~

Drishti ~ **Toes**

Comments - Do not think in terms of getting your nose to your knees while practicing **Paschimotanasana**. Leading with the nose tends to create a rounding in the back and a collapsing in the chest which gives the illusion of being deeper because of the closer proximity of the nose to the knees. This approach is a recipe for lower back pain. It is much safer and more effective to lead with the sternum keeping the spine long and the shoulders back. This will strengthen the lower back as you lengthen the hamstrings.

Paschimottanasana C

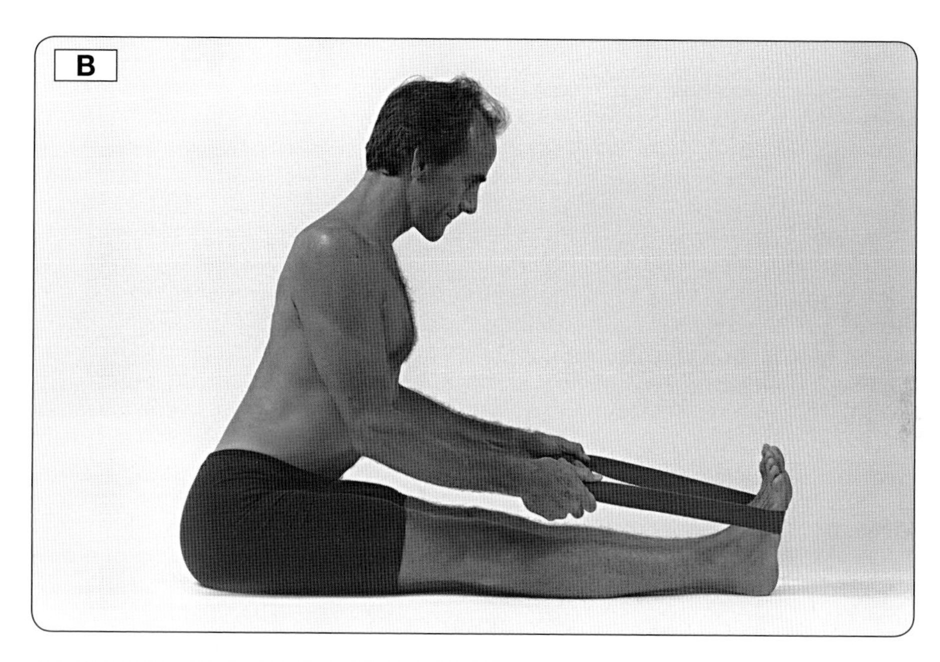

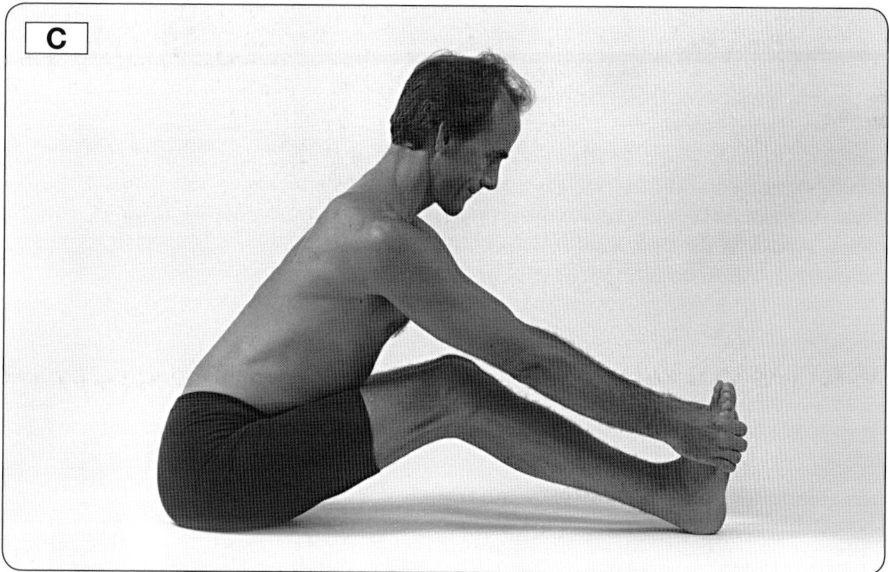

More about Vinyasa

"Dancing with Prana"

Here begins the first application of a jumping Vinyasa from a seated position. As with the **"flying"** options described earlier you may utilize whichever method feels most appropriate for you. Vinyasa is a benevolent aspect of Ashtanga Yoga. It now occurs after every posture as well as after every side of every posture. Whenever there is a vinyasa prescribed I will print the word **VINYASA**. You may then choose your favorite method and proceed into the next asana after completing it. You will find a variety of options in the following pages. If you choose the **"Waiting"** option you would simply omit the vinyasa and change sides or move into the next asana. It is important to move with your breath even when not jumping back. Even simply changing the position of your feet should be done with total awareness and in conjunction with the breath. Then you are applying the full principle of vinyasa. There is no need to choose only one option. You may find that it will be wonderful to insert a couple of one method and then apply another as you move along. Remember, this is **YOUR** practice! I have given a variety of choices in the asanas as well as the vinyasas so that you may build a personal practice. Your unique experience will grow and evolve over time. What is appropriate today may not be tomorrow. When you reach the parts of the series where it says **VINYASA**, make the appropriate choice and continue on. Feel the inherent flow. It is rooted in the breath. The main focus of Vinyasa is breathing with awareness. Whichever option you choose keep that in mind and it will deepen your experience. Enjoy the journey and do not fret about achieving postures. **There is a difference between doing yoga and simply making an asana of ourselves**. Yoga is a meditative experience which promotes inner calmness and tranquility. Making asanas of ourselves creates a competitive atmosphere which is counter-productive to the essence of yoga. Each practice is like a new day. Enter it with the eyes of a child. Find wonder in the practice of yoga. Feel joy in breathing fully. Vinyasa is more than simply moving the body on a physical level. Vinyasa is dancing with the energy of the universe. It is the external expression of the invisible movement of our subtle life-force.

Ride it with a smile on your face!

"It is good to have an end to journey toward;
but it is the journey that matters in the end."

Ursula K. LeGuin

Vinyasa Option #1

"Waiting"

When developing the endurance to practice Ashtanga Yoga some students have found that including all of the Vinyasas between postures is overwhelming. Rather than risk discouragement, I believe it is better to adjust the practice in such a way that each practitioner may grow with it at a personal rate. For this reason I am including the **"Waiting"** option in which you may delete some, or even all, of the Vinyasas and gradually incorporate them into the practice. If you choose to utilize the **"Waiting"** option it is crucial that full ujjayi breath is maintained while pausing. In this way your internal heat will be retained and the focus fixed upon the breath. This option may be inserted whenever you feel the need.

Vinyasa Option #2

"Take-It-Up-Asana"

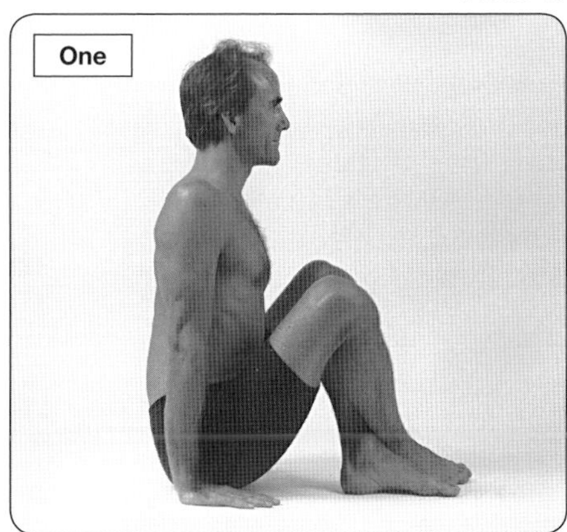

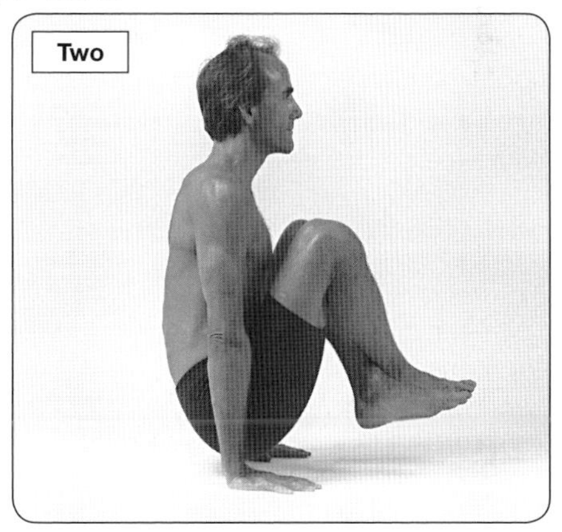

This is a great preparation for Vinyasa. One of the main challenges of vinyasa is the understanding and application of the bandhas. **"Take-It-Up-Asana"**, when performed properly, isolates the specific areas required to take the body on the journey from sitting to **Chaturanga Dandasana**, the plank pose. It is common for people to feel that their arms are too short to enable them to lift up. I have been asked about the idea of using blocks to elevate the hands to create greater clearance. That will create more clearance but then it is still possible to use solely the arms to lift the body while dangling the torso without utilizing the locks to lift. It is much more effective to keep the hands on the floor and develop the strength and control to "take it up" by shortening the mid-section rather than lengthening the arms. Even if "lift-off" is not achieved, **Do Not Worry!** As long as you feel the locks and abdominal muscles working then you are reaping the benefits and increasing your "take-it-up" abilities. It is imperative that your breath continues to flow. **"Take-It-Up-Asana"** may be used in conjunction with or instead of the other options.

Take-It-Up-Asana

One - **Exhale** cross your legs (alternate which one is on top). Place both hands flat on the floor (not on your finger-tips).

Two - **Inhale** draw the knees toward the chest. Lift the hips and feet up from the floor. Feel the bandhas working! Lift on an **inhale** and lower on an **exhale**. You're then ready for the next asana.

Vinyasa Option #3

"Jumping"

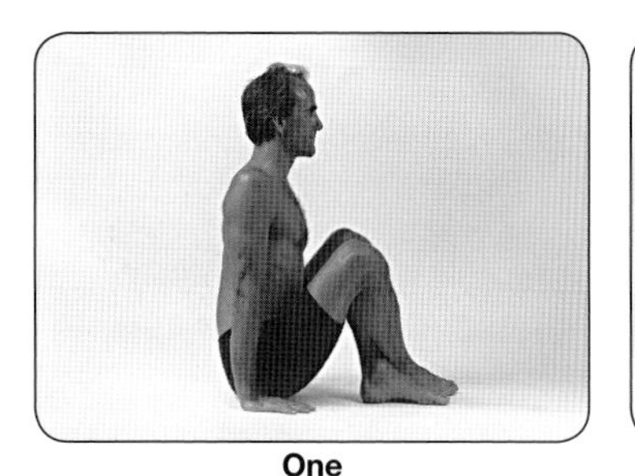

One

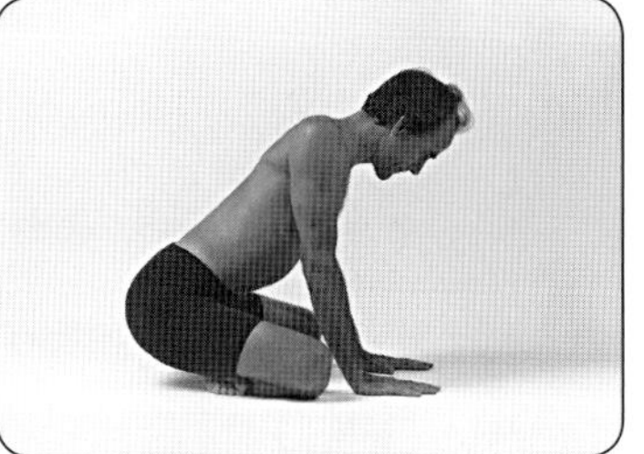

Two

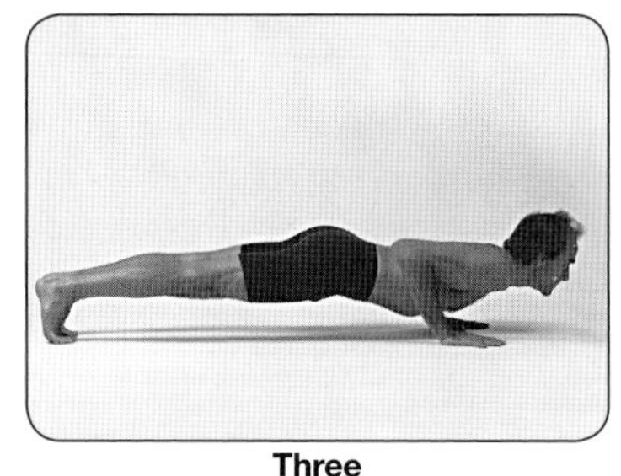

Three

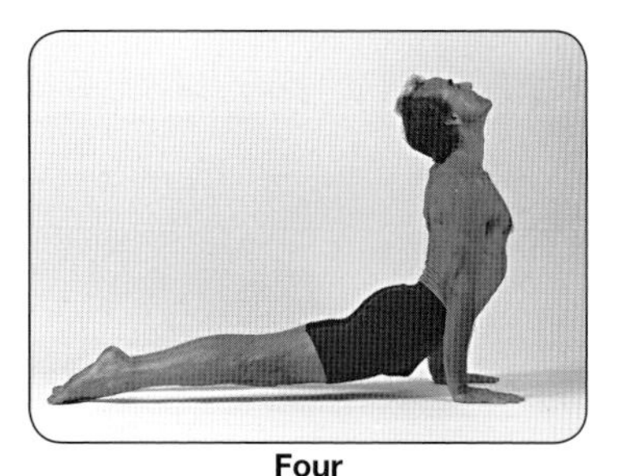

Four

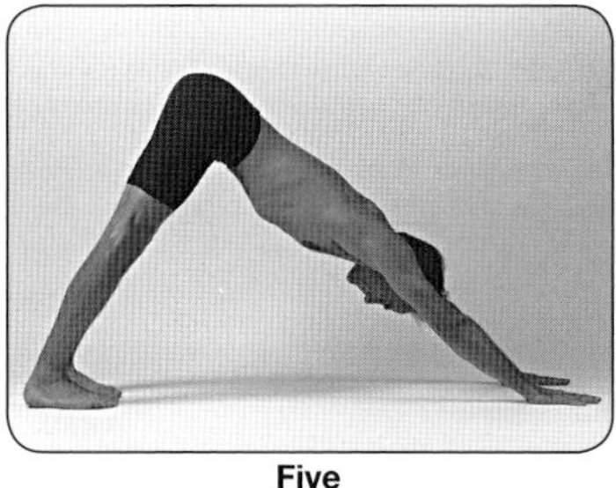

Five

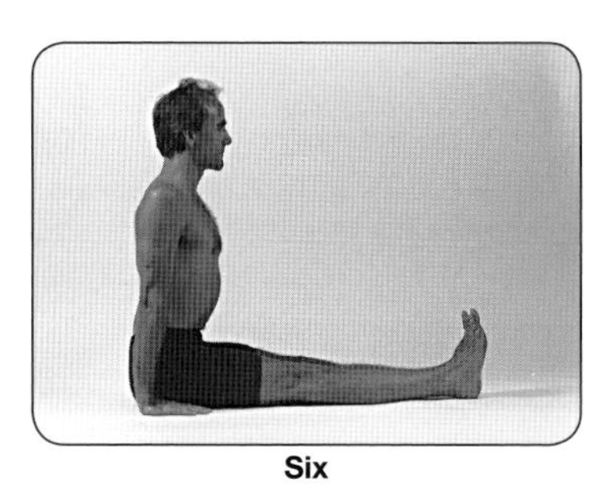

Six

This vinyasa option is probably the most popular method of jumping back. Instead of lifting the body up as in **"take-it-up asana"**, you will roll forward by placing the hands on the floor in front of the legs. Transfer weight into the arms while lifting the hips and then shoot or walk the feet back to **Chaturanga Dandasana**. In this way you may participate in the inherent flow of vinyasa without having to lift up. It is an effective way to maintain heat and initiate the etch-a-sketch effect, yet it is possible to neglect the bandhas and abdominal dynamic required in take-it-up-asana. I would therefore recommend that you either insert take-it-up-asana before each jump back or at least insert it periodically to develop the quality of your bandhas and move toward a lifting up version of this jump-back. As with all other vinyasa methods you must move with your breath in order to develop a fertile environment for exploration of the subtle realms of yoga.

Vinyasa Option #3

One - **Exhale** cross your legs and place the hands flat on the floor.

Two - **Inhale** lean forward and place your hands on the floor in front of your legs. Transfer weight into your hands and begin to lift your hips up while leaving the feet on the floor.

Three - **Exhale** as you either walk or jump your legs back into **Chataranga Dandasana**.

Four - **Inhale** and lift your chest and heart up high into the **Upward-Facing Dog** position while dropping the head back slightly with the gaze up. Keep the legs active.

Five - **Exhale** press your hips up toward the sky into the **Downward-Facing Dog** position.

Six - Do not pause in the **Downward Dog**. While **inhaling**, bend the knees and choose one of the options offered earlier in the "**Physics of Flight**" to bring you back through to sitting.

Vinyasa Option #4

"Floating"

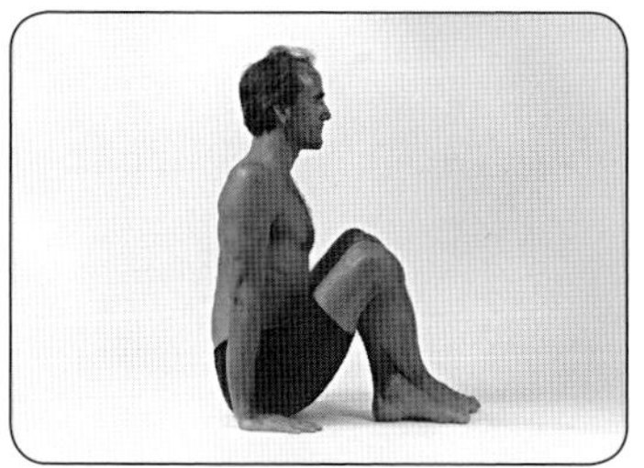

One

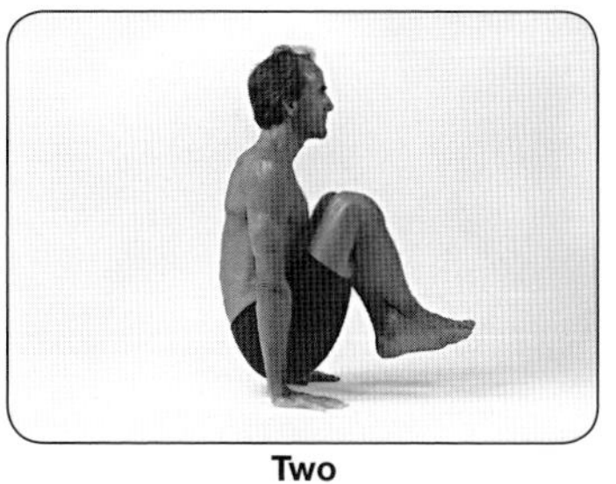

Two

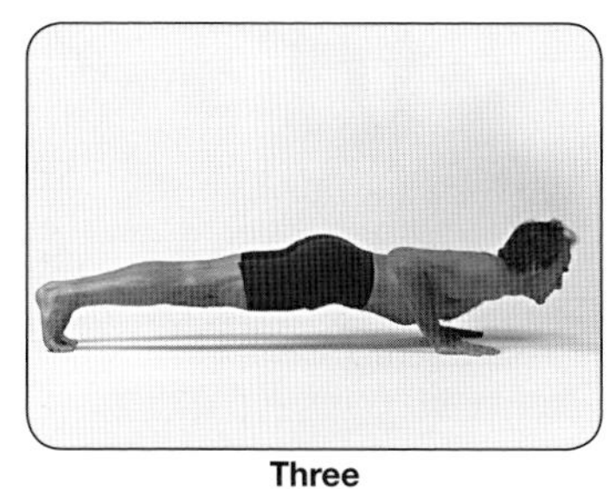

Three

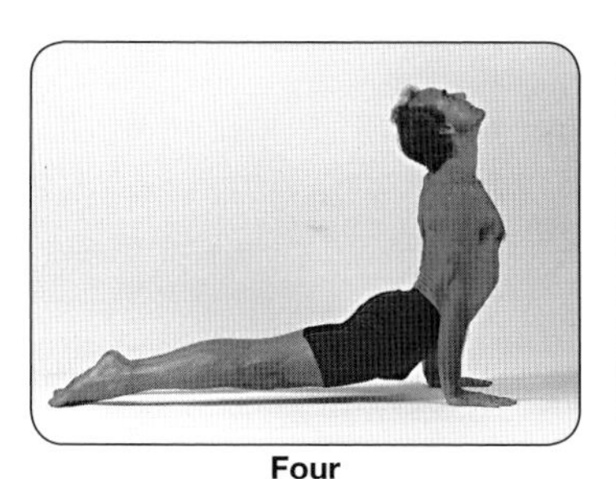

Four

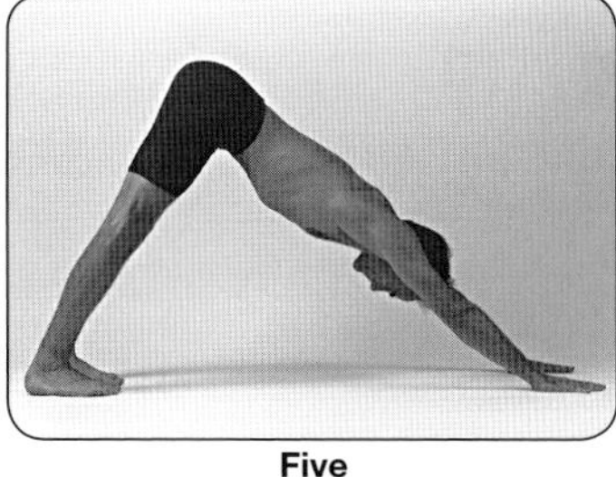

Five

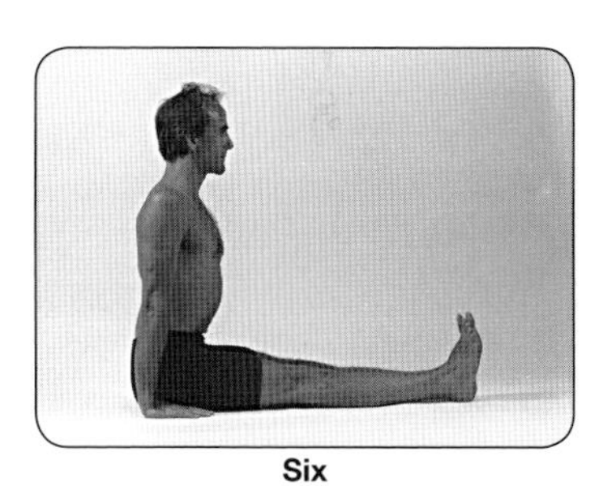

Six

This is the most difficult of the Vinyasa options. It requires a strong foundation within the bandhas in order to lift the body away from the floor and propel it back and through the arms. You may build your practice toward including this option. In the beginning it is wise to choose one of the preparatory methods so as not to wear yourself out from too much effort. Just as with finding depth in the asanas requires time so also the refinement of Vinyasa and the endurance it requires takes time. **Be Patient!**

Vinyasa Option #4

One - Release the asana from which you are exiting and cross your legs while exhaling.

Two - **Inhale** as you press your hands down and lift up as in take-it-up-asana.

Three - **Exhale** while swinging your legs back and through the arms into **Chaturanga Dandasana** without the feet touching the floor.

Four - **Inhale** lift your chest and heart. Drop the head back slightly. Keep the legs active.

Five - **Exhale** while pressing your hips up toward the sky into the **Downward-Facing Dog** position.

Six - Do not pause in the **Downward Dog**. While inhaling, bend the knees and jump forward, floating the legs back through the arms without the feet touching the floor and then lower into a seated position.

Purvottanasana

Purva = Eastern   Uttana = Intense Stretch

"Eastern Intense Stretch Posture"

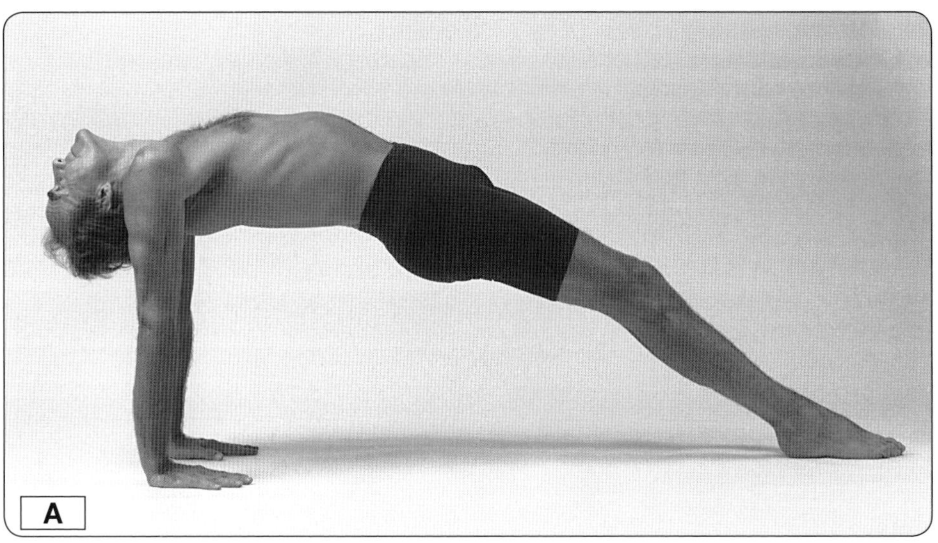

Note - Enter this asana after applying whichever Vinyasa method is most appropriate for you.

1) **Exhale** place the hands flat on the floor behind the hips with the fingers pointing toward the toes.

2) **Inhale** drop the head back. Push the hips up toward the sky. Keep both legs straight with the feet touching and the soles of the feet on the floor. Both arms are straight and fully engaged **(A)**. If it is too intense to practice this with straight legs then before lifting the hips you may bend your knees and bring the feet half way in toward the buttocks. Place the feet hip-width apart and then lift **(B)**. A third option is to leave the hips on the floor and lift only the chest while dropping the head back **(C)**.

Remain Here For 5 Deep Breaths

3) **Exhale** as you lower the hips to release the asana.

~VINYASA~

Drishti ~ **Nose**

Comments - Be aware of the position of your hands in relation to the shoulders after you lift the hips. The wrists should be directly below the shoulders with the arms straight. If you start with them too close to the hips then when lifting you will have the sensation that you are being pulled from behind and it will be difficult to find your point of balance. If on the other hand you start with the hands too far behind the hips it will put undue strain on the shoulders and wrists. Seek the point of balance in order to find the correct spatial relation between the hands, hips and shoulders. Maintain a slight inward rotation of the thighs.

Purvottanasana

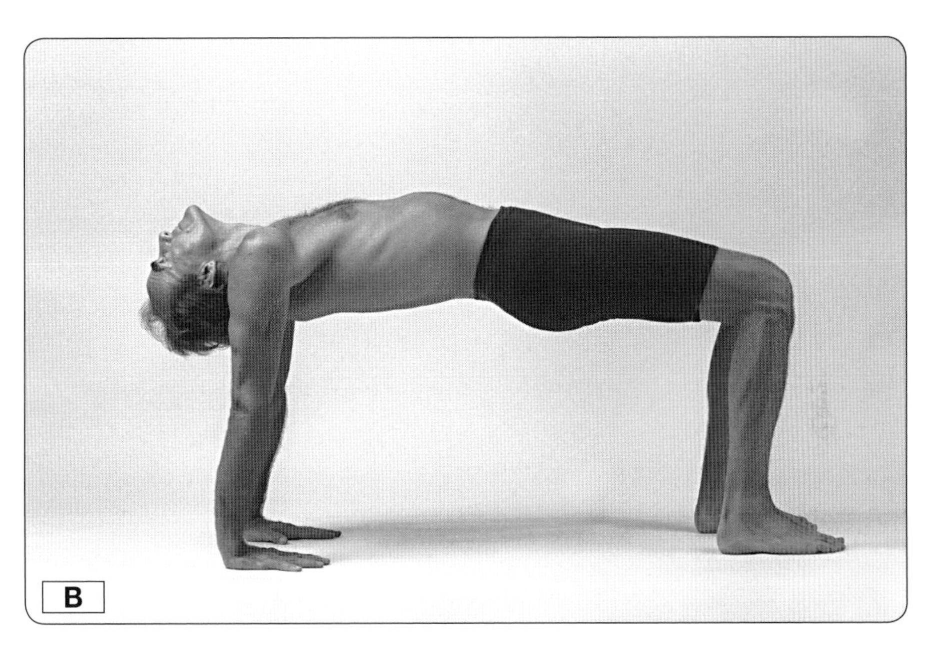

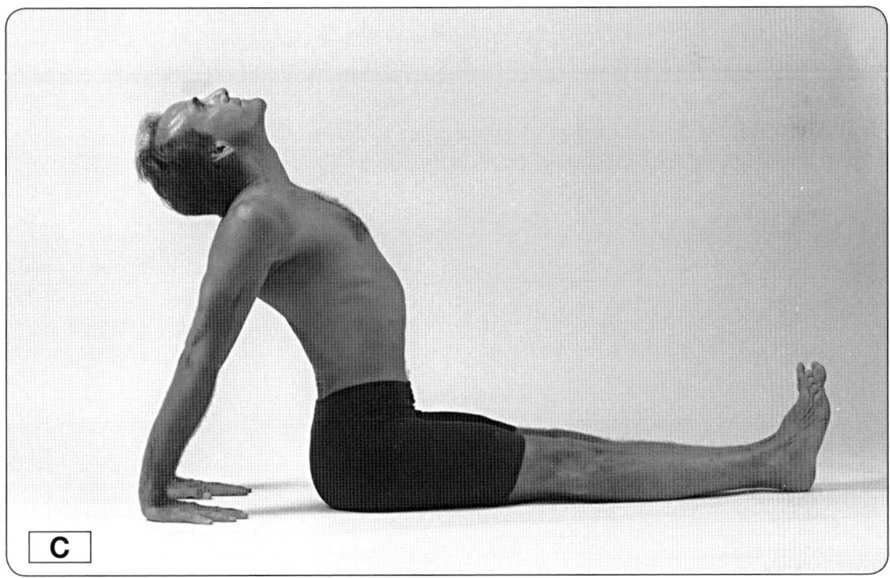

Ardha Baddha Padma Paschimottanasana

Ardha = Half Baddha = Bound Padma = Lotus
Paschima = Western Uttana = Intense Stretch
"Half Bound Lotus Western Intense Stretch Posture"

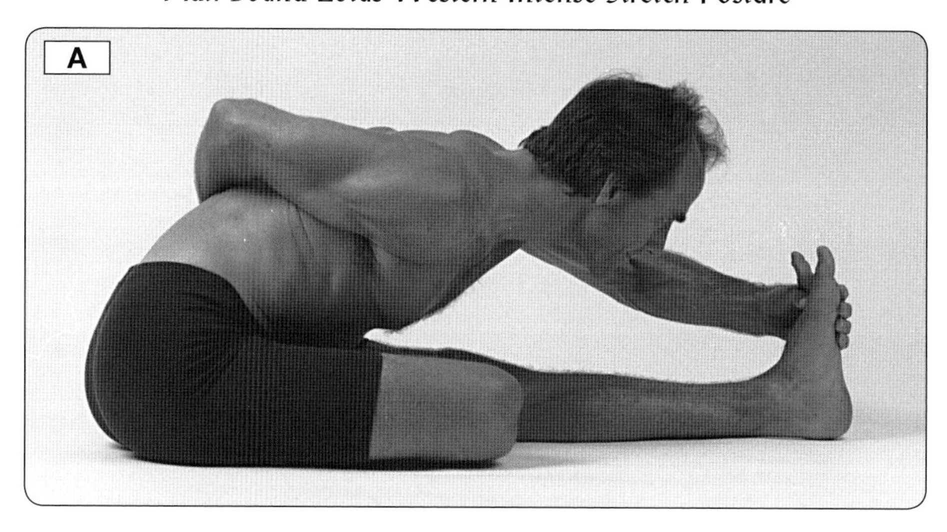

1) **Exhale** take the right foot in the left hand. Lift it up and bring it across to the upper left thigh while supporting the right knee in your right hand. Reach behind the back with the right hand and clasp the right foot. Hold the left foot with the left hand. Knees close together **(A)**. If it is too much to clasp the right foot when reaching behind the back then hold it with the left hand and use the right hand to clasp the left elbow **(B)**. If you use props, wrap a strap around the foot or feet that you are having difficulty reaching **(C)** or you may leave the right foot on the floor instead of taking it on top of the left thigh **(D)**.

2) **Inhale** lift the head and lengthen the spine.

3) **Exhale** and lower into whichever level is appropriate for you.

Remain Here For 5 Deep Breaths

4) **Inhale** lift the head and lengthen the spine.

5) **Exhale** release the foot and straighten both legs.

~VINYASA~

Repeat Steps 1-5 On the Left Side

~VINYASA~

Drishti ~ **Toes**

Comments - ***Be aware of your knees!*** Open from the hip. Take the right knee in the right hand and the left foot in the left hand to fully support the leg as you approach the half-lotus. Choose the appropriate option.

Ardha Baddha Padma Paschimottanasana

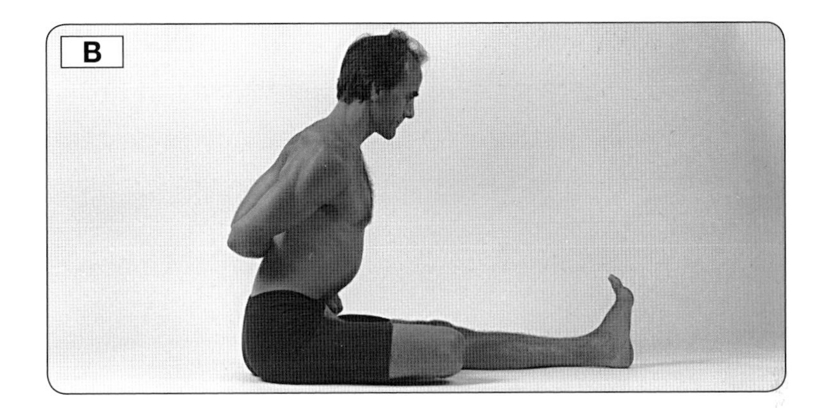

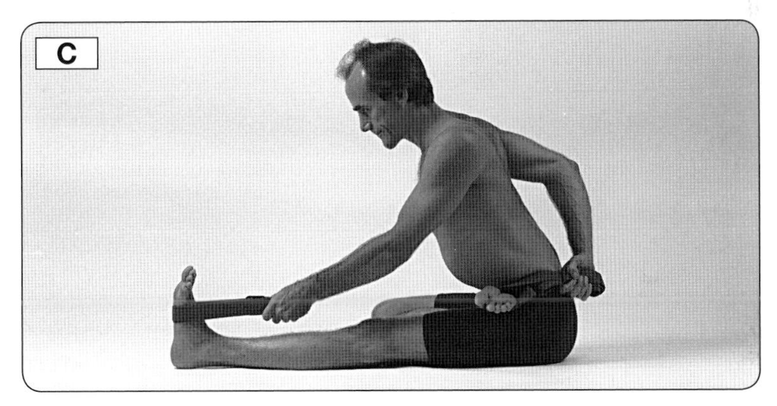

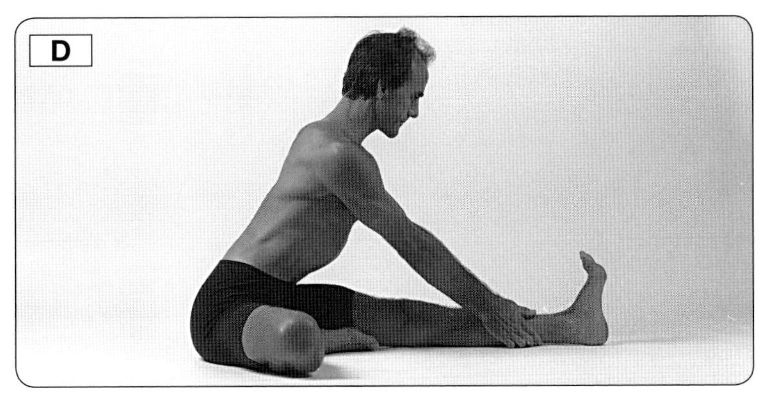

Trianga Mukhaikapada Paschimottanasana

Tri = Three Anga = Limb Mukha = Face Eka = One Pada = Foot
Paschima = Western Uttana = Intense Stretch

"Three Limbs Face One Foot Western Intense Stretch Posture"

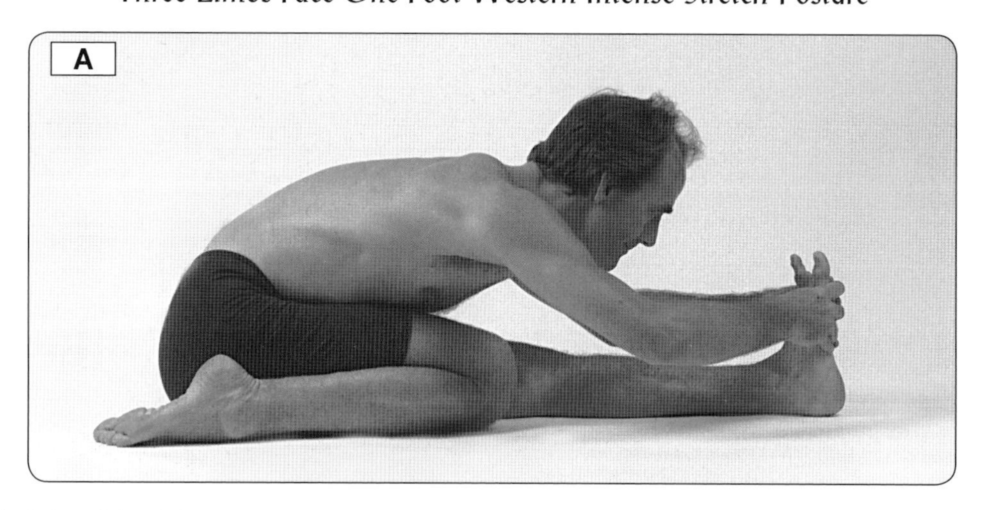
A

1) **Exhale** bend the right knee placing the right foot outside the right hip with the top of the foot touching the floor. Left leg straight. Both hands clasping the left ankle or foot **(A)**. If you feel like you are falling over or it is too much stretch on the right knee then elevate the left hip with a prop **(B)**. If it is still too extreme then you may approach this asana by sitting with your buttocks between the heels as in **(C)** or sit on top of the heels as in **(D)**. **Use a pad under the top of the feet if you feel discomfort**.

2) **Inhale** lengthen the spine and take your gaze to the horizon

3) **Exhale** move into whichever option is most appropriate for you.

Remain Here For 5 Deep Breaths

4) **Inhale** lift the head and lengthen the spine.

5) **Exhale** release the asana and straighten both legs.

~VINYASA~

Repeat Steps 1-5 On the Left Side

~VINYASA~

Drishti ~ **Toes**

Comments - If you feel as though you are going to tip over to one side in option **(A)** or **(B)**, check the position of your shoulders. Make sure that they are on an even plane. Lengthen both sides of the torso equally. If you feel discomfort on top of the foot then place a thin cushion under it. Be sure the foot that is beside the hip is placed with the top of the foot touching the floor with the toes pointing straight back. **Do *NOT* point the toes out to the side with the inner ankle on the floor**. That would be dangerous for the knee.

Trianga Mukhaikapada Paschimottanasana

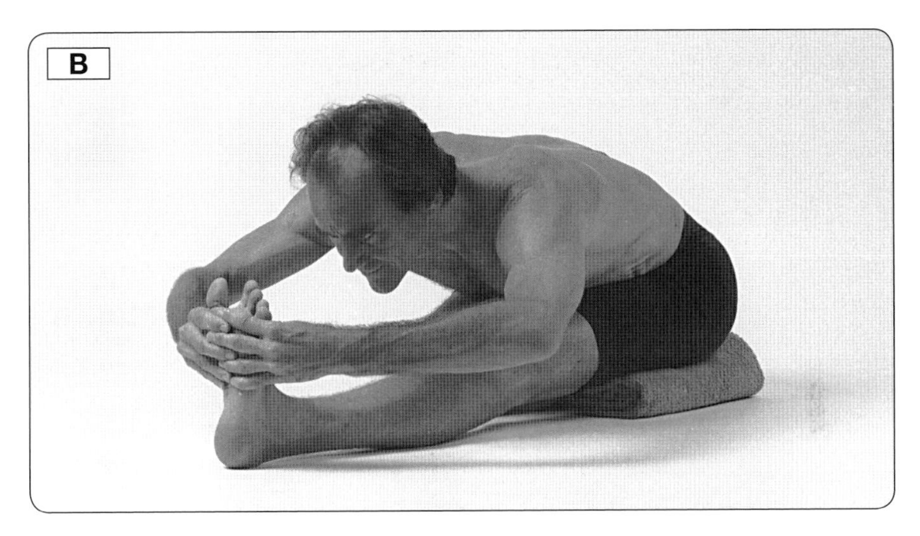

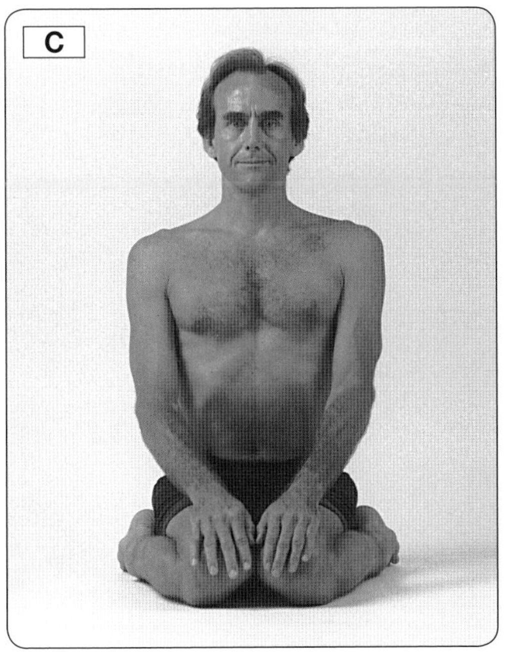

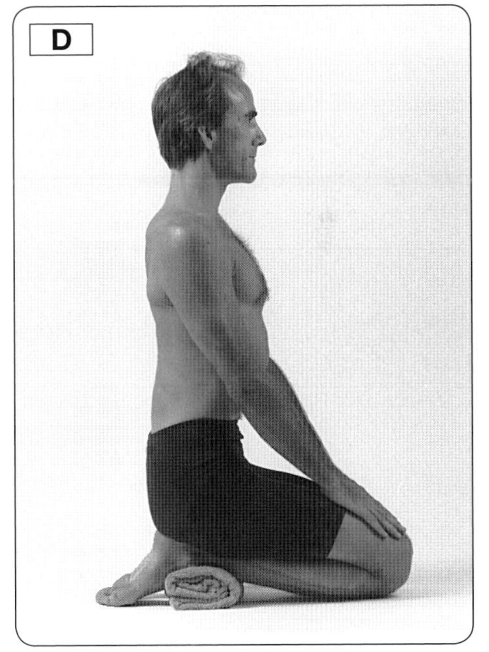

Janu Sirsasana A

Janu = Knee   Sirsa = Head

"Head to Knee Posture"

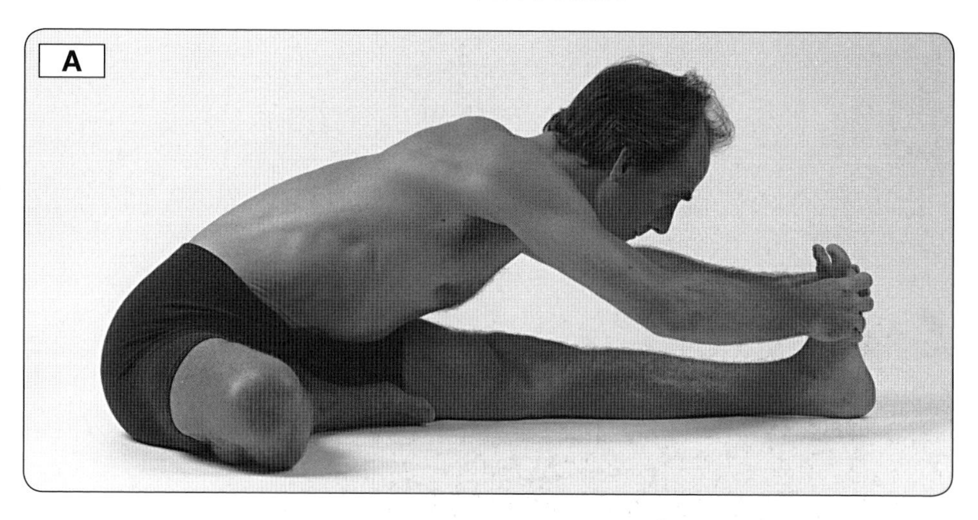

1) **Exhale** bring the right foot into the inner left thigh. Create a **ninety-degree angle** between the knees with the left leg straight. Clasp the the left foot with both hands **(A)**. If it is too extreme to reach the left foot then clasp near the ankle or shin **(B)**. You may also use a strap to wrap around the foot **(C)**.

2) **Inhale** lengthen the spine and take your gaze to the horizon

3) **Exhale** fold forward into whichever option is most appropriate for you.

Remain Here For 5 Deep Breaths

4) **Inhale** lift the head and lengthen the spine.

5) **Exhale** release the asana and straighten both legs.

~VINYASA~

Repeat Steps 1-5 On the Left Side

~VINYASA~

Drishti ~ **Toes**

Comments - Even though this is called the head-to-knee posture the focus should really be the extension of the sternum toward the knee so as not to encourage a rounding of the back. Keep the elbows away from the floor. If you feel discomfort in the bent knee you may place a towel under it for a slight elevation. This will take some pressure off. You may also bring the foot closer to the left knee instead of the inner left thigh.

Janu Sirsasana A

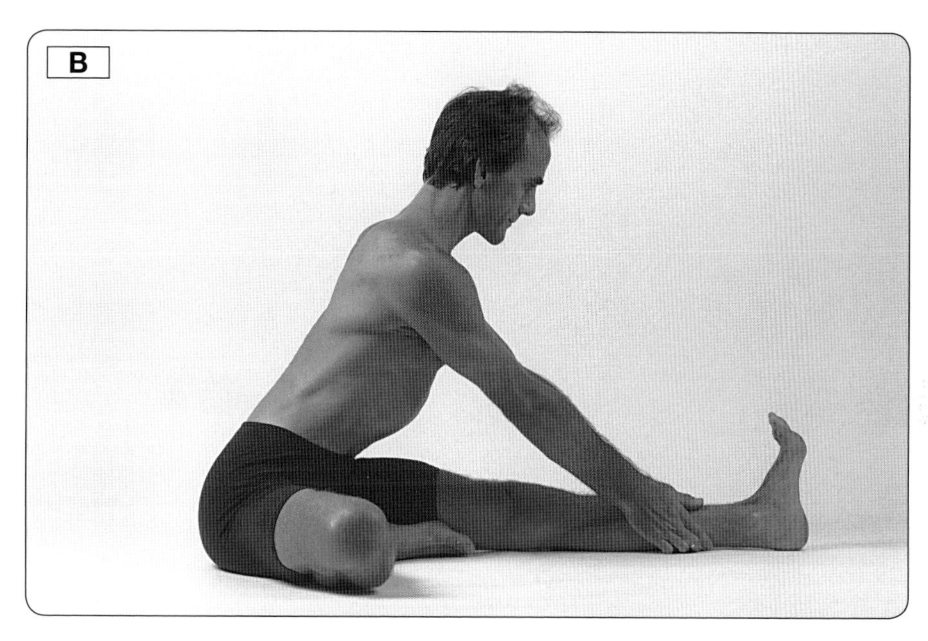
B

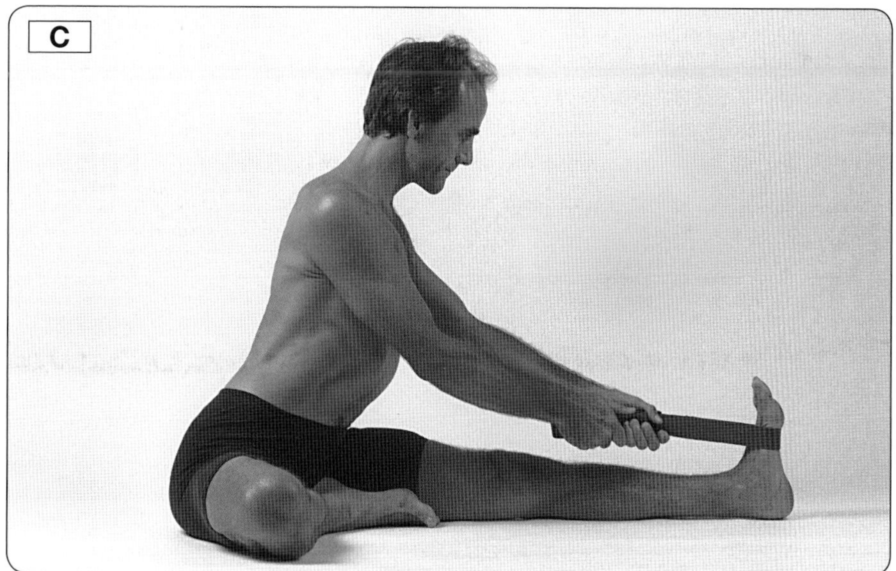
C

Janu Sirsasana B

Janu = Knee Sirsa = Head

"Head to Knee Posture"

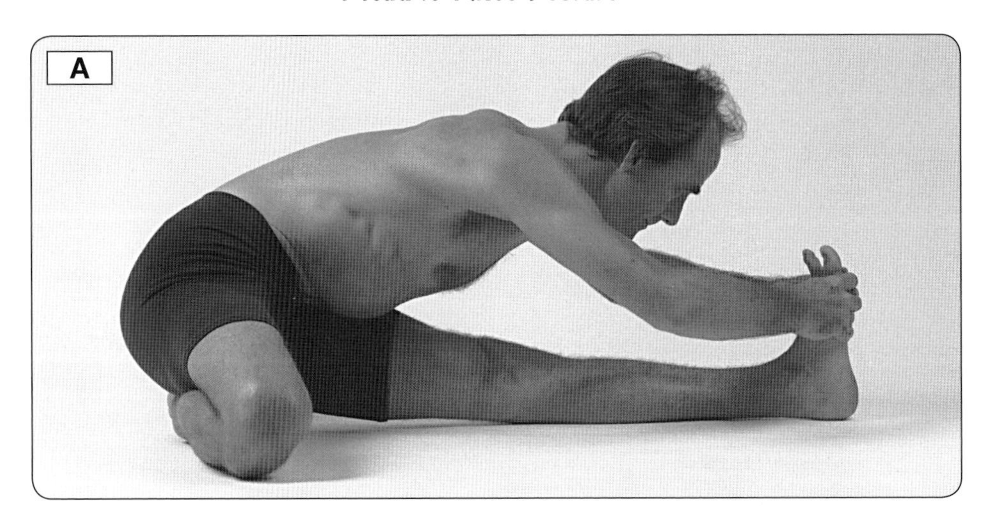

1) **Exhale** as you sit on the right heel. Place the heel at the location of the perineal muscle in front of the anus and behind the genitals. The right foot should be positioned so that the toes point directly out to the left and the top of the foot is resting on the floor with an **eighty-five degree angle** between the knees. The left leg is straight. Clasp the left foot with both hands **(A)**. If you cannot reach the left foot then hold the ankle **(B)** or use a strap **(C)**. If you find this asana to be too much then repeat **Janu Sirsasana A**.

2) **Inhale** lengthen the spine and take your gaze to the horizon

3) **Exhale** fold forward into whichever option is most appropriate for you.

Remain Here For 5 Deep Breaths

4) **Inhale** lift the head and lengthen the spine.

5) **Exhale** release the asana and straighten both legs.

~VINYASA~

Repeat Steps 1-5 On the Left Side

~VINYASA~

Drishti ~ **Toes**

Comments - This posture is meant to stimulate **mulabandha** by the placement of the heel on the perineal muscle. Move into it slowly by keeping your hands on the floor for support. If the top of the foot hurts from pressing into the floor then place a thin cushion under it. If your knee is bothered you may repeat **Janu Sirsasana A** instead or omit this asana for now. **Be Patient!**

Janu Sirsasana B

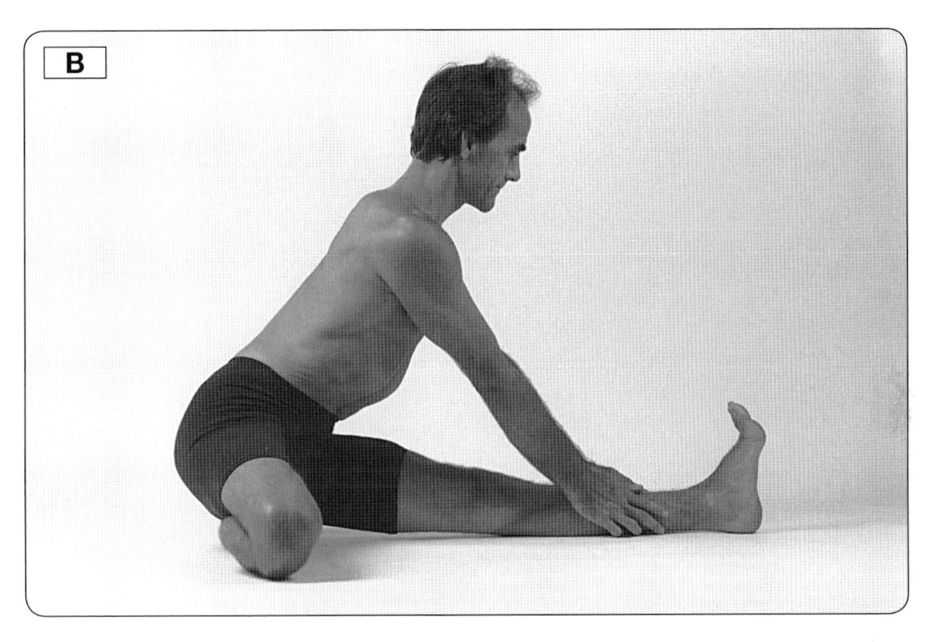

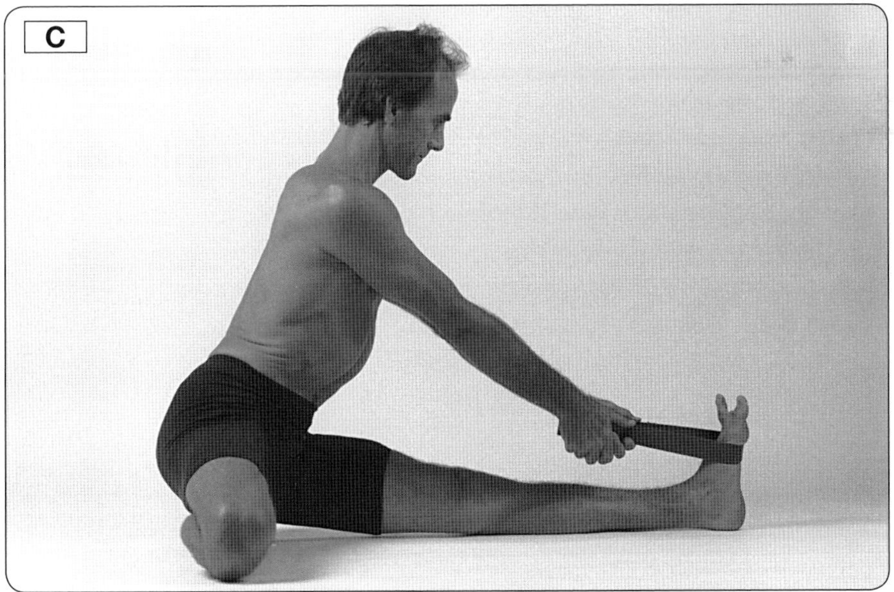

Janu Sirsasana C

Janu = Knee Sirsa = Head

"Head to Knee Posture"

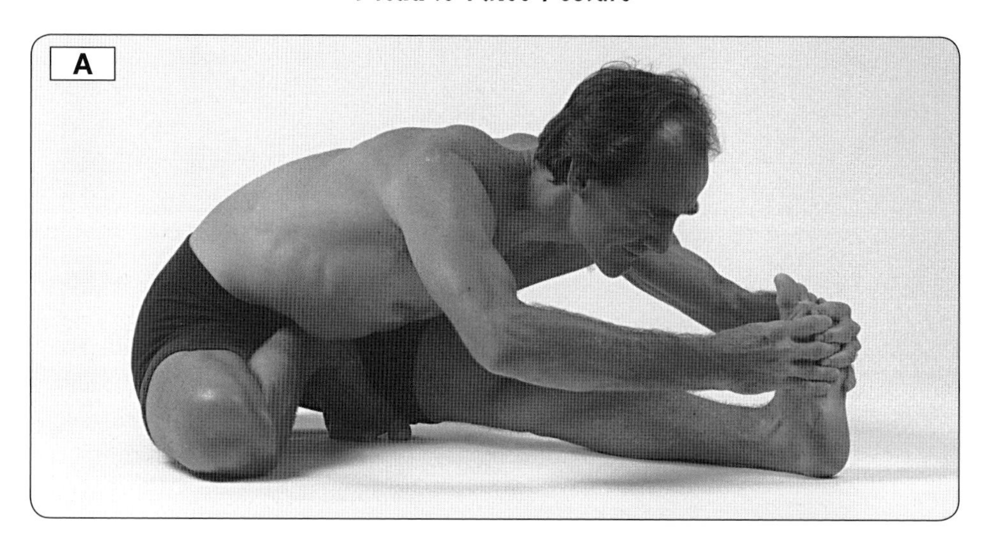

1) **Exhale** take the right heel in the left hand. Keep the foot flexed. Reach the right hand under the right ankle and grab the foot. Rotate it so that the ball of the foot is touching the floor and the heel is pointing straight up with the arch of the right foot resting on the inner left thigh. Keep the left leg straight with a forty-five degree angle between the knees. Clasp the left foot or ankle with both hands **(A)**. You may find it helpful to elevate the hips with a prop **(B)** or sit up straight and rotate the foot in a preparatory phase without placing it on the floor **(C)**. If this is too extreme then repeat **Janu Sirsasana A** or **B**.

2) **Inhale** lengthen the spine and take your gaze to the horizon

3) **Exhale** and move into whichever option is most appropriate for you.

Remain Here For 5 Deep Breaths

4) **Inhale** lift the head and lengthen the spine.

5) **Exhale** release the asana and straighten both legs.

~VINYASA~

Repeat Steps 1-5 On the Left Side

~VINYASA~

Drishti ~ **Toes**

Comments - ***Proceed with great caution and awareness in this asana***. There is no hurry! If you feel discomfort in your knee, back off. It is important to rotate from the hip so as not to take undue strain in the knee. Find the best option for you. Remember it is fine to leave an asana out and move toward it later.

Janu Sirsasana C

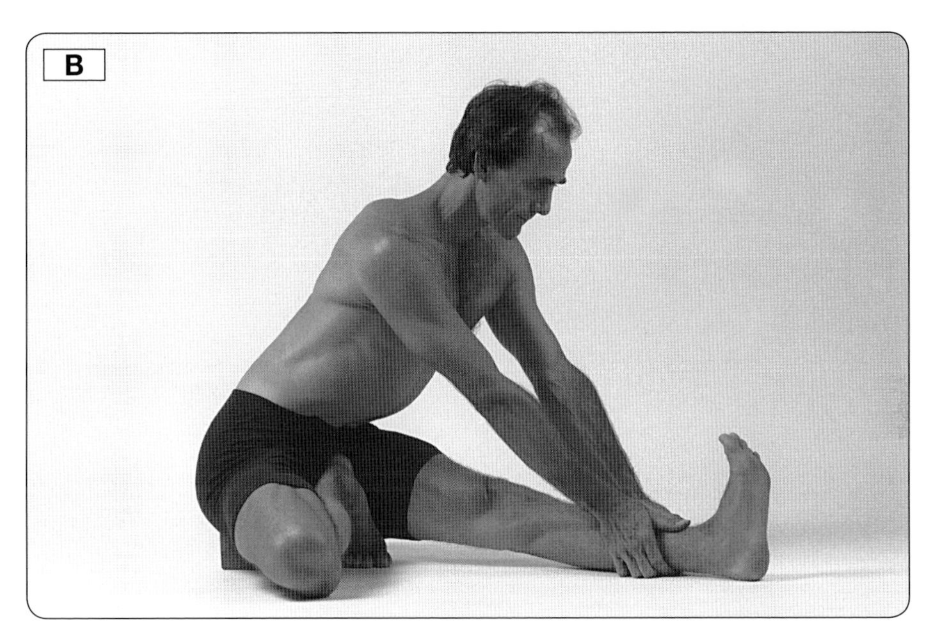

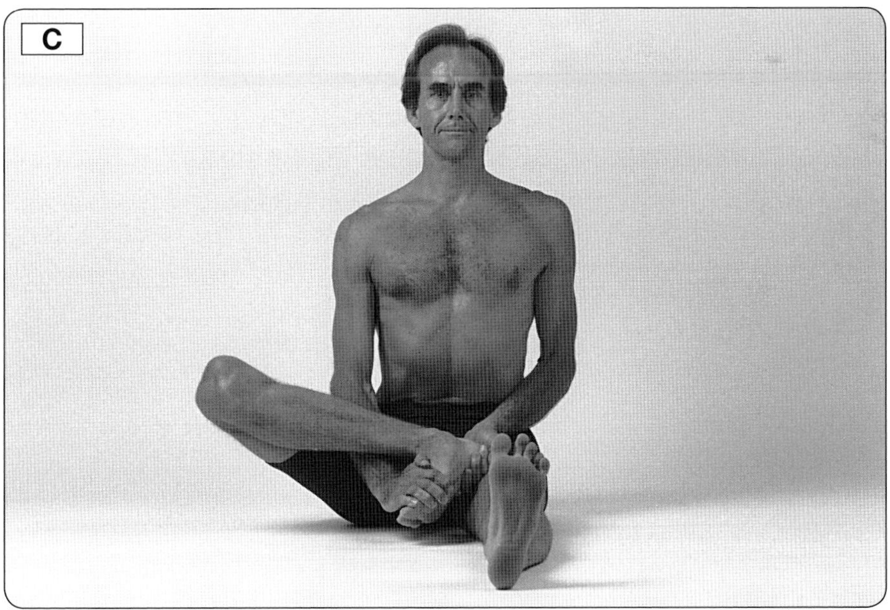

Marichyasana A

Marichi = A great sage and son of Brahma

"Dedicated to Marichi"

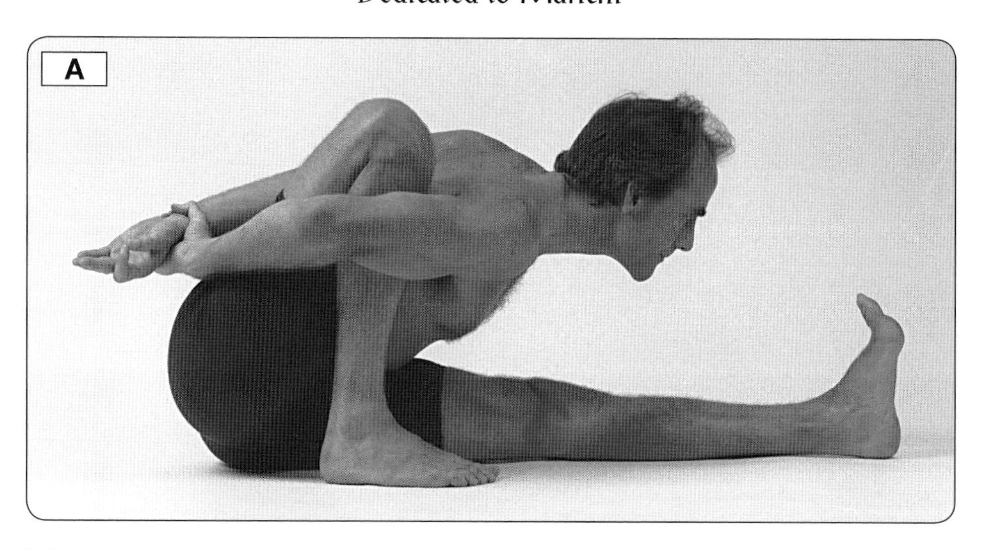

1) **Exhale** bend the right leg placing the heel near the right sit-bone with the right knee pointing toward the sky. Wrap the right arm around the right leg using equality of opposition as leverage. Clasp both hands behind the back. Fold forward **(A)**. If you are not clasping the hands then leave them on the floor **(B)** or hold the left leg with both hands **(C)** or use a strap to connect the hands behind the back **(D)**.

2) **Inhale** lengthen the spine and take your gaze to the horizon.

3) **Exhale** and fold forward into whichever option is most appropriate for you.

Remain Here For 5 Deep Breaths

4) **Inhale** lift the head and lengthen the spine.

5) **Exhale** release the asana and straighten both legs.

~VINYASA~

Repeat Steps 1-5 On the Left Side

~VINYASA~

Drishti ~ **Toes**

Comments - A key factor to moving into this asana is the dynamic force created between the arm and the bent knee for options **A, B** and **D**. Here you may press the arm back in order to draw the chest forward. In **C** pull the shoulders back as you extend forward with the chest. In all options lead with your sternum and not with the nose. Encourage length in the spine. The extended leg should remain active. Whenever clasping the hands behind the back **"the wrapper is the grabber"**; use the arm that wraps the leg to grab with.

Marichyasana A

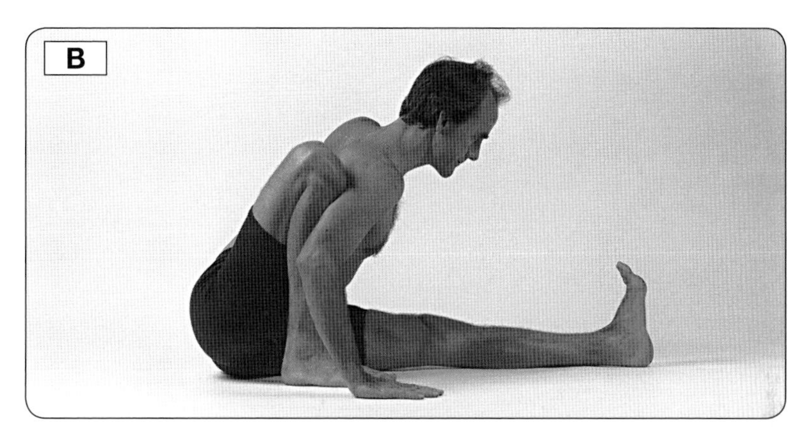

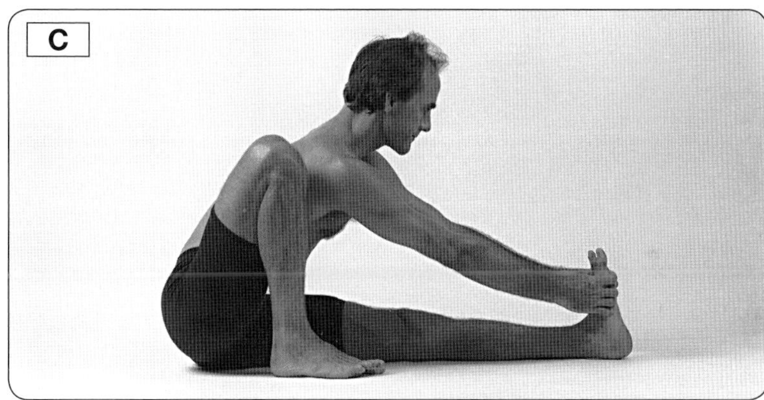

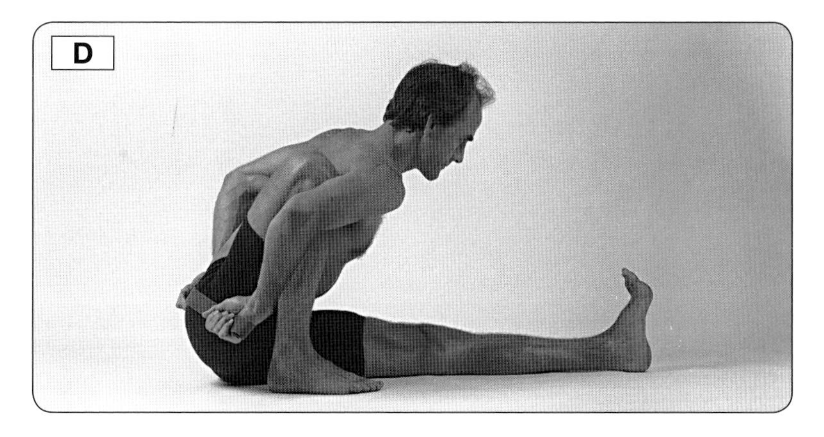

Marichyasana B

Marichi = A great sage and son of Brahma

"Dedicated to Marichi"

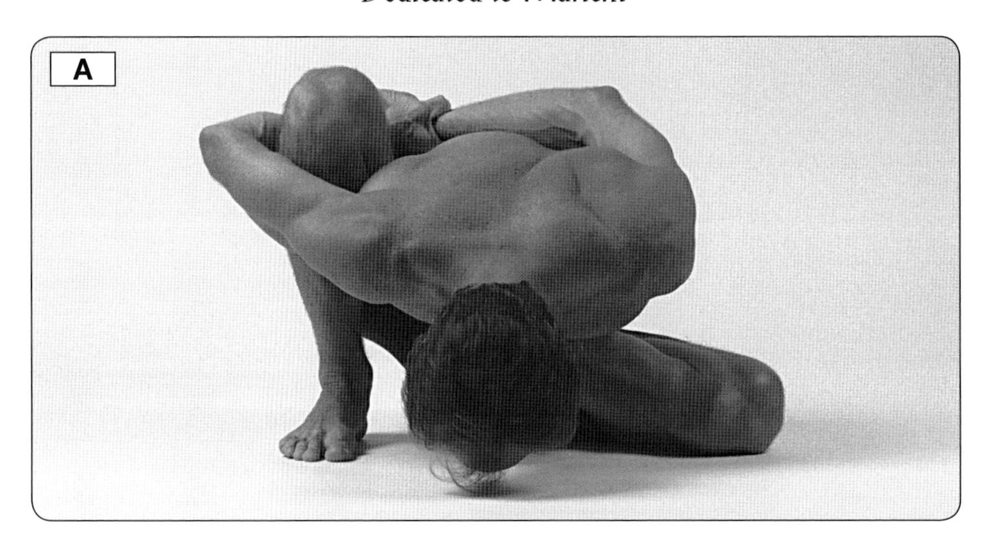

1) **Exhale** and place the left leg in half-lotus. Raise the right knee placing the right heel in line with the right sit-bone. Open the space between the left knee and the right foot. Wrap the right arm around the right leg and clasp the hands behind the back. Fold forward **(A)**. If folding forward is too intense then sit up straight and hold the right knee with both hands **(B)**. If half-lotus is too much then leave the left foot on the floor behind the right heel **(C)**. Another option is to repeat **Marichyasana A**.

2) **Inhale** lengthen the spine and take your gaze to the horizon.

3) **Exhale** and fold forward into whichever option is most appropriate for you.

Remain Here For 5 Deep Breaths

4) **Inhale** lift the head and lengthen the spine.

5) **Exhale** release the asana and straighten both legs.

~VINYASA~

Repeat Steps 1-5 On the Left Side

~VINYASA~

Drishti ~ **Nose**

Comments - ***Proceed with caution when placing the leg in half-lotus!*** In the West our knees are inherently tight due to centuries of sitting in chairs and on western-style toilets. Use the option which most suits you. Lead with your chest and encourage the heart to open. Listen to your body and breathe with awareness.

Marichyasana B

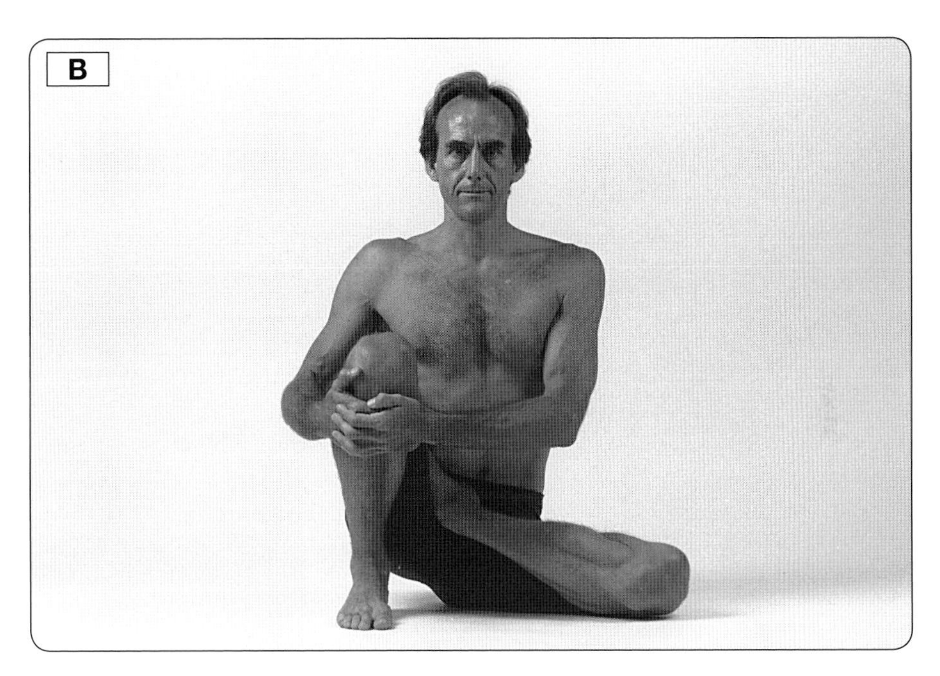

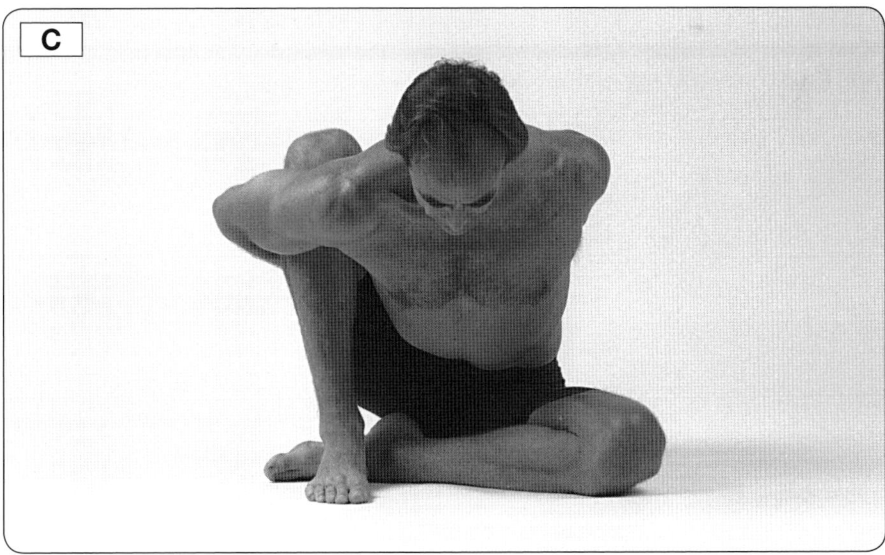

Marichyasana C

Marichi = A great sage and son of Brahma

"Dedicated to Marichi"

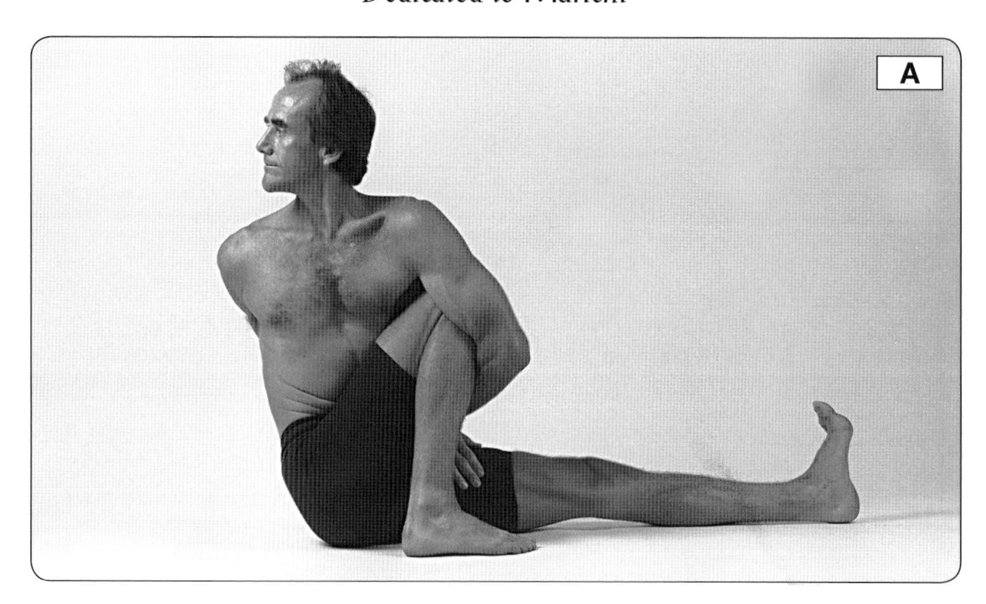

1) **Exhale** bend the right leg. Place the heel near the right sit-bone or slightly to the outside of it. Bring the left arm across between the chest and the right knee. Wrap the left arm around the right knee. Take the right arm behind the back and clasp your hands or wrist. **(A)**. If you are not clasping the hands behind your back yet, then leave the right hand on the floor behind you, left arm bent with the elbow pressing against the outer right knee **(B)** or hold the right knee with the left hand and place the right hand on the floor **(C)**.

2) **Inhale** lengthen the spine and take your gaze over the right shoulder.

3) **Exhale** and move into whichever option is most appropriate for you.

Remain Here For 5 Deep Breaths

4) **Inhale** and gaze to the front.

5) **Exhale** release the asana and straighten both legs.

~VINYASA~

Repeat Steps 1-5 On the Left Side

~VINYASA~

Drishti ~ **Over the Shoulder**

Comments - Twisting requires length. The greater length you create in the spine the easier it will be to breathe deeply. Elongate the spine in a spiraling motion. Use the arm and knee opposition to assist in both the lengthening and twisting process to create the desired spiraling effect. Keep the extended leg active.

Marichyasana C

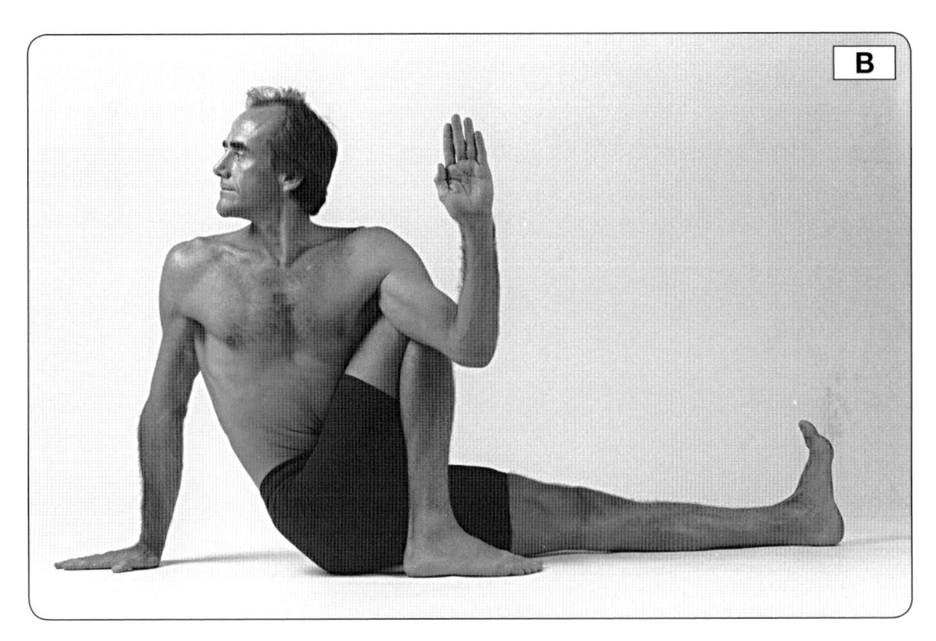

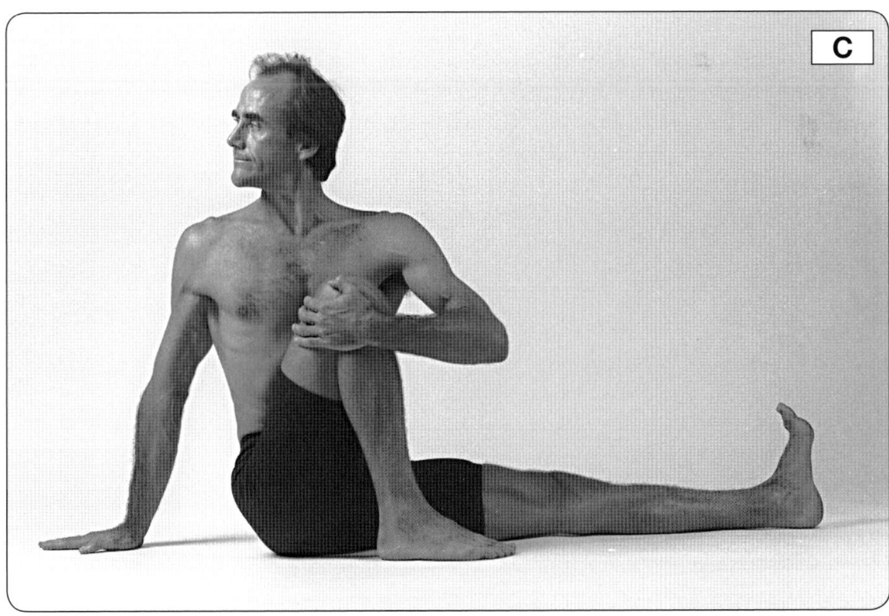

Marichyasana D

Marichi = A great sage and son of Brahma

"Dedicated to Marichi"

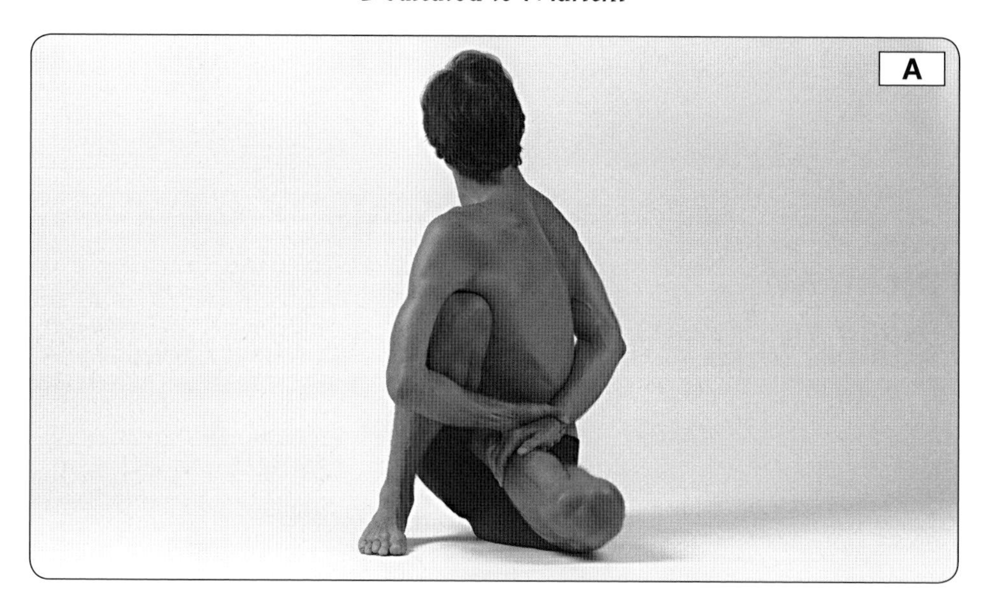

1) **Exhale** place the left leg in half-lotus. Raise the right knee placing the right heel in line with the right sit-bone or slightly wider. Draw the left knee across toward the right foot. Wrap the left arm around the right knee and clasp your hands behind the back **(A)** or leave the left foot on the floor instead of in half-lotus **(B)**. If you cannot clasp the hands behind the back then sit up straight and hold the right knee instead **(C)**. Another option is to leave the left foot on the floor behind the right heel. Place the left elbow outside the right knee with the right hand on the floor behind you **(D)**. You may repeat **Marichyasana C**.

2) **Inhale** lengthen the spine and take your gaze over the right shoulder.

3) **Exhale** and move into whichever option is most appropriate for you.

Remain Here For 5 Deep Breaths

4) **Inhale** gaze to the front.

5) **Exhale** release the asana and straighten both legs.

~VINYASA~

Repeat Steps 1-5 On the Left Side

~VINYASA~

Drishti ~ **Over the Shoulder**

Comments - ***Proceed with extra caution when practicing this asana!*** As in **Marichyasana B** bring additional awareness to your knees. Follow your breath. Choose the appropriate level and listen internally.

Marichyasana D

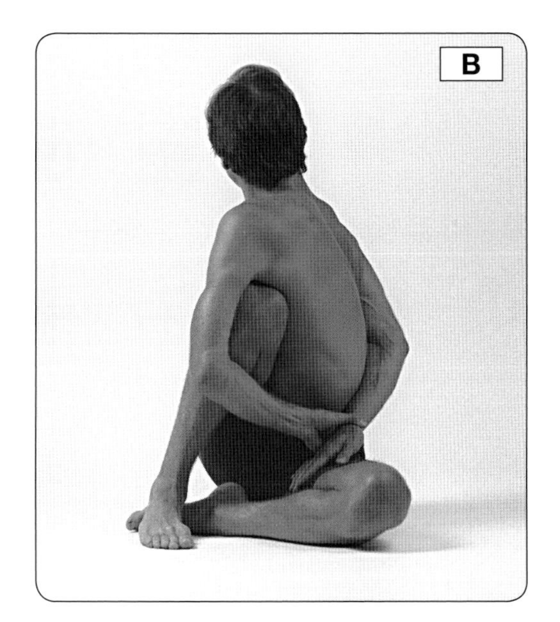

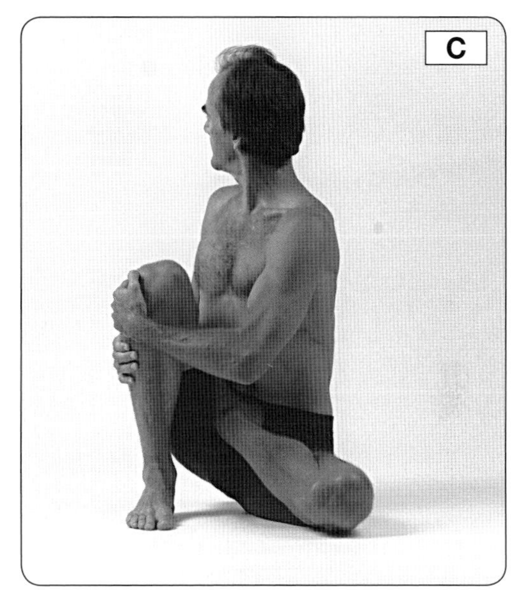

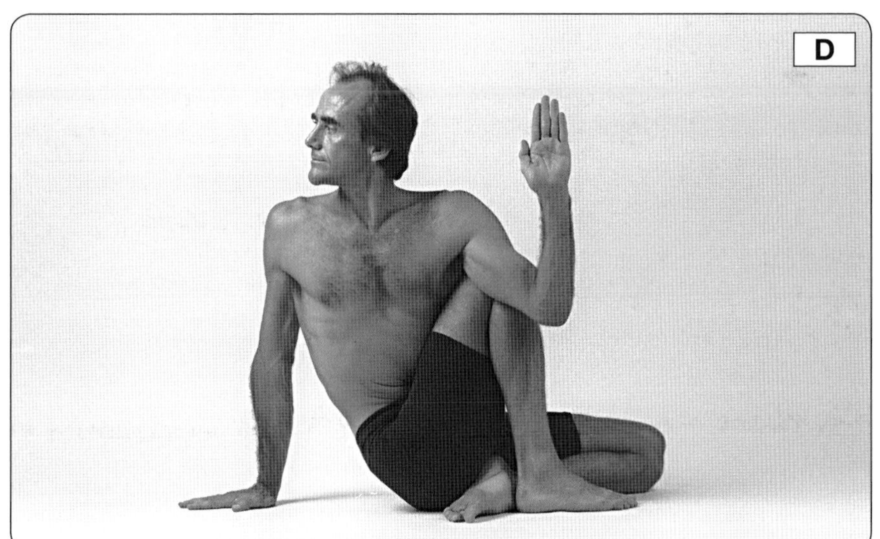

Navasana

Nava = Boat

"Boat Posture"

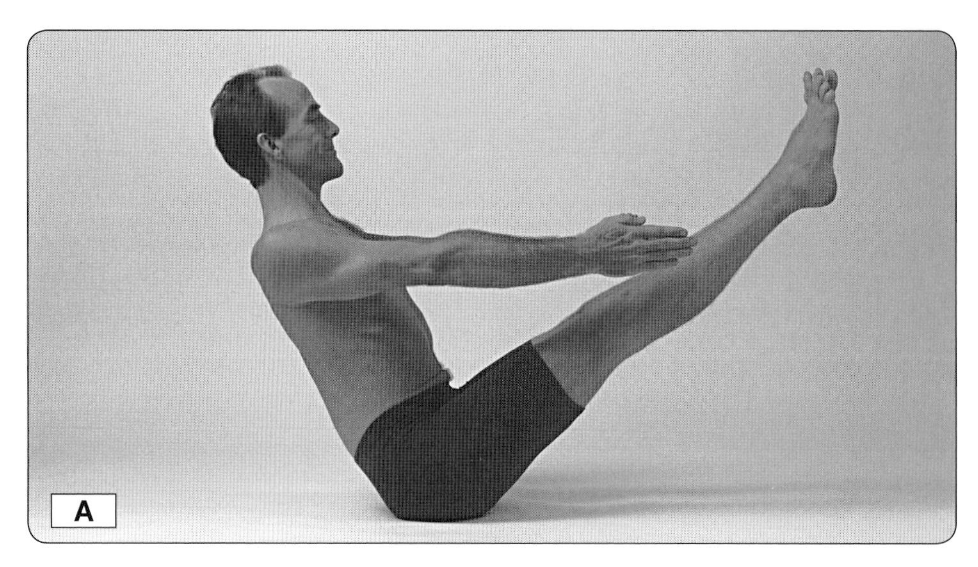

1) **Inhale** lift and straighten both legs with the feet together and the toes pointed at eye level. Arms straight and parallel to the floor with the palms facing each other **(A)** or bend the legs with the shins parallel with the arms **(B)**. You may also hold the back of the knees for support **(C)**.

Remain Here For 5 Deep Breaths

2) **Exhale** hands to the floor beside the hips.

3) **Inhale** lift up into **"take-it-up-asana" (D)** or **Handstand (E) & (F)**.

3) **Exhale** lower to the floor again.

Repeat Steps 1-3 Four More Times For a Total of Five Repetitions

~VINYASA~

Enter the next asana from Downward Dog

Drishti ~ **Nose**

Comments - The greatest challenge of this asana is to keep the lower back lifting. There is a tendency for it to sag toward the floor. Use the abdominal muscles and bandhas to create greater support. That is where you will find stability in the lower back. Draw the shoulders back. If you choose to work with the handstand option you may practice by facing a wall. Be sure it is clear of obstructions. After each set of five breaths you may then kick the feet up on an inhale using the wall for support. Come down on the next exhale in preparation for the next boat. When lowering use control in the abdominal area. If five repetitions is too much then choose fewer to suit your needs. You may also leave out the lifting part and work toward it over time.

Navasana

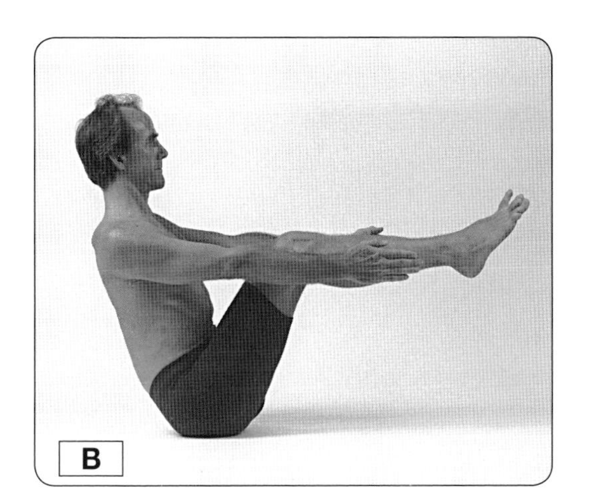

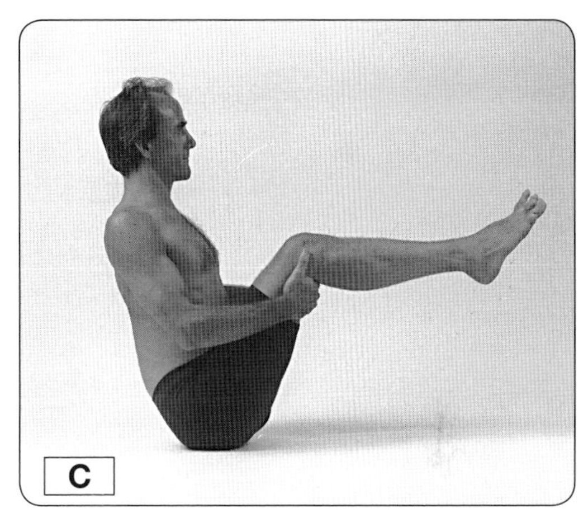

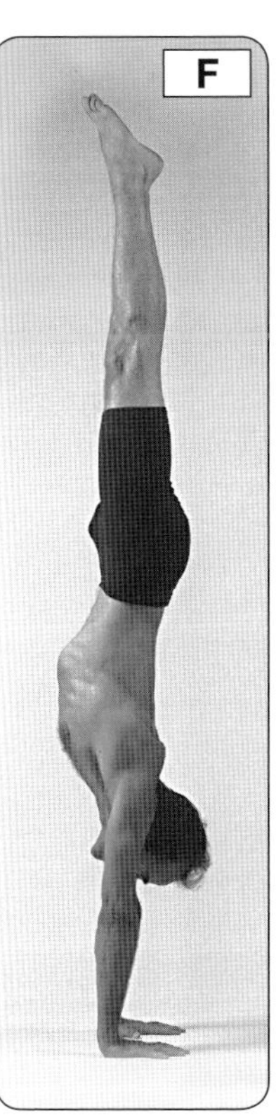

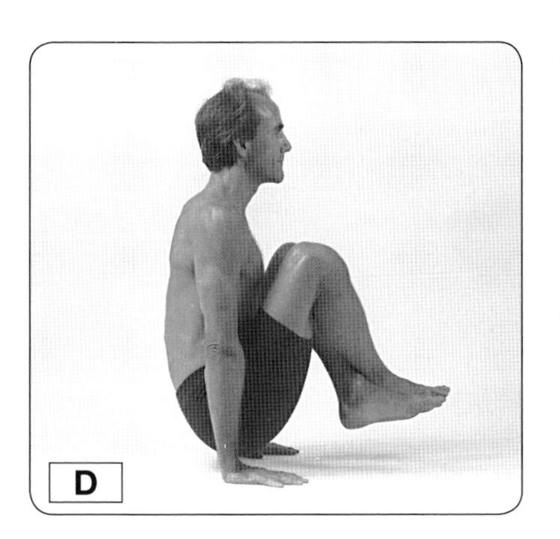

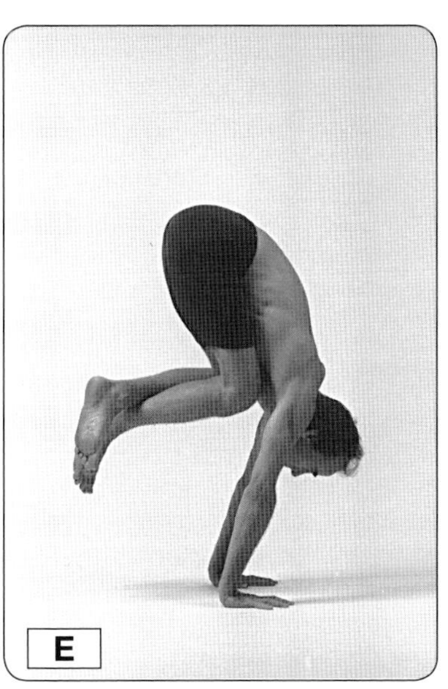

Bhujapidasana

Bhuja = Arm or Shoulder Pida = Pressure

"Arm Pressure Posture"

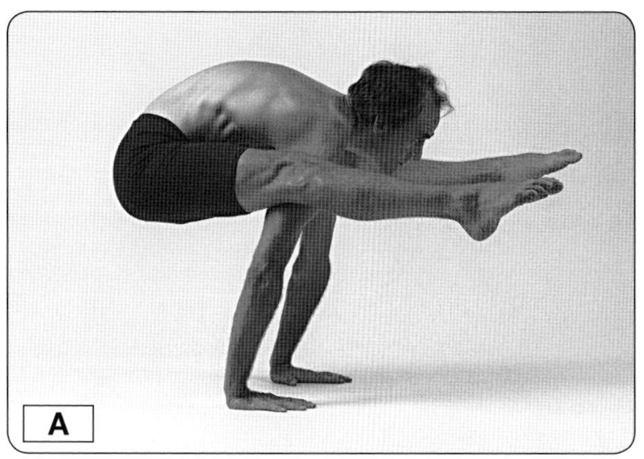

This is an entry transition. Do not remain here.

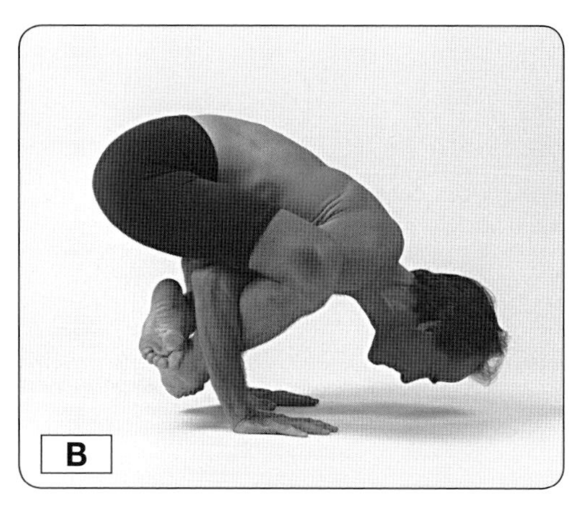

1) **Inhale** jump from **Downward-Dog** and land with the legs on the upper arms with the toes pointed **(A)**.

2) **Exhale** bend the legs and cross the ankles. Pull the feet back through the arms. Lower the head until the feet and head are both hovering just above the floor **(B)** or rest the head on the floor **(C)**. It is quite difficult to jump into this asana as described in **(A)** so an alternative is to jump the feet forward just outside of the hands **(D)**. Then lower the hips toward the floor and bend the elbows until the hips rest upon them. Wriggle your feet toward each other until you are able to cross them. Keep the feet in front of the hands and slightly lifted away from the floor with the elbows bent **(E)**. Another option is to leave the feet near the hands and drop the hips while bending the elbows and then remain in that position **(F)**.

Remain Here For 5 Deep Breaths

3) **Inhale** release the ankles and straighten the legs as in **(A)**.

4) **Exhale** and if you were in option **(A)** exit by bending the knees and point the feet back. Then jump to the plank pose. In the other options you may take the feet to the floor and then step or jump back.

~VINYASA~

Enter the next asana from Downward Dog

Drishti ~ **Nose**

Comments - To practice this asana with the least amount of strength required, you must bend the arms so that the elbows are directly above the heels of your hands. The backs of the thighs may rest on top of the elbows. In this way you may support your weight with the bones of the forearms rather than relying fully on the muscles. If you choose an option that requires you to lean forward then you must feel the distribution of weight transfer as the head comes forward and the feet go back. Keep the forearms perpendicular to the floor.

Bhujapidasana

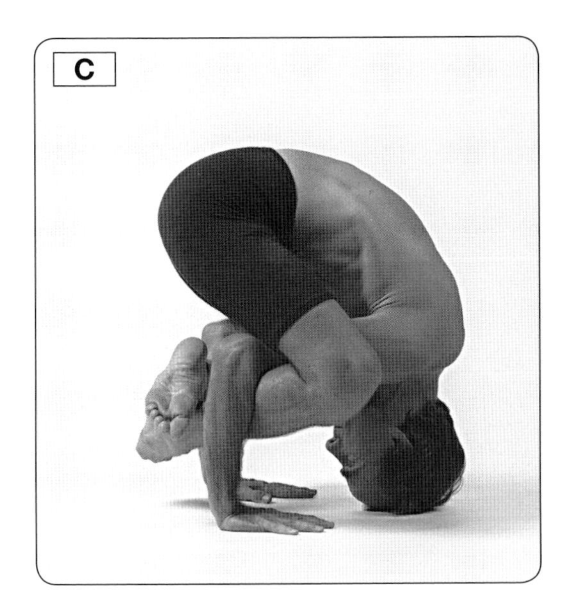

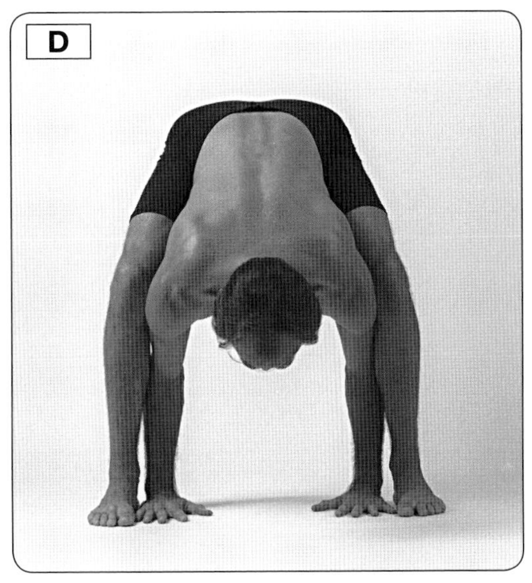

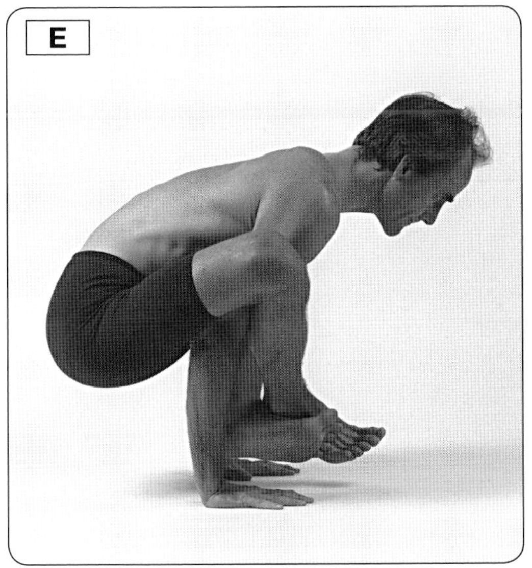

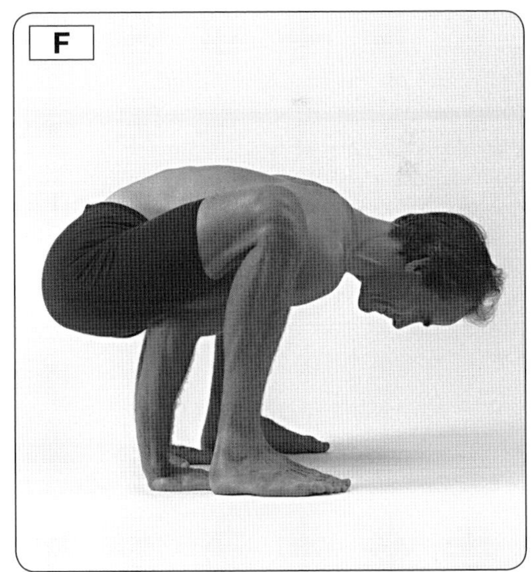

Kurmasana

Kurma = Tortoise

"Tortoise Posture"

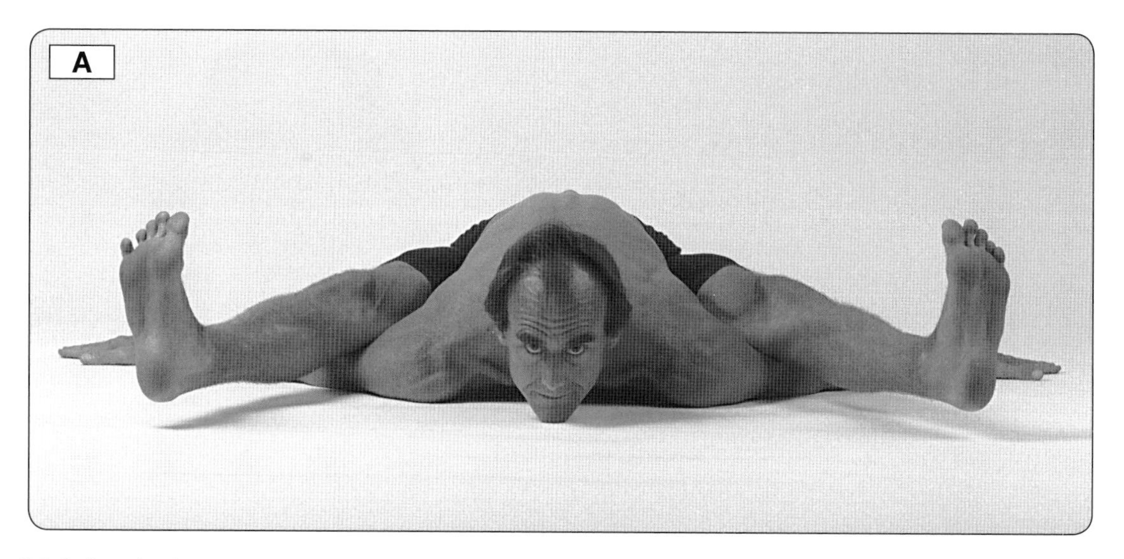

1) **Inhale** take the same entry as in **Bhujapidasana** by either jumping from **Downward Dog** and landing with the legs on the arms and the feet hovering in the air or resting on the floor outside the hands. You may also choose your favorite Vinyasa option and come all of the way through the hands to a sitting position.

2) **Exhale** if you jumped onto the arms with the feet hovering then keep the legs straight with the feet in the air and lower your chest down to the floor. Flex the feet. Engage the quadriceps until the heels lift **(A)**. If jumping onto the arms was too much then hop the feet outside the hands and sit down. Fold forward with the chest and take the arms back under the knees at a forty-five degree angle from the shoulders. Slide the feet forward without straightening the legs **(B)**. You may also take your Vinyasa through to a sitting position and extend forward with the chest. Clasp the ankles with your hands and gently pull the chest forward without creating discomfort in the lower back or hamstrings **(C)** or hold the knees and lengthen the spine as you extend forward **(D)**.

Remain Here For 5 Deep Breaths

Enter The Next Asana From Here

Drishti ~ **Third Eye**

Comments - If you feel a strain in the back or discomfort in the hamstrings then back off until you reach a level that is appropriate. Lead with the sternum. If you are flexible enough to place your chest and shoulders on the floor then you may work toward engaging the quadriceps and lifting the heels up. ***Do not put pressure on the back of the elbows.*** Keep the shoulders under the knees.

Kurmasana

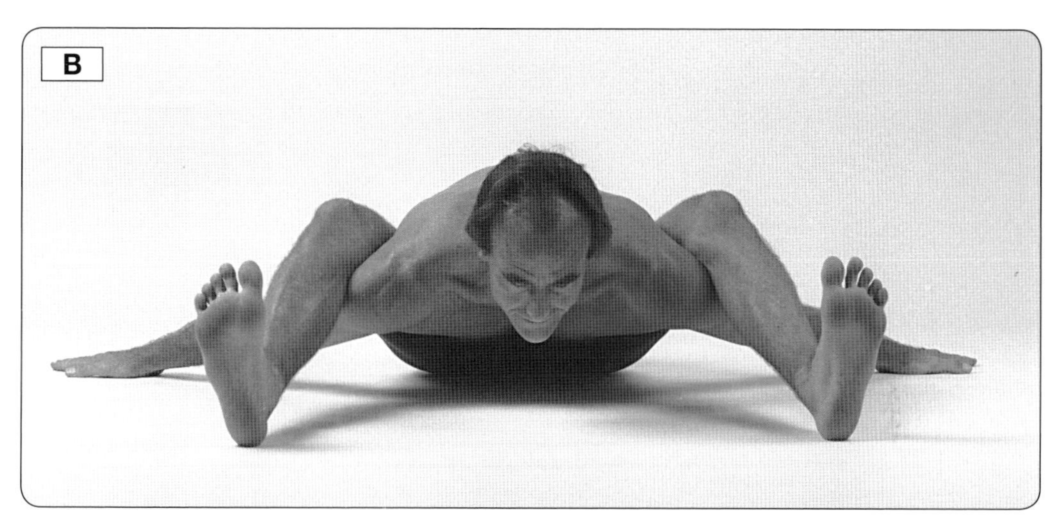

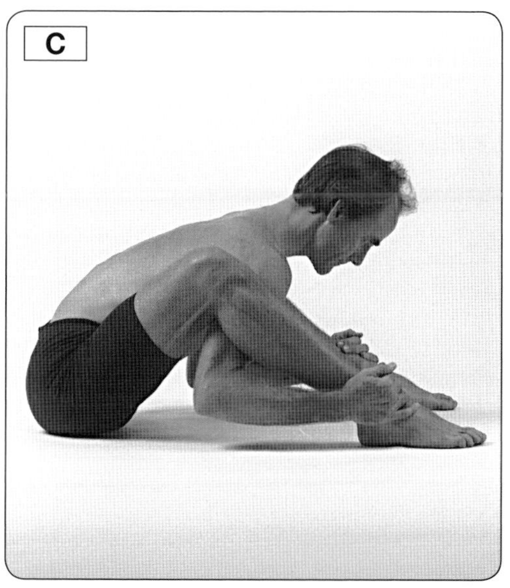

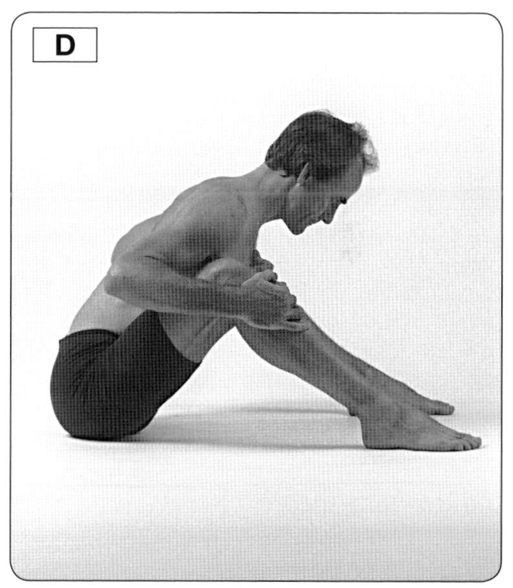

Supta Kurmasana

Supta = Sleeping Kurma = Tortoise

"Sleeping Tortoise Posture"

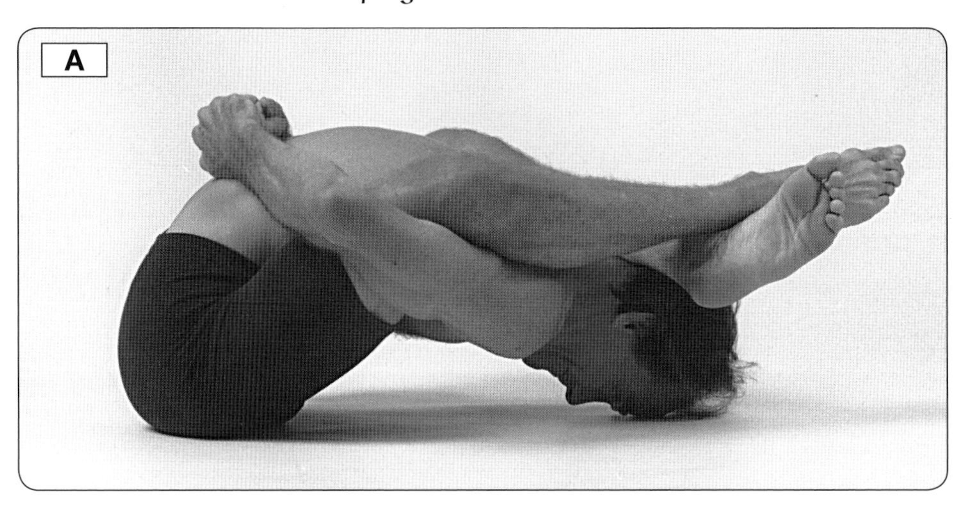

1) **Inhale** and look up. Bend the knees and bring the feet in slightly.

2) **Exhale** and if you are extremely flexible you may sit up and place the legs behind the head and then put the forehead on the floor and clasp the hands behind the back **(A)**. This first option is quite extreme and takes years of practice. An alternative is to draw the feet in toward each other and cross the ankles on top of one another leaving the feet on the floor. Then clasp the hands behind the back **(B)**. If it is too intense to cross the ankles you may bring the soles of the feet together instead. If the hands do not reach behind your back you may leave them on the floor beside the hips **(C)** or use a strap to connect the hands **(D)**. You may also choose to repeat the previous asana or leave this phase of **Kurmasana** out for now.

Remain Here For 5 Deep Breaths

~VINYASA~

(For this Vinyasa you may either lift up with straight legs on top of the arms and then shoot the feet back as seen in **(E)**, **(F)** and **(G)** or choose another of your favorite Vinyasa options to jump back or wait.)

Drishti ~ **Third Eye**

Comments - In order to take the hands behind the back it is imperative that the shoulders move under the knees. You may then rotate the shoulders which will enable the elbows to bend freely. If you choose to cross your ankles you may find discomfort in the one on the bottom due to its pressing against the floor. If this is true then place a towel or cushion under it. Externally rotate the hips when crossing the ankles.

Supta Kurmasana

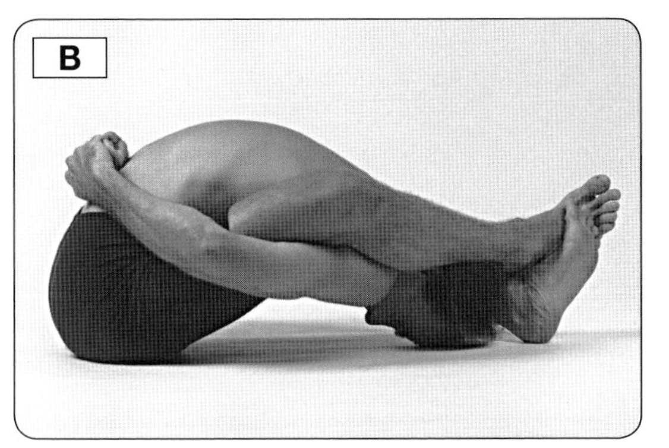

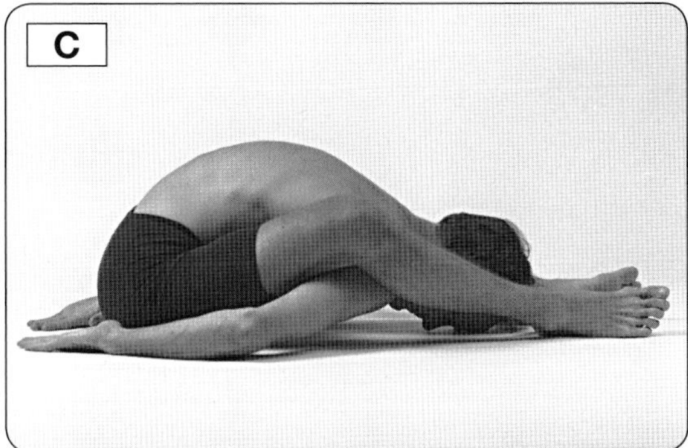

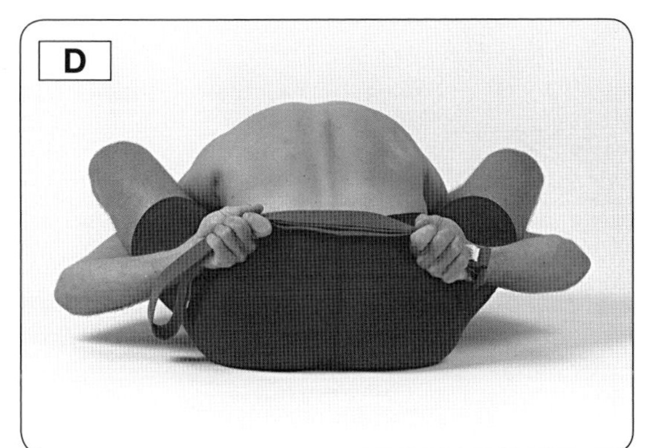

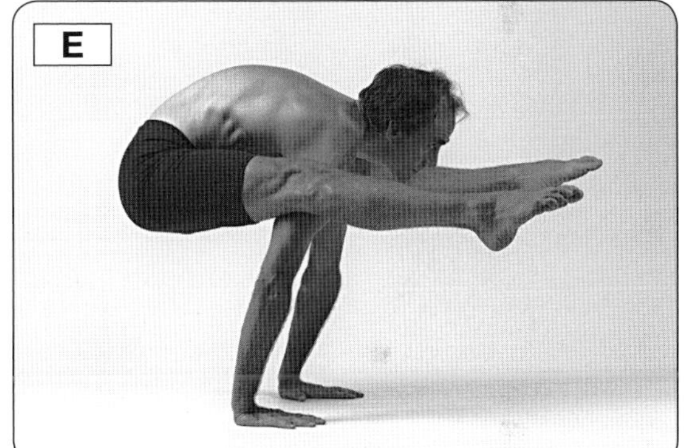

Transition. Do Not Hold.

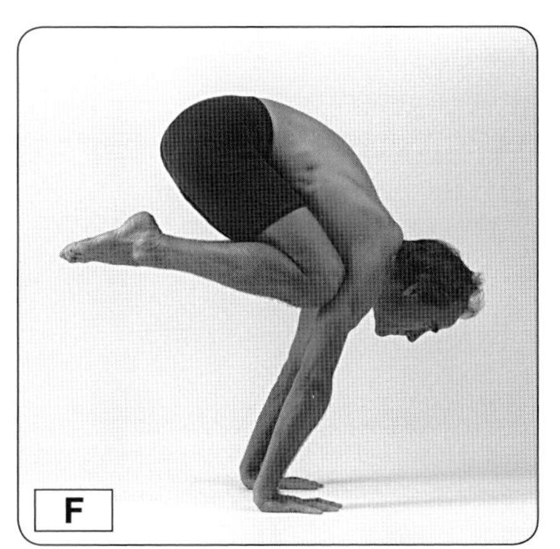

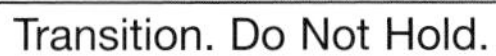
Transition. Do Not Hold.

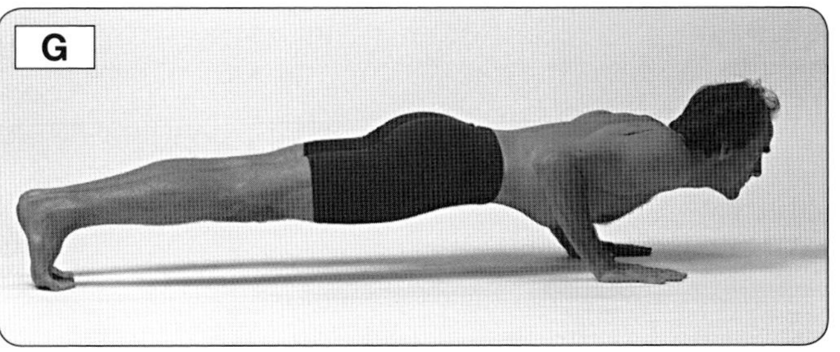

Transition. Do Not Hold.

Garbha Pindasana

Garbha = Womb   Pinda = Embryo

"Womb Embryo Posture"

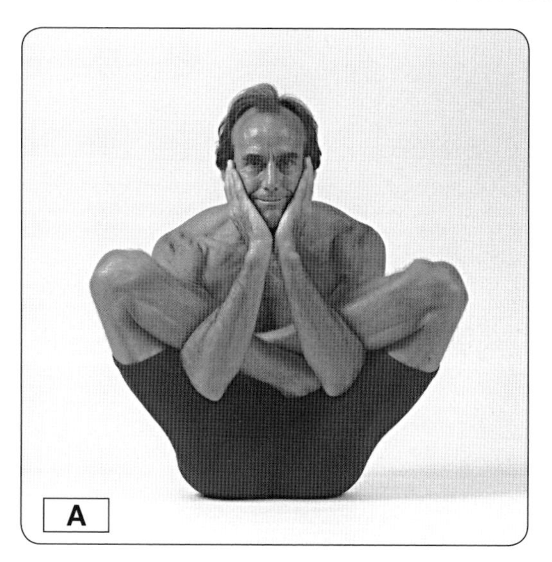

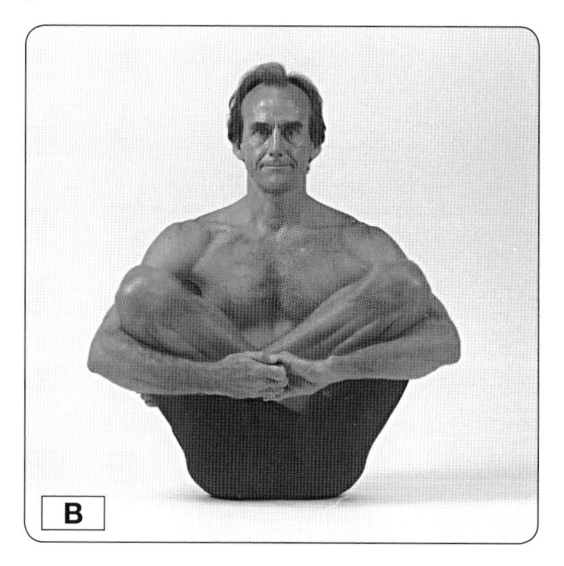

1) **Exhale** place your legs in full-lotus. Slip the arms through the legs in front of the feet. Rest your chin in your hands **(A)**. If it is too much to slip the hands through the legs then reach around the outer thighs and clasp your hands **(B)**. If full lotus is too much then place the right foot on top of the left thigh in the half-lotus position. Reach the arms around the thighs **(C)**. If half-lotus is too much, cross the legs **(D)**.

2) **Inhale** sit up straight in the option which is most appropriate for you.

Remain Here For 5 Deep Breaths

3) **Exhale** as you roll back and inhale as you roll forward moving with a slight rotation with each roll so that you progress in a clockwise circle. Roll eight times progressing back to the front.

4) **Inhale** as you roll up and balance on your hands. This is called **Kukkutasana**. Choose option **(A1)**, **(B1)**, **(C1)** or **(D1)** to correspond with the rolling option that you chose in the first phase of this asana

Remain Here For 5 Deep Breaths

5) **Exhale** release the asana and straighten your legs.

~VINYASA~

Drishti ~ **Nose**

Comments - When rolling back and forth it is important to roll on the muscles on each side of the spine rather than the spine itself. If you still find discomfort then you may double up your mat behind you or use a blanket. Use your breath to assist in the rolling action. ***Be aware of the space around you before rolling.***

Garbha Pindasana plus Kukkutasana

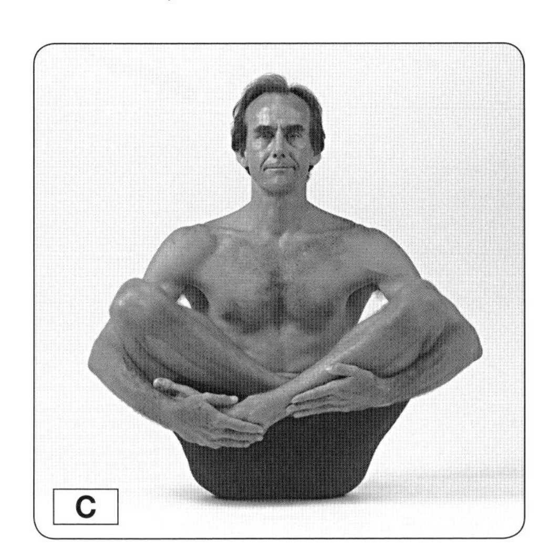

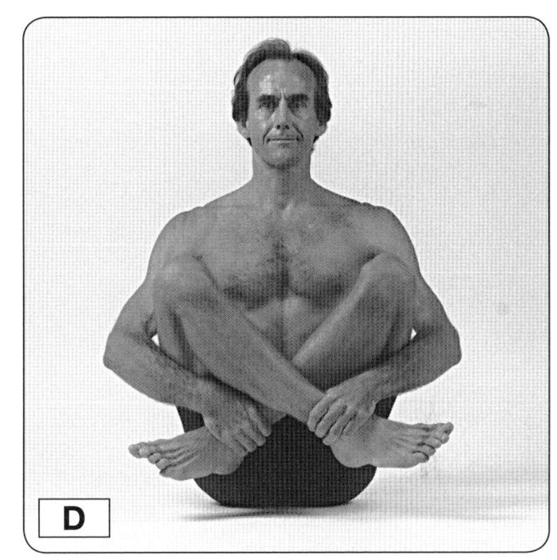

Kukkutasana / Kukkuta = Cock

A1 through D1

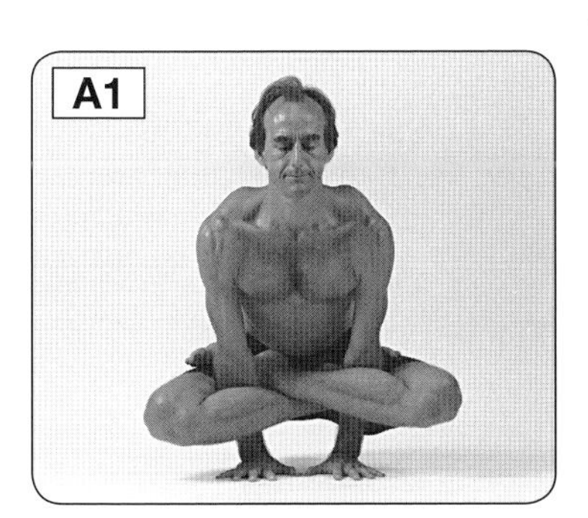

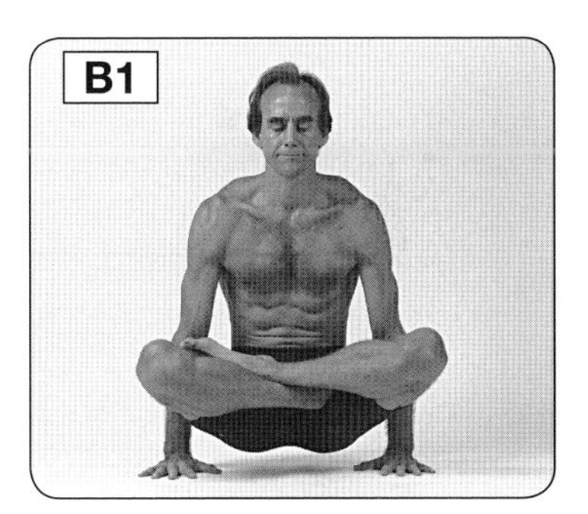

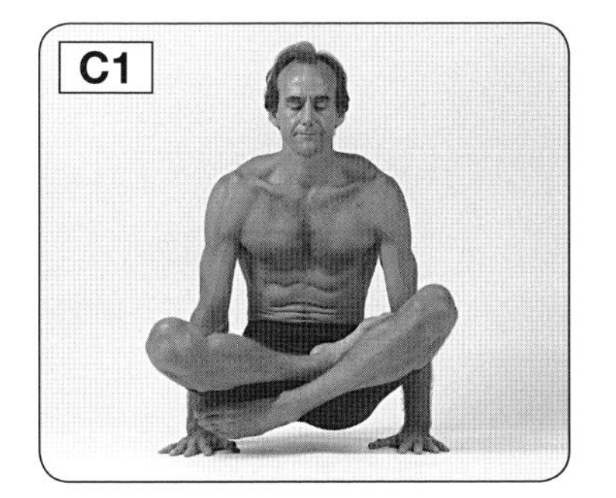

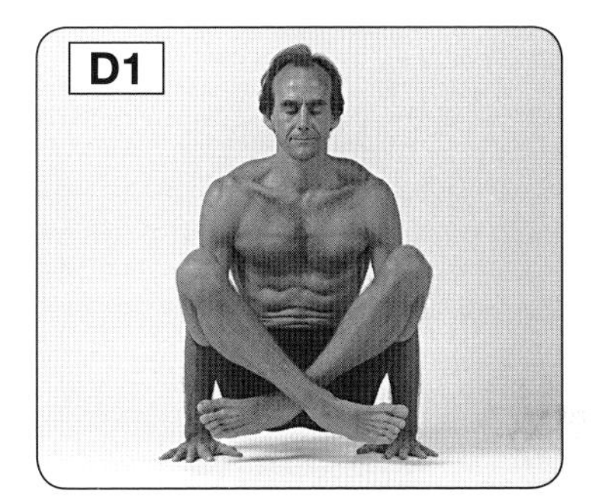

Baddha Konasana

Baddha = Bound Kona = Angle

"Bound Angle Posture"

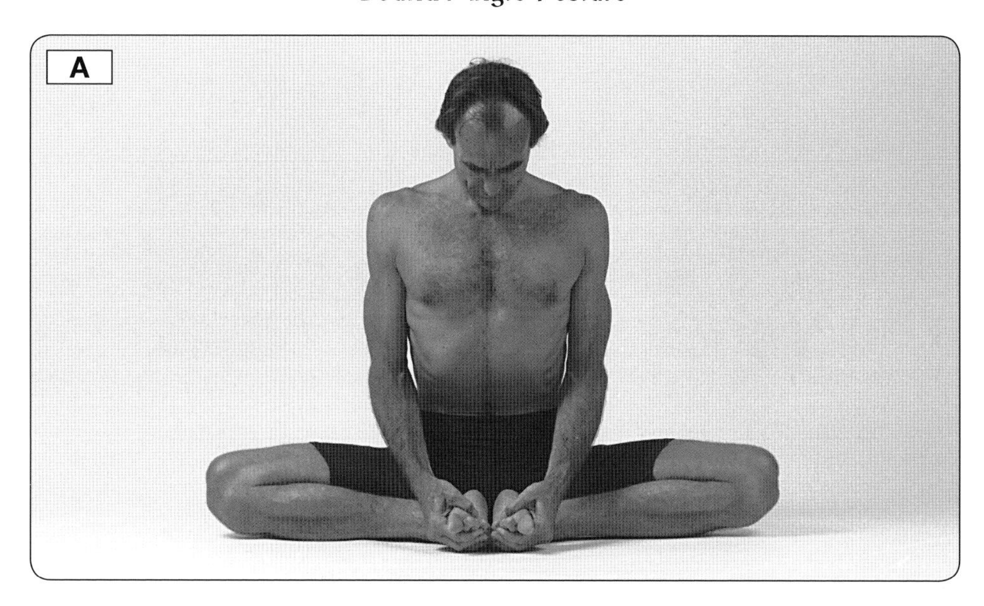

1) **Exhale** draw both feet in toward the groin. Hold the feet with the fingers on top and the thumbs in the soles. Open the feet and lower the knees toward the floor **(A)** or if you find it to be too intense to open the feet or lower the knees then leave the soles of the feet touching and hold the tops of the feet **(B)**. You may also elevate the hips with a prop **(C)**. In all options drop your chin to your chest and sit up straight.

Remain Here For 5 Deep Breaths

2) **Inhale** and lift your chin. Gaze to the horizon.

3) **Exhale** fold forward. Bring the chest toward the feet and the chin toward the floor **(D)** or extend only part of the way forward toward the floor **(E)** or repeat **(A)**, **(B)** or **(C)**.

Remain Here For 5 Deep Breaths

4) **Inhale** as you sit up.

5) **Exhale** release the feet and straighten the legs.

~VINYASA~

Drishti ~ **Nose**

Comments - The opening of the feet works as a symbiosis with the opening of the hips. The lowering of the knees is initiated from the movement of the hips. This cooperative movement allows more freedom with less effort. There is another symbiosis in the relationship between the hands which are pulling against the feet and the lifting of the chest to lengthen the lower back. Avoid the tendency to collapse in the lower spine.

Baddha Konasana

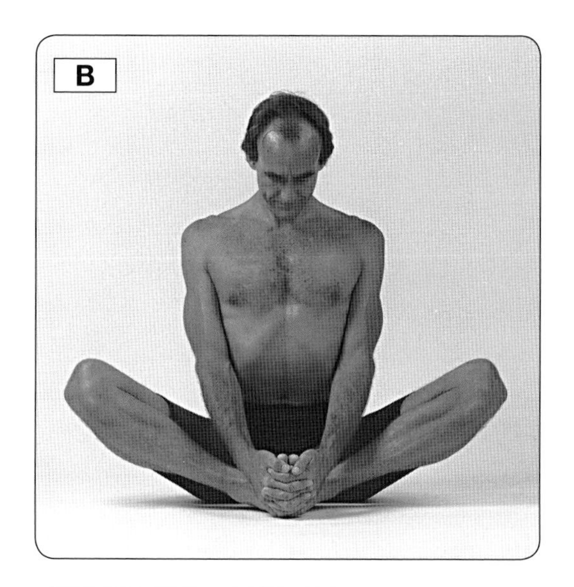

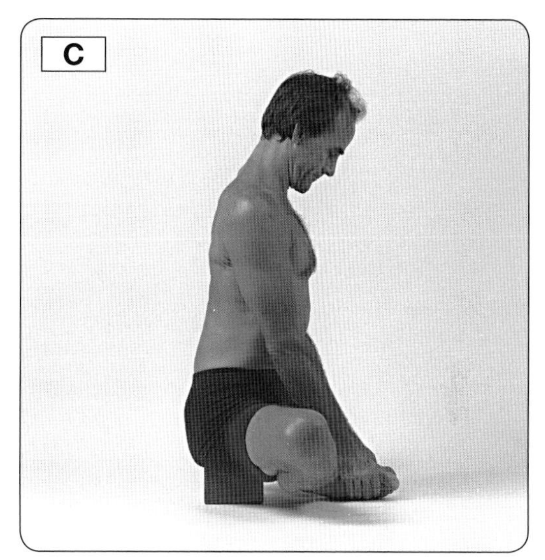

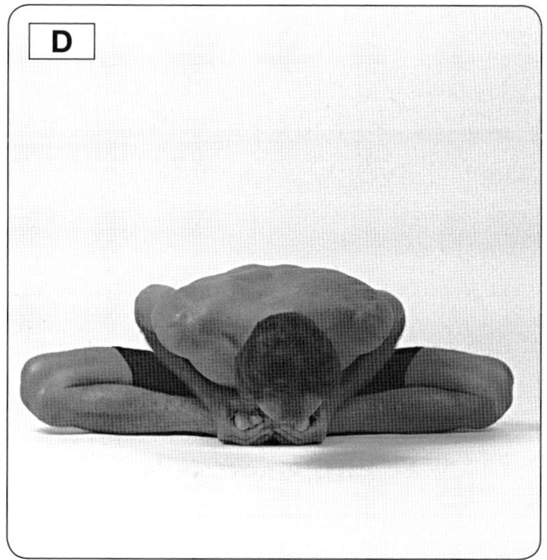

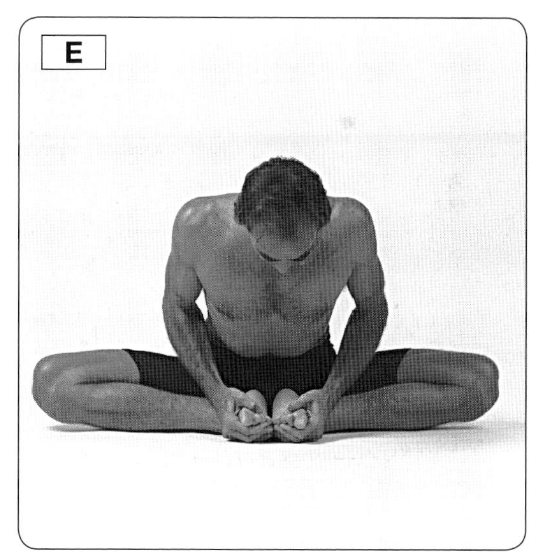

Upavishta Konasana

Upavishta = Seated Kona = Angle

"Seated Angle Posture"

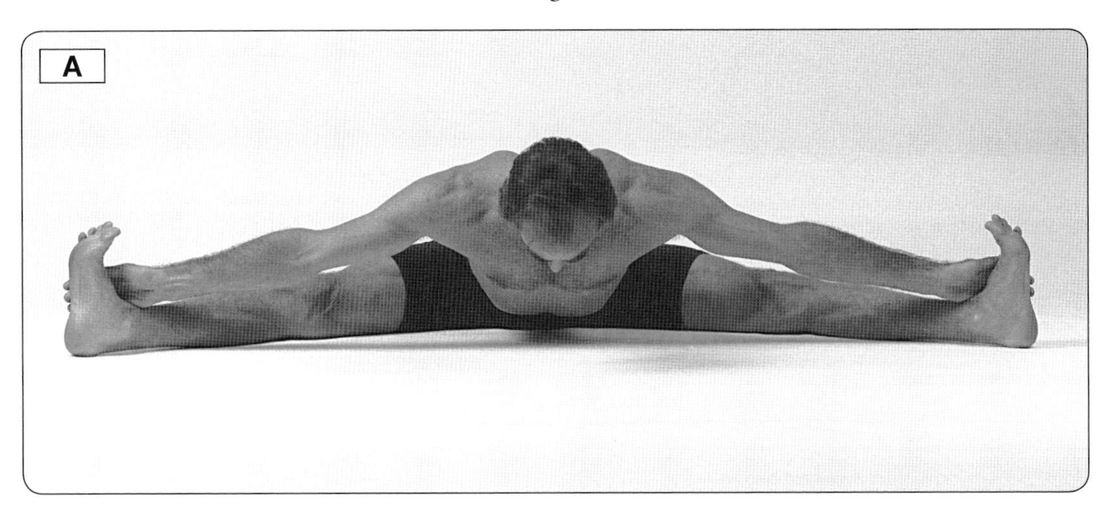

1) **Exhale** open the feet wide with the legs straight. Hold the feet with your hands. Fold forward and take the chest and chin to the floor **(A)**. If it is too much to hold the feet then hold the shins or ankles **(B)**. You may also place the hands on the floor between the legs for support **(C)** or use straps to hold the feet **(D)**.

2) **Inhale** lengthen the spine and gaze to the horizon.

3) **Exhale** and move into whichever option is most appropriate for you.

Remain Here For 5 Deep Breaths

4) **Inhale** look up to the horizon.

5) **Exhale** change your grip to the big toes with legs straight if you are practicing option **(A)** or bend your legs until you can reach your toes if you are practicing option **(B)**. If in **(C)** release the asana.

6) **Inhale** pop up to a point of balance on your sit-bones by pushing the floor away with the feet and legs. At the same time lift the head and torso up toward the sky. Keep holding onto the feet **(E)**.

Remain Here For 5 Deep Breaths

7) **Exhale** release the asana and take the feet to the floor.

~VINYASA~

Drishti ~ **Third Eye**

Comments - When folding forward in option **(A)** it is important to keep the knees pointing toward the ceiling and resist the temptation to allow them to roll in toward the floor. In all options the legs should remain active. The sternum is your headlight. Shine it straight ahead. Be joyful in the option that you choose.

Upavishta Konasana

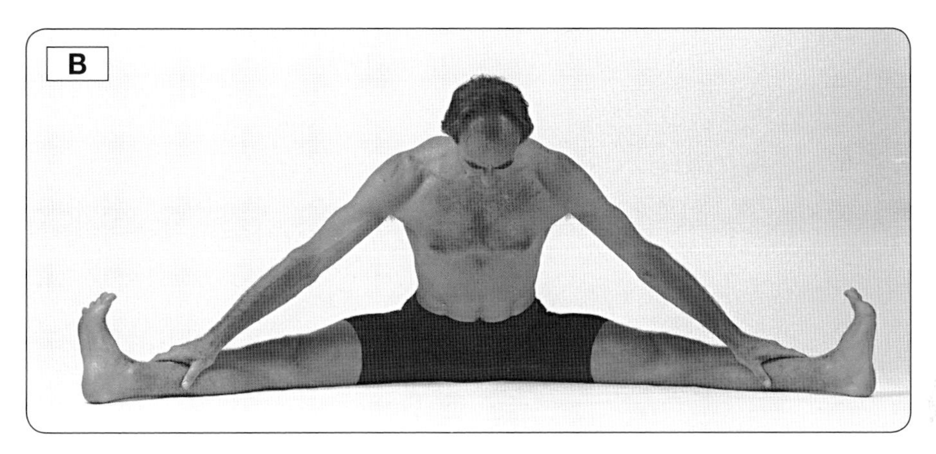

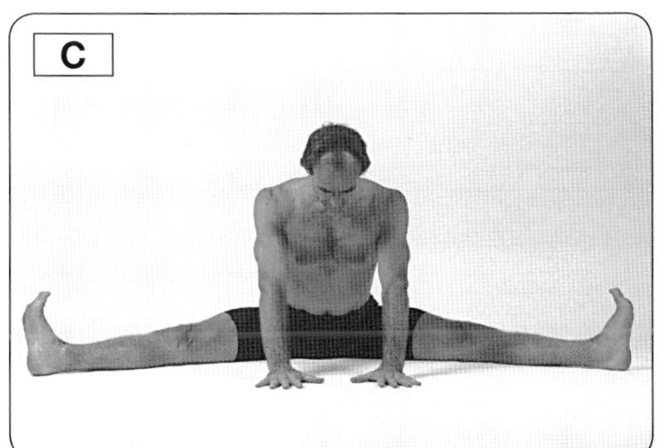

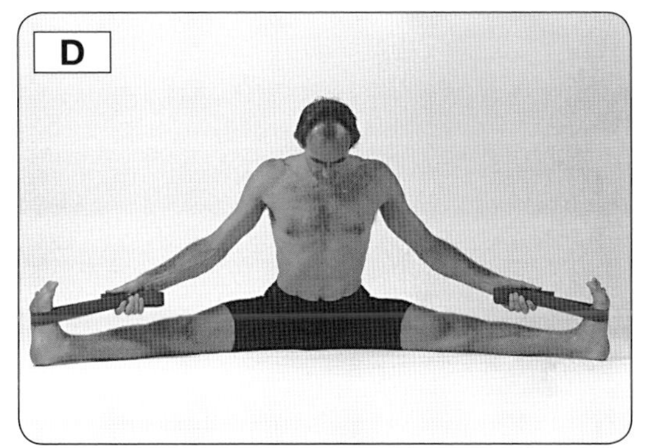

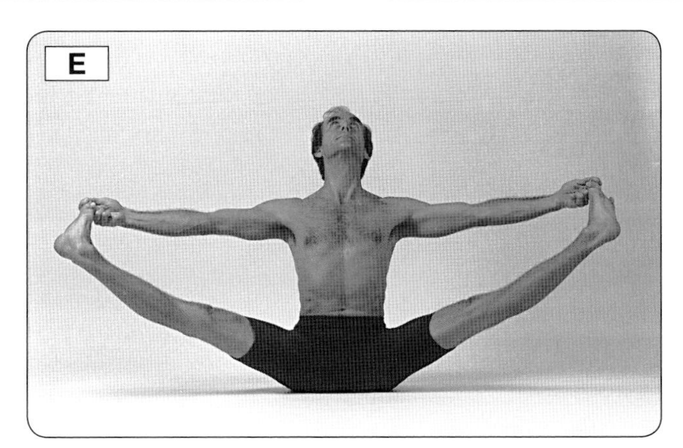

Supta Konasana

Supta = Sleeping Kona = Angle

"Sleeping Angle Posture"

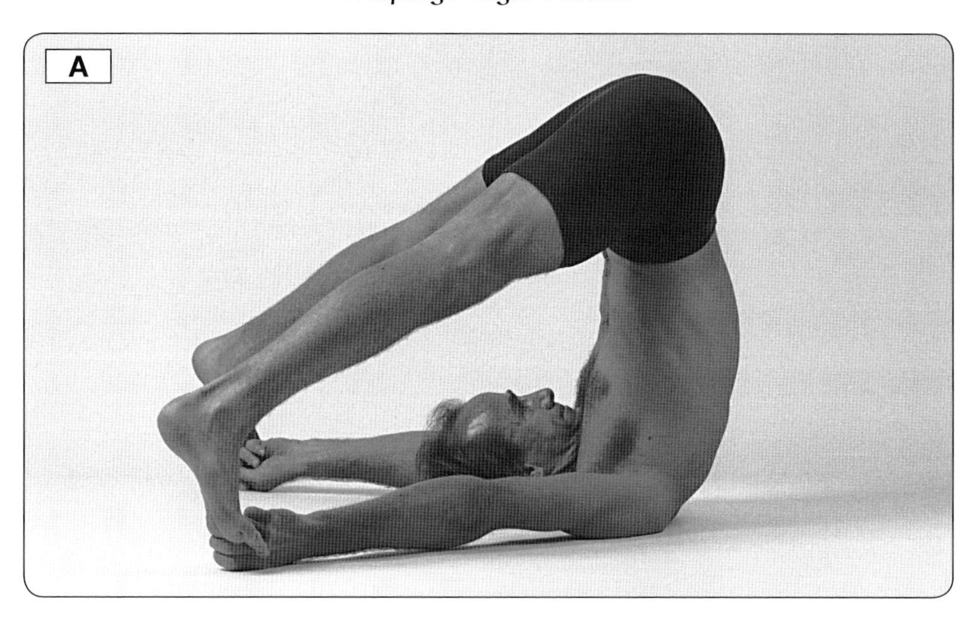

1) **Exhale** roll back onto your shoulders with the feet spread wide on the floor above your head. Hold the big toes with two fingers of each hand. Keep the legs straight **(A)**. If you are unable to hold the toes with the feet on the floor then hold the ankles with the feet in the air **(B)** or leave the hips on the floor and raise only the legs. Hold the ankles or toes **(C)** or raise the hips and bend the knees as in **(D)**.

Remain Here For 5 Deep Breaths

2) **Inhale** roll up. Balance on your sit-bones **(E)**. You may need to bend the knees to assist in coming up.

3) **Exhale** and fall forward so that the calf muscles land on the floor and not the heels **(F)**.

Note - This method of falling forward requires great flexibility in the hamstrings in order to avoid crashing the heels onto the floor. In the beginning it is more effective and safer to bend the knees and lower the feet slowly with control or to release the feet altogether and take the feet down that way.

4) **Inhale** look up to the horizon.

5) **Exhale** release the asana.

~VINYASA~

Drishti ~ **Nose**

Comments - Be aware of pressure on your neck in this asana. In options **(A)** and **(B)** keep the back lifting and the shoulders drawing in toward each other. This will assist in keeping the neck free from the floor. It will also protect the lower back. Engage your bandhas to find extra support.

Supta Konasana

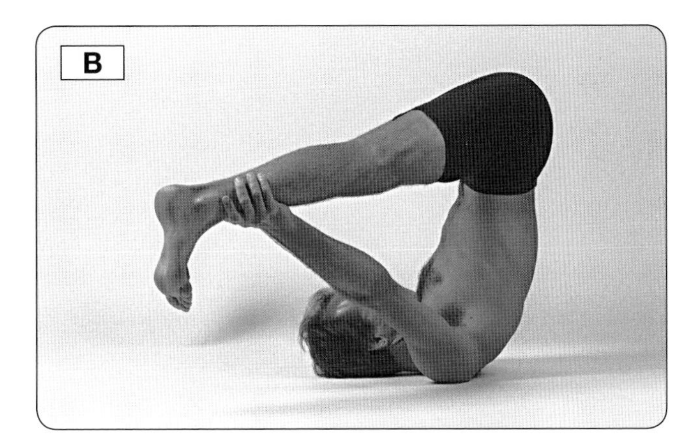

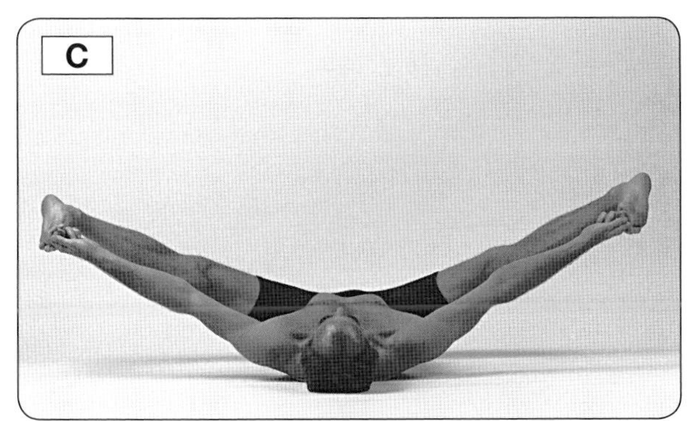

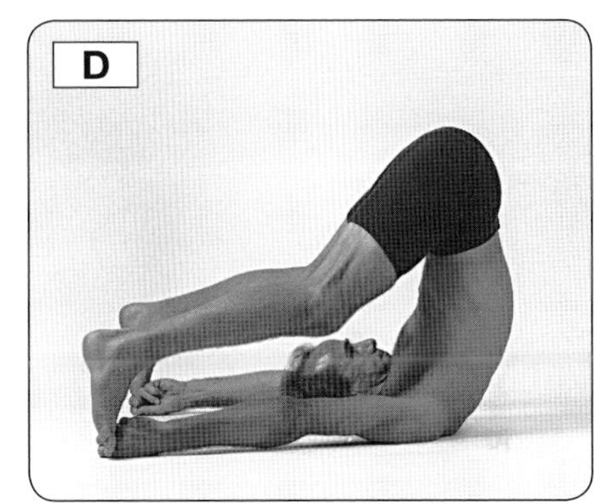

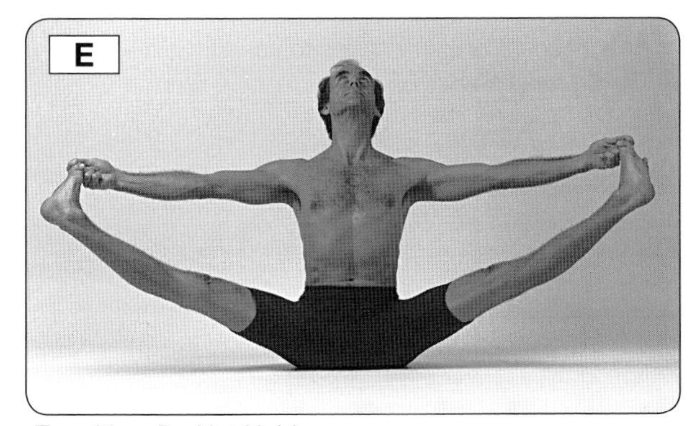

Transition. Do Not Hold.

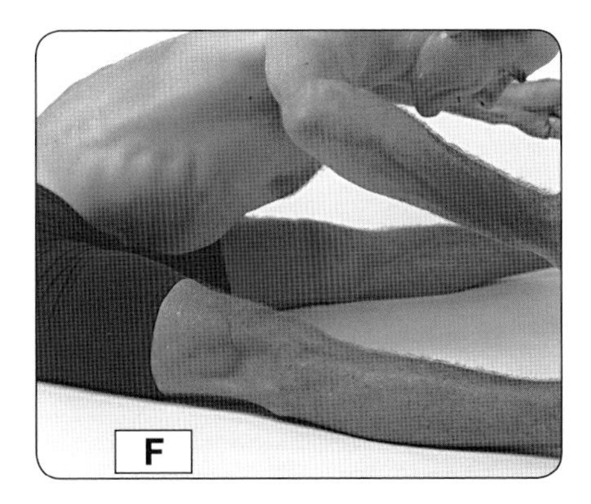

Supta Padangusthasana A

Supta = Sleeping Pada = Foot Angustha = Big Toe

"Sleeping Big Toe Posture"

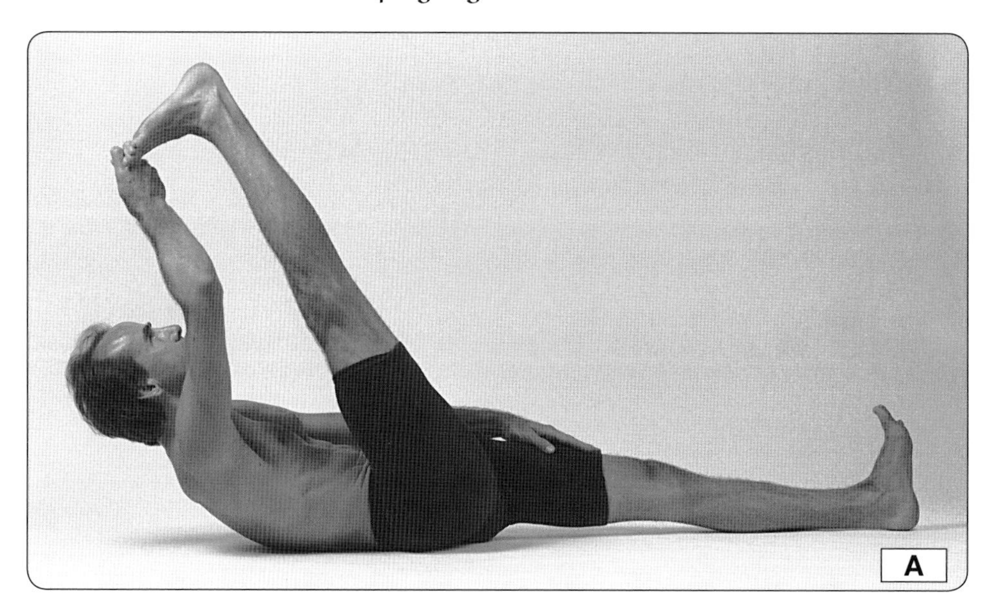

1) **Exhale** as you lie down on your back.

2) **Inhale** raise your right leg and grab the big toe with two fingers keeping both legs straight. Place the left hand on the left thigh **(A)** or if it is too much to reach the toe you may hold the ankle **(B)**. You may also use a strap to hold the foot **(C)**. In all options the left hand should slide toward the left knee.

3) **Exhale** lift the chest toward the leg with the head away from the floor. Use whichever method of holding the leg is most appropriate for you, choosing from options **(A)**, **(B)** or **(C)**.

Remain Here For 5 Deep Breaths

4) **Inhale** lower the head and shoulders to the floor.

Enter Supta Padangusthasana B From Here

Drishti ~ **Toes**

Comments - This asana progresses in three phases. In this first phase the purpose of lifting the chest and raising the head away from the floor is to engage the abdominal muscles and to encourage the bandhas. There are two actions working simultaneously. The chest and head are lifting but also the leg is being drawn in toward the upper body. The left leg should remain fully active. Press through both heels and pull the toes back while slightly moving the balls of the feet forward. The quadriceps should be working as well to release the hamstrings. Keep the breath flowing. When engaging the abdominal area you need to keep the area above the navel supple enough to draw in a full breath.

Supta Padangusthasana A

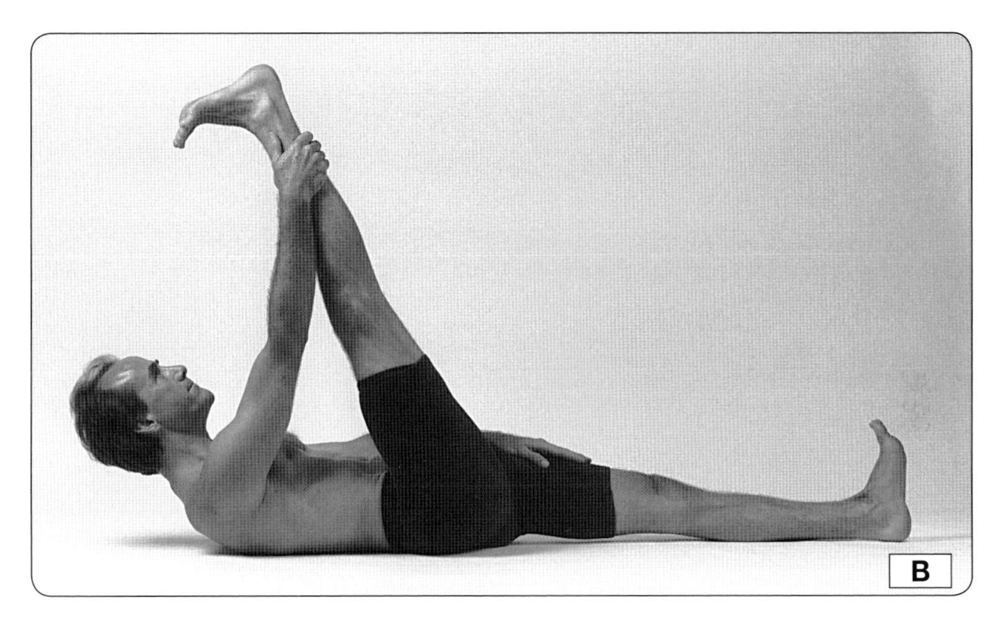

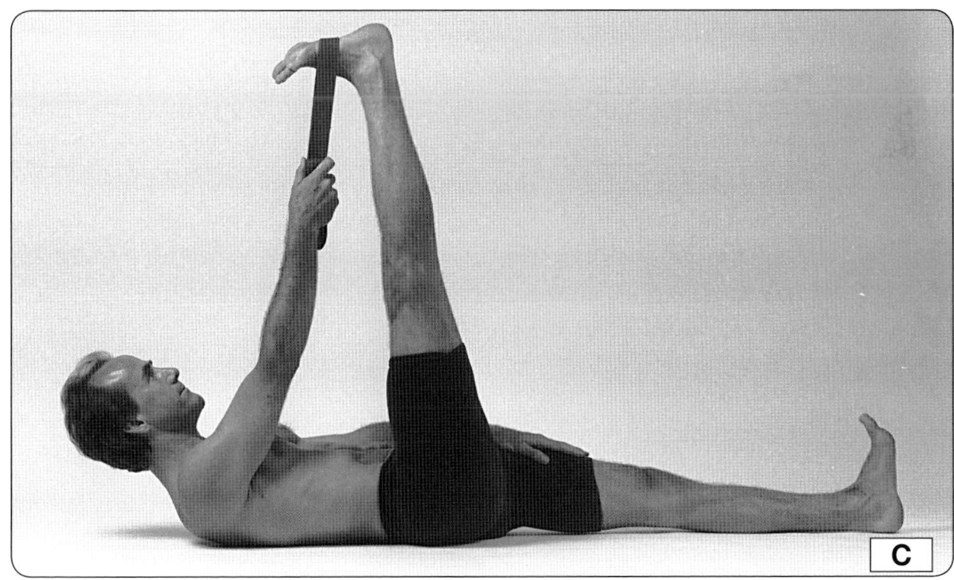

Supta Padangusthasana B

Supta = Sleeping   Pada = Foot   Angustha = Big Toe

"Sleeping Big Toe Posture"

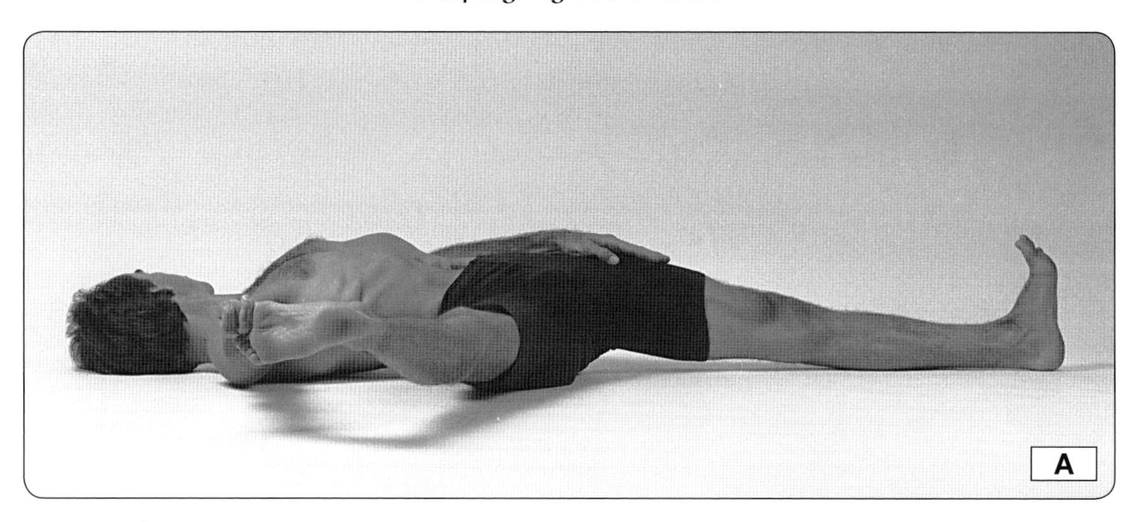
A

1) **Exhale** open the hips by lowering the right leg toward the floor to the right. Continue to hold the toes with the leg straight. Leave the left hand on top of the left thigh and turn your gaze the opposite direction **(A)**. If you were holding your ankle in the first phase of this, you could now bend the right leg and hold the knee as you open to the right **(B)**. If you were using a strap then continue holding it as you lower the leg **(C)**.

Remain Here For 5 Deep Breaths

2) **Inhale** return the leg to the center.

Enter Supta Padangusthasana C From Here

Drishti ~ **Side**

Comments - If you recall the standing sequence of **Utthita Hasta Padangusthasana** you will notice that **Supta Padangusthasana** is simply the same procedure in a reclining position. This means that the same criteria apply for certain aspects of both. When lowering the leg to the side, your hips should remain on an even plane, so that one is not lifting higher than the other. Extend through the heel to emphasize the opening of the inner groin. On the opening leg, avoid the knee rolling in. Work toward both shoulders remaining on the floor. The opposing hip will have a tendency to rise as the leg lowers. Lower the leg only as far as you may maintain contact with the floor with both hips.

Supta Padangusthasana B

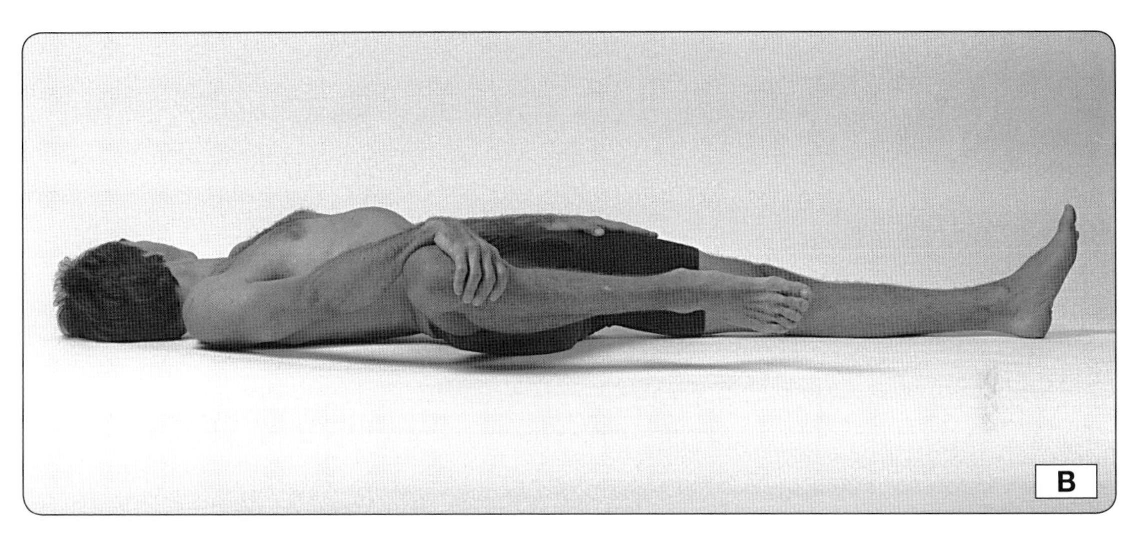

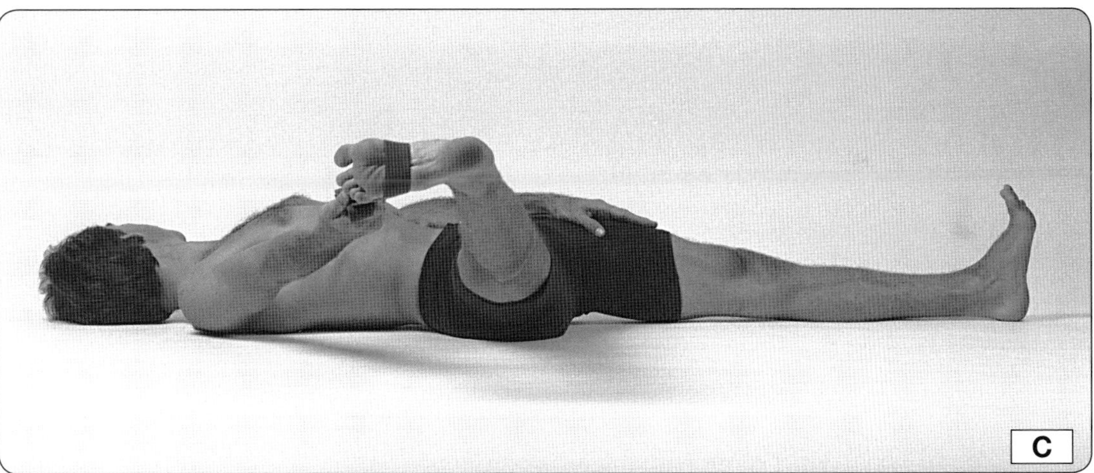

Supta Padangusthasana C

Supta = Sleeping Pada = Foot Angustha = Big Toe

"Sleeping Big Toe Posture"

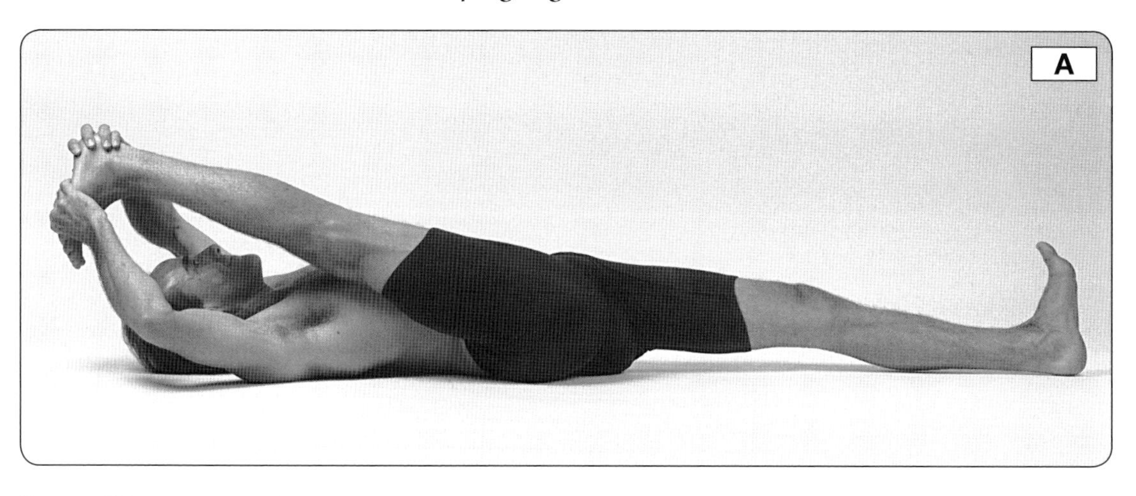

Note - This version of Supta **Padangusthasana C** is sometimes omitted from the Primary Series or substituted with a touch of the nose to the knee before proceeding on to the next asana. (It is also called **Supta Trivikramasana** and is present in the Advanced Series).

1) **Exhale** leave your head on the floor and grab the right foot with both hands. Keep the left leg active and pull the right leg toward the floor outside your right ear **(A)**. The first option requires a great deal of flexibility in the hamstrings so you may choose to hold the ankle or behind the knee as in **(B)** or bend the leg and pull the knee into your chest **(C)**. If using a strap, hold it with both hands **(D)**.

Remain Here For 5 Deep Breaths

2) **Inhale** and slightly release the pulling action.

3) **Exhale** and lower the right leg to the floor beside the left.

Repeat All Phases of Supta Padangusthasana A, B and C, on the Left Side

~CHAKRASANA~

(Chakrasana is a specialized VINYASA.
Refer to its description on pages 120-121 before proceeding)

Drishti ~ **Toes**

Comments - Instead of lifting the chest and head as in Supta Padangusthasana A you now leave the head on the floor and bring the leg to you. In order to keep the stretch directly in the hamstrings, it is important to avoid outward rotation of the hip. Keep the right knee pointing directly at the floor or shoulder. As in the previous postures keep the quadriceps working on both legs and push through the heels with the toes pulling back. Even though the chest is not lifting to engage the abdominal area you must keep the bandhas functioning fully. This will help to support the lower back. Keep the chest open and the breath flowing freely.

Supta Padangusthasana C

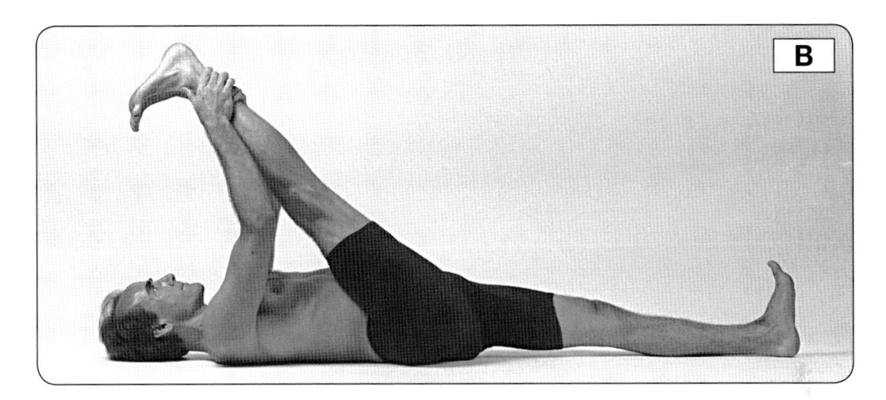

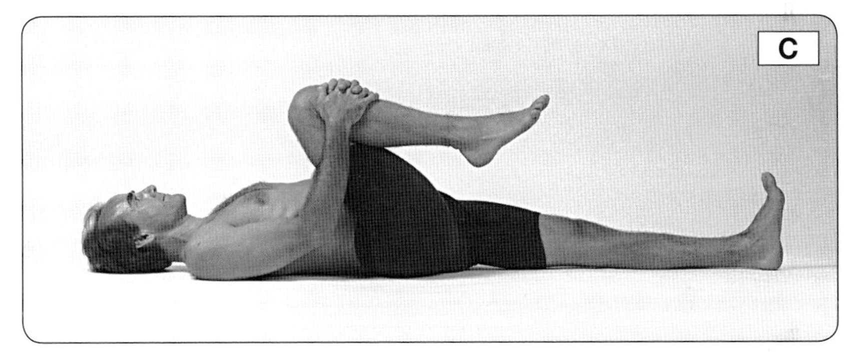

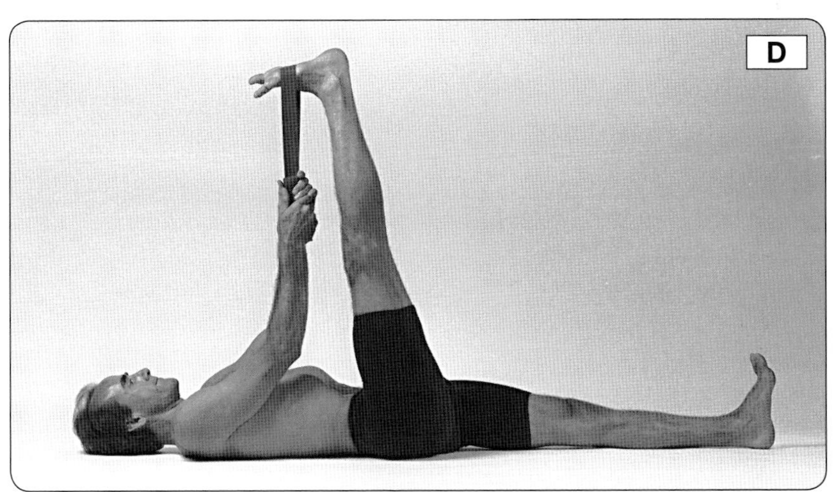

Chakrasana

Chakra = Circle or a Wheel

"Wheel Posture"

If you have never attempted Chakrasana before or if you have any neck problems then you should leave this method of vinyasa out and apply one of the other seated variations of jumping back described earlier in this text.

Chakrasana occurs twice in the Primary Series. The first is after **Supta Padangusthasana** and the second after **Setu Bandhasana**. There is also a **Chakrasana** in the finishing sequence after **Uttana Padasana.** This method of vinyasa requires timing, confidence, momentum and a sense of adventure. ***It should be learned under the guidance of a competent teacher. If Chakrasana is new to you or if it is too difficult, you may substitute your favorite jumping Vinyasa from the options offered earlier.*** For those of you that have already practiced it with supervision, I am offering some additional details which you may find beneficial in the refinement of Chakrasana. This maneuver is basically a backward rolling somersault combined with breath and bandhas. Remember, when you find **~CHAKRASANA~** listed you may either use the method described here or apply the standard **~VINYASA~** options.

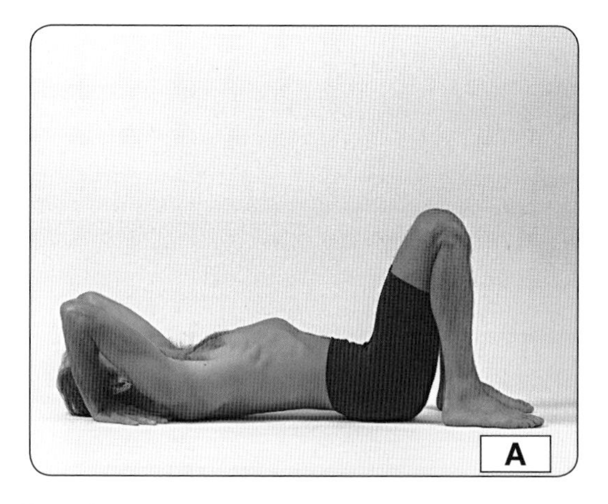
A

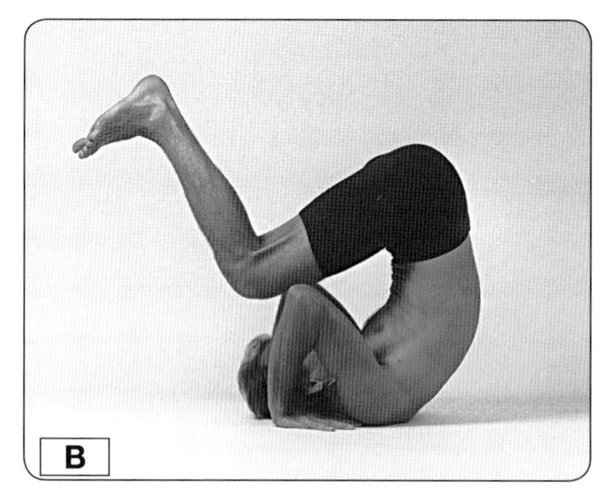
B

Step One - Lay on your back. Hands under the shoulders, palms down, fingers toward the feet. Draw the heels in toward the buttocks as though you were preparing to do a back bend **(A)**.

Step Two - Draw the knees in toward the chest as your hips lift. Direct the feet toward the floor over your head. Keep the chin tucked into the chest **(B)**. ***Do not turn the head to one side***.

Step Three - As you feel the weight moving over your shoulders, press the hands firmly into the floor and push. ***This is the most important phase of Chakrasana.*** This pushing action will take the weight into your hands and away from the neck **(C)**.

Step Four - Let the feet land in a shortened downward dog position with the knees bent **(D)**.

Step Five - Either hop **(E)** or walk **(F)** your hands forward into **Chaturanga Dandasana (G)**.

Continue as usual through Upward Dog, Downward Dog and come back to sitting

Chakrasana

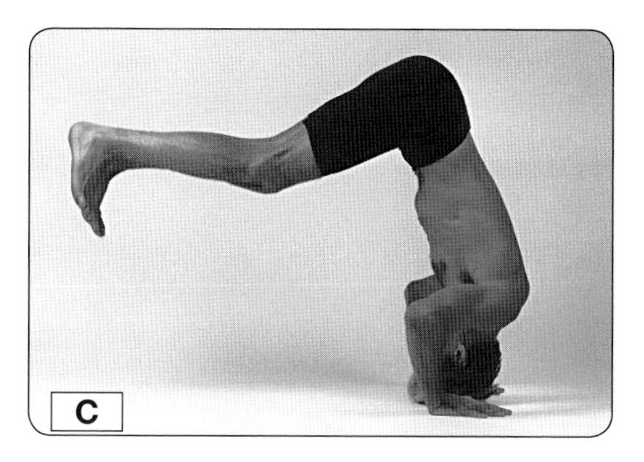

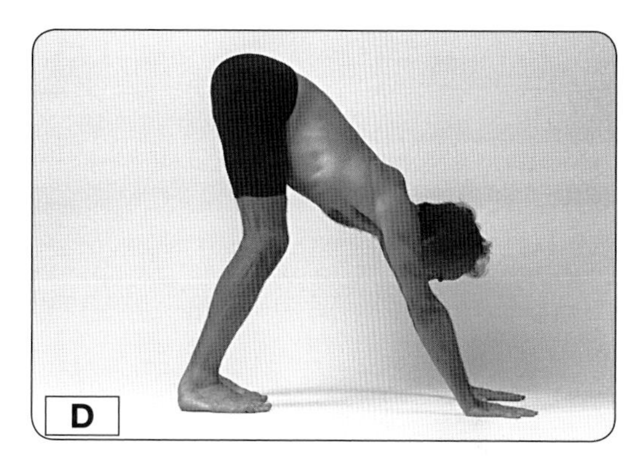

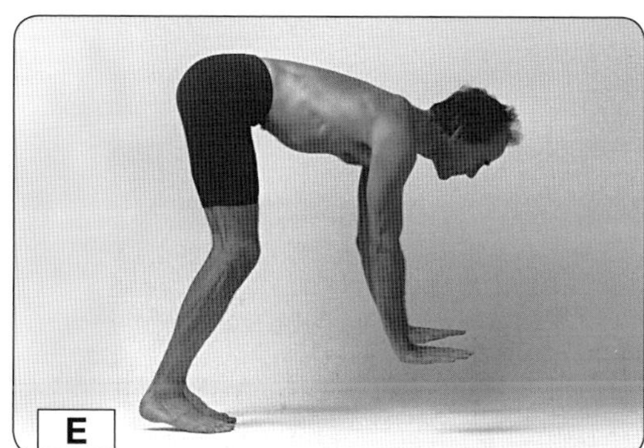

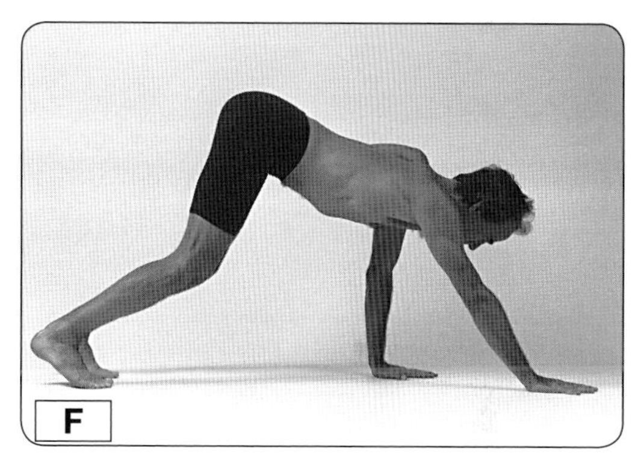

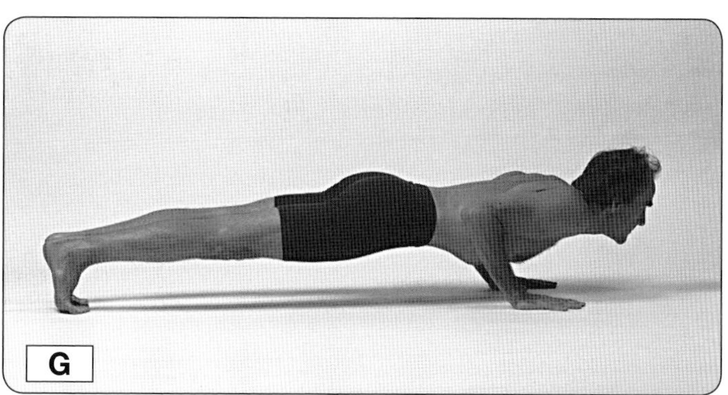

Ubhaya Padangusthasana

Ubhaya = Both   Pada = Foot   Angustha = Big Toe

"Both Feet Big Toe Posture"

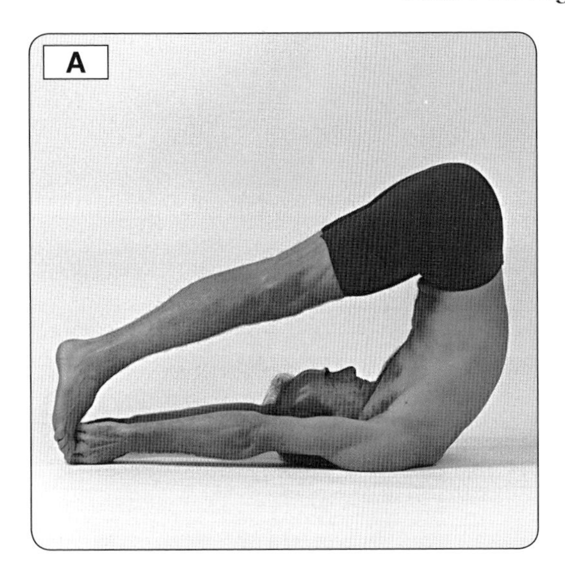

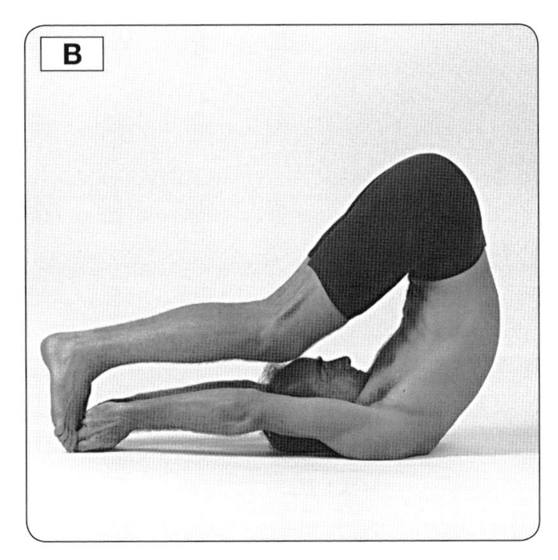

1) **Exhale** roll back onto your shoulders and take the feet to the floor above your head. Lift your hips toward the sky. Clasp the big toes with two fingers of each hand while keeping the feet together **(A)**. If maintaining straight legs is too intense then bend them slightly and clasp the toes **(B)** or use a strap to hold the feet **(C)**. If lifting the hips away from the floor is too intense, then leave them down and bend the legs **(D)**.

2) **Inhale** roll up from one of the positions above and balance on your sit-bones. You may balance here with the legs and arms straight while clasping the toes **(E)** or with the legs slightly bent as in **(F)** or holding the feet with a strap **(G)**.

Remain Here For 5 Deep Breaths

3) **Exhale** release the asana and lower the feet to the floor.

~VINYASA~

Drishti ~ **Nose**

Comments - When rolling up use opposition between the feet and hands to draw you forward. Push with the feet a bit more than you pull back with the hands and this will create a force that you may ride forward. As you reach the sit-bones decrease the momentum until you find your balance. This is difficult to do with the legs straight. You may bend them slightly or even pull the heels down toward the buttocks to assist. Once you are balanced the next challenge is to avoid collapsing in the lower back. You may utilize the same dynamic tension between the hands and feet yet this time create an equality of opposition in order to find your point of stillness. This action coupled with engagement of the bandhas and pulling back of the shoulders will lift the lower back. To further support the lumbar area, it is best to lead with the sternum.

Ubhaya Padangusthasana

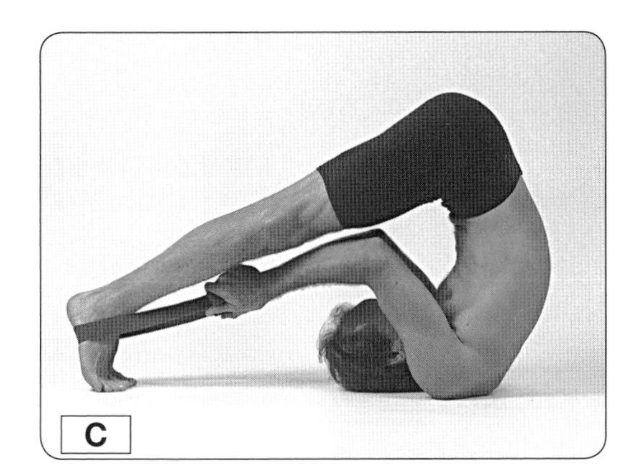
C

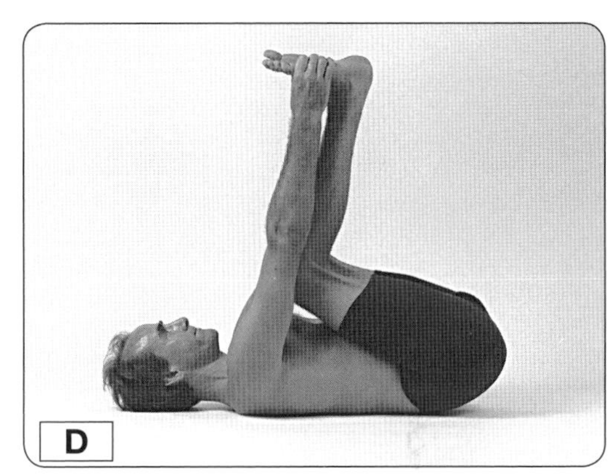
D

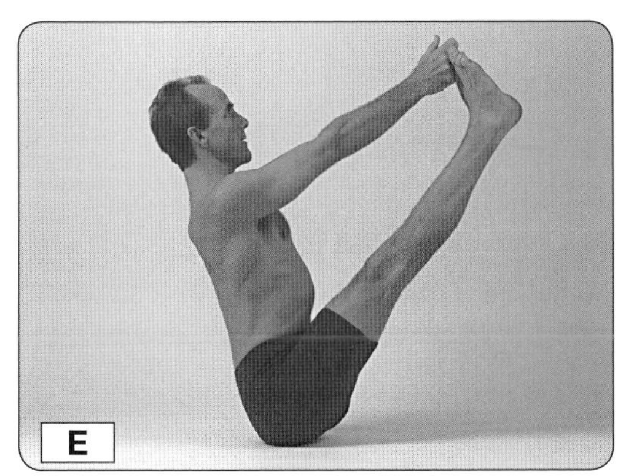
E

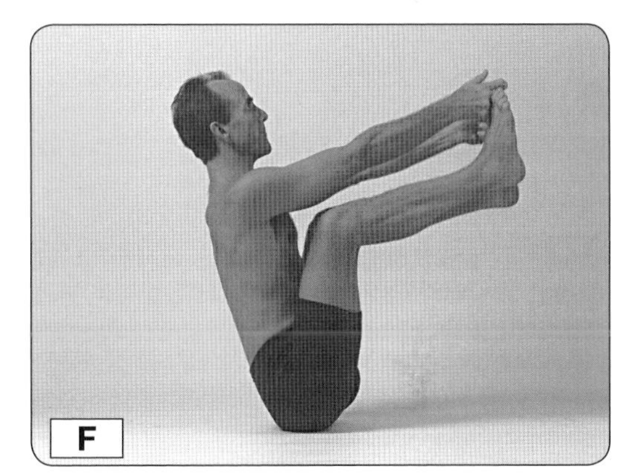
F

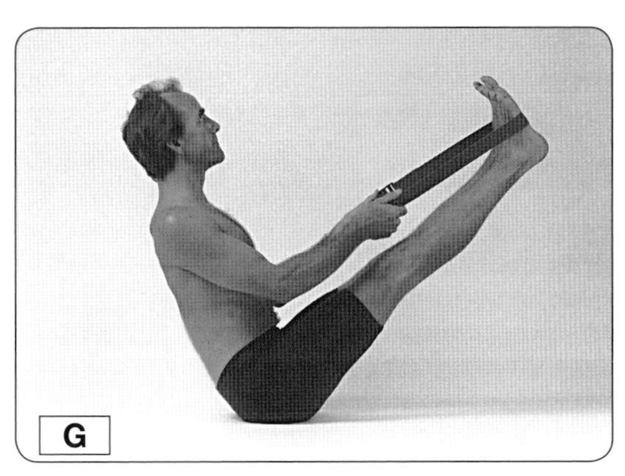
G

Urdhva Mukha Paschimottanasana

Urdhva = Upward Mukha = Face
Paschima = Western Uttana = Intense Stretch
"Upward Facing Western Intense Stretch Posture"

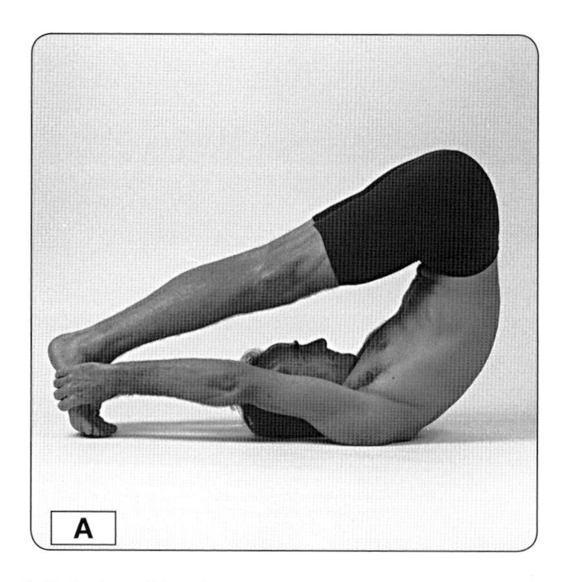

A

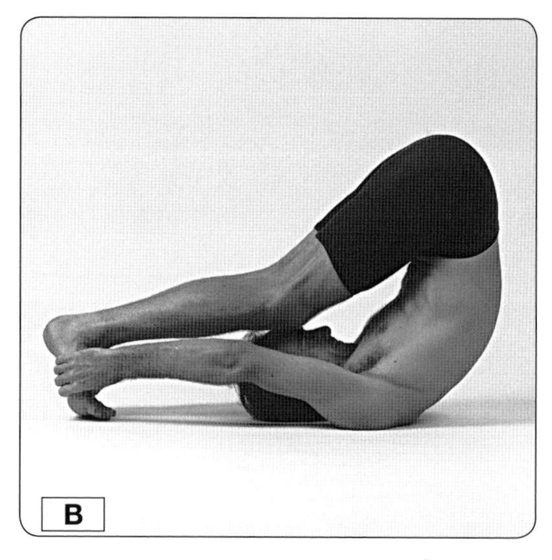

B

1) **Exhale** roll back onto your shoulders in the same manner as in **Ubhaya Padangusthasana**. This time instead of holding the toes you will hold the outer edges of the feet as in **(A)**. If keeping the legs straight is too intense then bend them slightly **(B)** or use a strap to hold the feet **(C)**. If lifting the hips away from the floor is too much then leave them down and bend the legs while holding the feet **(D)**.

2) **Inhale** roll up from one of the positions above and balance on your sit-bones. Bring the chest and legs together like a diver in pike position with the toes pointed **(E)** or hold behind the legs **(F)** or hold the feet with a strap **(G)**.

Remain Here For 5 Deep Breaths

3) **Exhale** release the asana and lower the feet to the floor.

~VINYASA~

Drishti ~ **Toes**

Comments - When rolling forward you may use the same approach as in the previous posture with either the legs straight or bent. The same dynamics also apply when balancing. The difference here is that now the chest and legs move toward each other. This will intensify the stretch. If you find it to be too much then back off and repeat an option from **Ubhaya Padangusthasana**. Engage the bandhas fully and pull with the hands. Lift the sternum. Draw the shoulders down the back away from the ears. When taking your gaze to your toes it is not necessary to drop the head back extremely. Use your eyes rather than solely the neck.

Urdhva Mukha Paschimottanasana

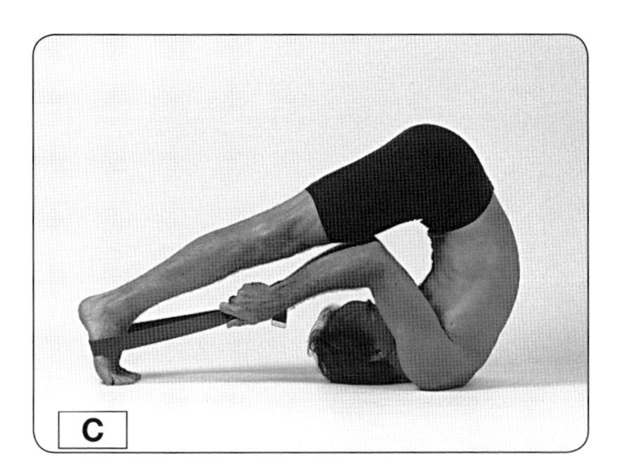

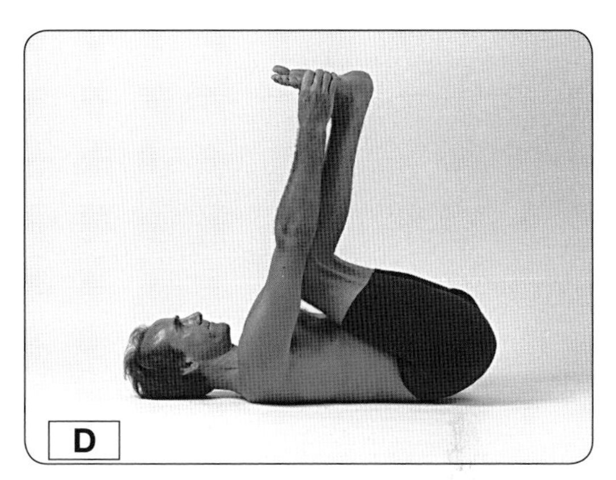

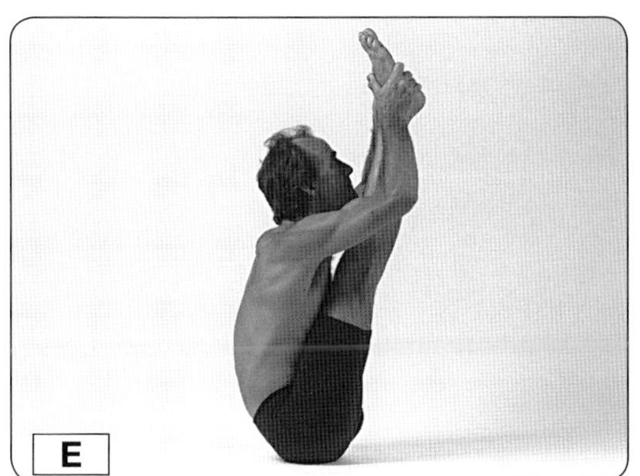

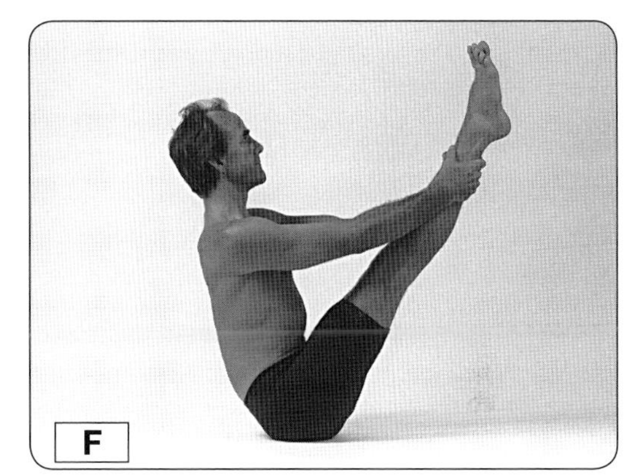

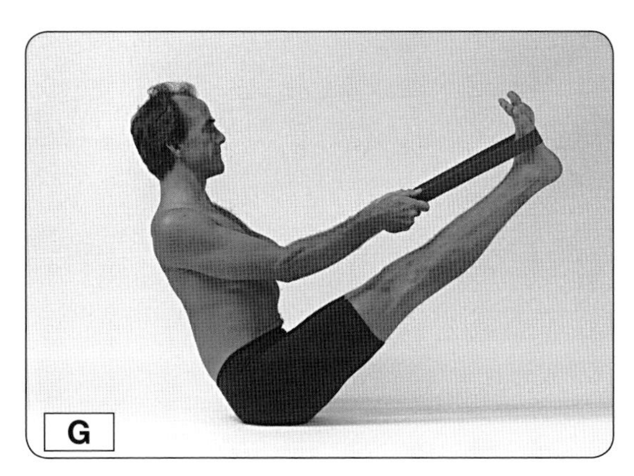

Setu Bandhasana

Setu = Bridge   Bandha = Bondage or Contraction

"Bridge Posture"

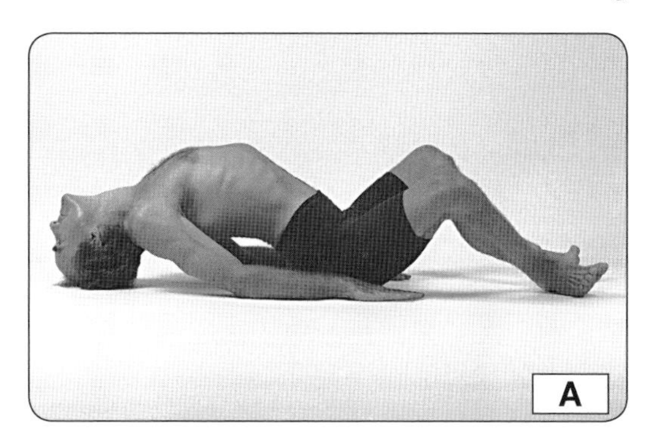

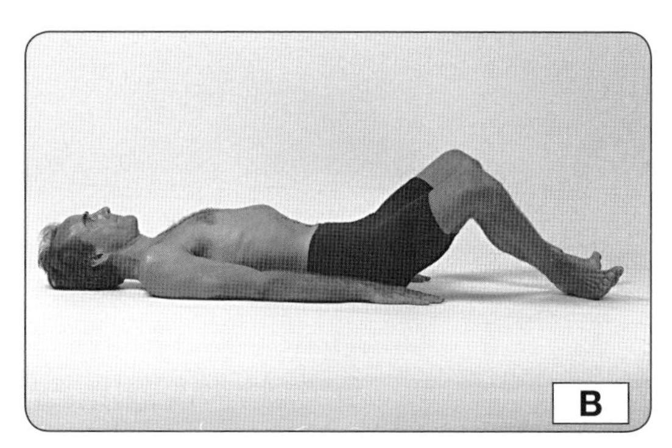

1) **Exhale** lie on your back. Bend your knees and bring them one-third of the way in toward your buttocks. Keep the heels touching and let the feet turn out like **"Charlie Chaplin"** so that the outer edges of the feet are touching the floor. Let the knees drop toward the floor. Press the elbows into the floor and arch your back by lifting the chest. Take the head back so that the top of the head is on the floor **(A)** or leave the head and the back flat on the floor instead of arching up **(B)**.

2) **Inhale** from position **(A)**. **Push** with the feet and raise the hips away from the floor. Roll onto the top of your head or even all of the way to the forehead. Cross the elbows across the chest with the hands on opposite shoulders for the full asana **(C)** or take the hands to the floor beside your head for support **(D)**. Instead of raising onto your head, you could enter from position **(B)** and leave your shoulders down and raise only the hips and then interlace the fingers and press the arms against the floor **(E)** or use the hands to support the hips **(F)**.

Remain Here For 5 Deep Breaths

3) **Exhale** release the asana and lower to the floor by taking the elbows down. **Pull** with the feet. Draw the chin into the chest as the hips move toward the heels.

~CHAKRASANA~

Remember your options from pages 120-121 or apply your favorite jumping Vinyasa

Drishti ~ **Nose**

This is the final asana of the Primary Series.
It completes the "filling" of the Ashtanga "sandwich".
From here proceed to the Finishing Sequence on page 206.

Comments - ***Proceed with caution in this asana!*** This posture requires strength and stability in the neck. If you have neck problems it is best to skip this asana for now or use the options with the shoulders on the floor. If you choose to move fully into it, use the hands for support to build confidence and strength as shown in **(D)**. Be patient. Listen to your body.

Setu Bandhasana

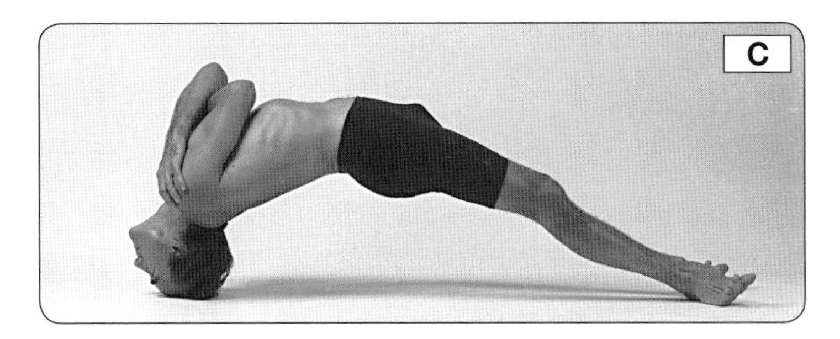

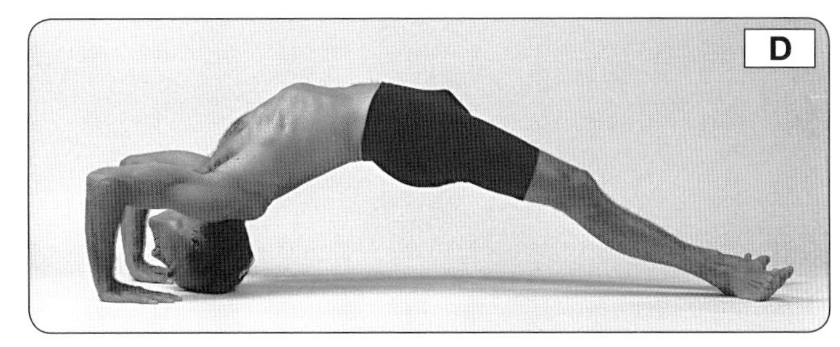

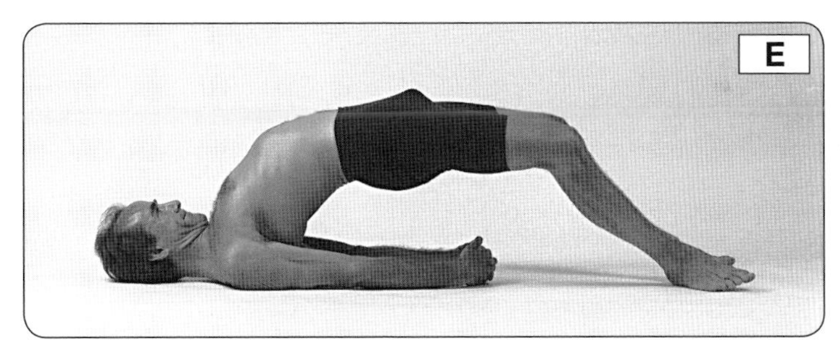

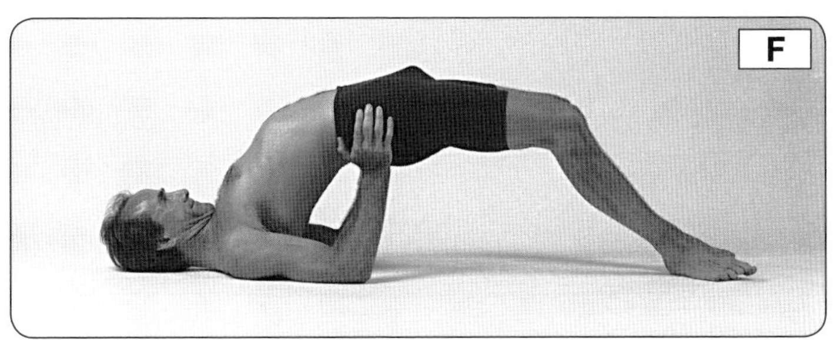

Focus

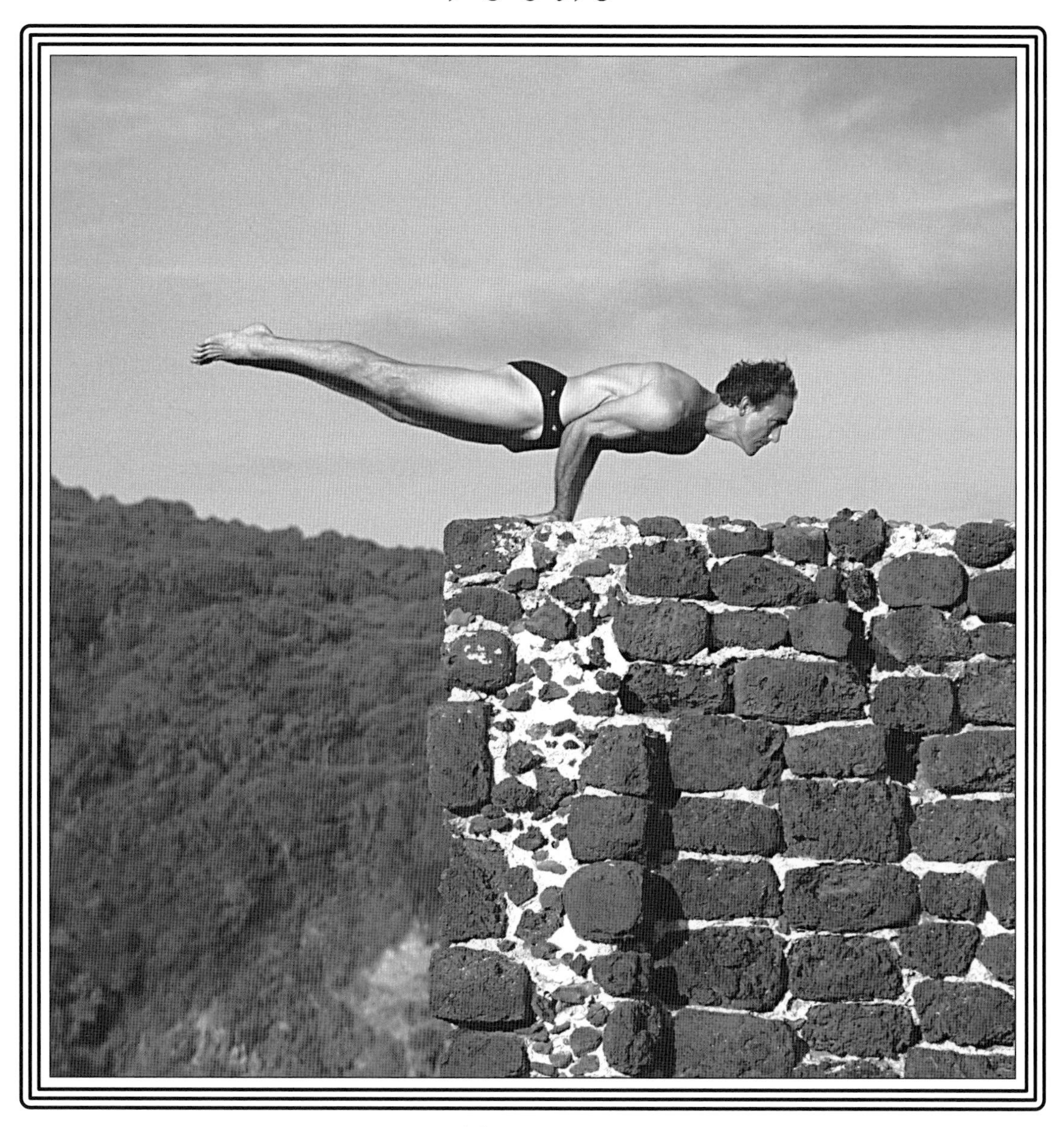

Mayurasana
Intermediate Series
David Swenson ~ Maui, Hawaii

Nadi Shodana

"Nerve Cleansing"

The Intermediate Series of Ashtanga Yoga is known as Nadi Shodana, which means **"nerve cleansing"**. The term, **"nerve cleansing"**, is applied in the Intermediate Series due to the focus on backward-bending asanas. Our spine is the housing for our nerve center. By bending and twisting the spinal column we are encouraging and maintaining suppleness on a physical level as well as opening energy channels to allow prana to flow freely on the subtle plane. This cleansing and toning occurs in each of the four series of Ashtanga Yoga. The Intermediate Series is particularly focused in the energetic regions of the spine, pelvis and hips. The Primary Series builds the foundation to continue into the Intermediate Series and the Intermediate Series prepares one for the Advanced Series. In this way the entire Ashtanga system is set up like a yogic "lasagne". Each step prepares the practitioner for the next, layer by layer.

There are many asanas within the Intermediate Series which are readily accessible for the practitioner that is coming to it for the first time. As the Intermediate Series is explored, it will become apparent that there is a logic to the arrangement of asanas. Sometimes people ask me if it is necessary to "master" the Primary Series before proceeding into the Intermediate Series. There is never a point in which any of us may master an asana, series or system. Whether one has been practicing for ten days, ten years or an entire lifetime, we are each engaged in what we refer to as our "practice". There is no ceiling to the knowledge available unless we choose to seal our mind from learning. Once we shut down to the possibility of growth, we are unable to assimilate new information or insights, and knowledge will simply run down the sides of our tight-knit exterior.

The general criterion I offer for entering the Intermediate Series is that one should have a sufficient knowledge of the flow of the Primary Series so that it is not necessary to refer to any external source, such as a video, book, tape or diagram, to prompt the mind as to which asana is next in the sequence. It is also logical that one should be able to continue through the entire Primary Series, from beginning to end, without stopping. The depth of the asanas is not as important as the knowledge of how to approach them at a personal level. This means following your intuition. Maintain full awareness within the breath. Remain cognizant of your purpose in doing yoga. If you remain fixed within those realms, then whichever series you practice will fill you with insights and internal knowing. Practice grows a breath at a time just as a painting is created within a series of single brushstrokes. Find joy in each breath as you practice and take pleasure in observing your personal portrait unfold.

Note - There are numerous Vinyasas in the Intermediate Series in which you will not come all of the way through to a sitting position from Downward Dog. Each of these instances is described fully. If there is no mention of a unique entry or exit, then take your vinyasa as usual and follow it all of the way through to a seated position, in preparation for the next asana.

Pashasana

Pasha = Noose

"Noose Posture"

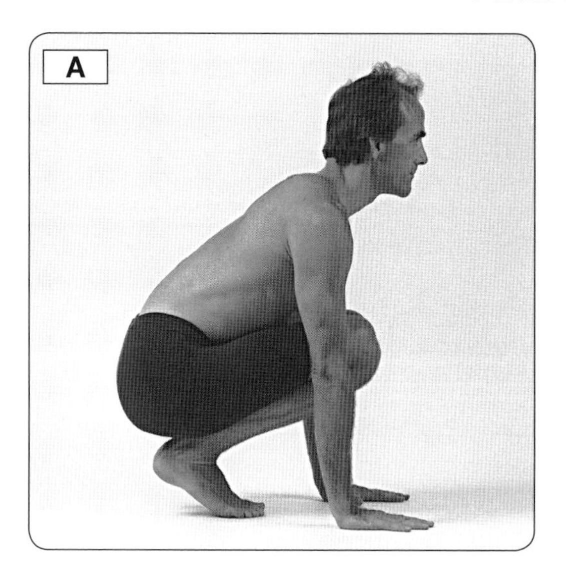

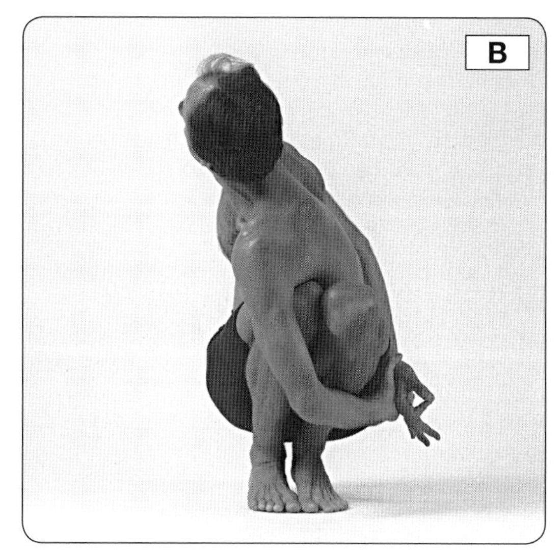

Enter the Intermediate Series after completing the final posture of the Standing Sequence on page 59

1) **Inhale** from **Downward Dog** and bring the feet forward into a squatting position **(A)**.

2) **Exhale** bring the left elbow outside the right knee and wrap the arm around it. Clasp both hands behind your back and press the heels toward the floor **(B)**. If you are unable to balance with the heels on the floor then roll up a mat and place it under them. Clasping the hands behind the back may be too difficult. In which case, you may use a strap to assist in making the connection, as in **(C)**. Instead of taking the elbow outside of the outer leg you could take it in between the knees and wrap around only one leg **(D)**. Another option is to keep the heels hovering above the ground and place the left elbow outside the right knee and then press the palms together and twist from that position, as in **(E)**.

Remain Here for 5 Deep Breaths

3) **Inhale** turn your gaze to the center.

4) **Exhale** repeat step 2 on the other side. (There is no VINYASA between sides for this asana)

Remain Here for 5 Deep Breaths

5) **Inhale** gaze to the center.

6) **Exhale** release the asana.

~VINYASA~

Drishti ~ **Side**

Pashasana

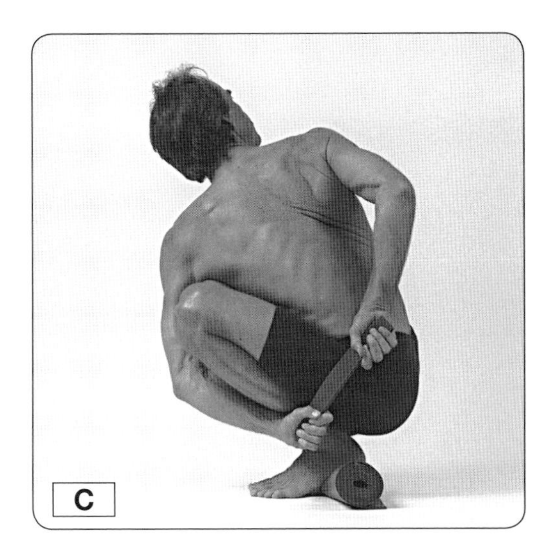

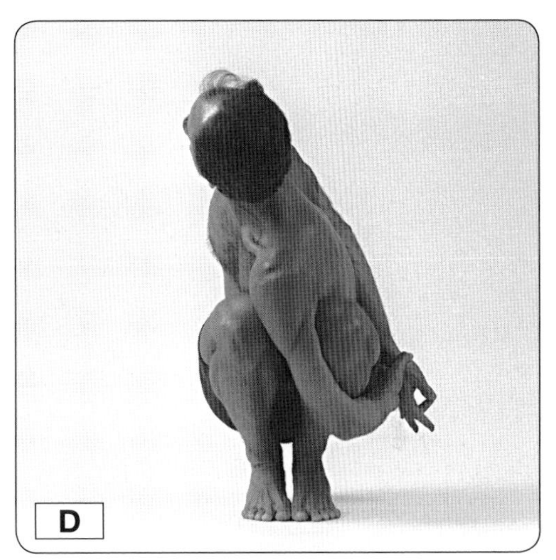

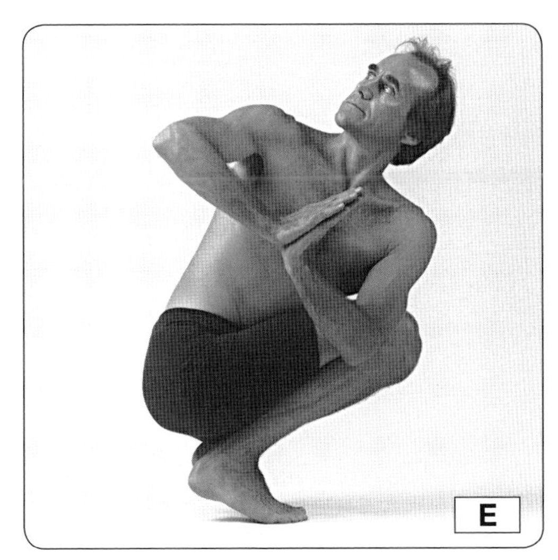

Comments - Create length in the spine by using opposing forces between the outer knee and the wrapping arm or elbow. Drop the sit-bones and extend up through the top of your head. The gaze should follow the direction of the stretch. Look far out over the shoulder which is behind. Length is crucial for full breathing.

Krounchasana

Krouncha = Heron

"Heron Posture"

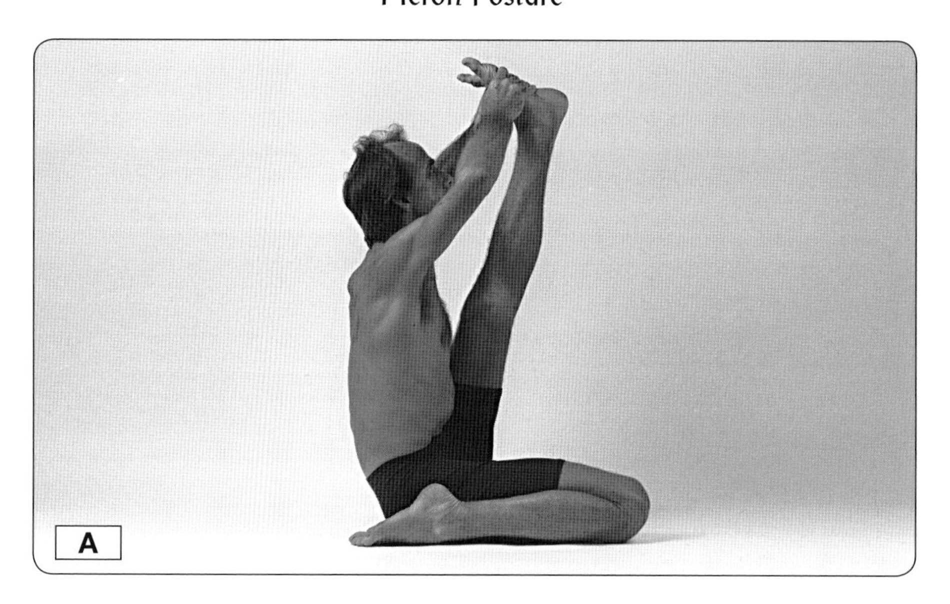

1) **Exhale** bend the right leg back with the top of the foot on the floor and the toes pointing back.

2) **Inhale** grab the left foot with both hands and straighten the leg with the toes pointing up.

3) **Exhale** lift the chest and draw the shin toward your chin **(A)**. If it is too much to straighten the leg you may practice it with the leg slightly bent as in **(B)**. You may also elevate the hips to take the pressure off of the outer leg by sitting on a block or cushion **(C)**.

Remain Here for 5 Deep Breaths

4) **Inhale** as you slightly release the stretch.

5) **Exhale** release the asana fully and straighten both legs.

~VINYASA~

Repeat Steps 1-5 On the Left Side

~VINYASA~

Enter the Next Asana from Downward Dog

Drishti ~ **Toes**

Krounchasana

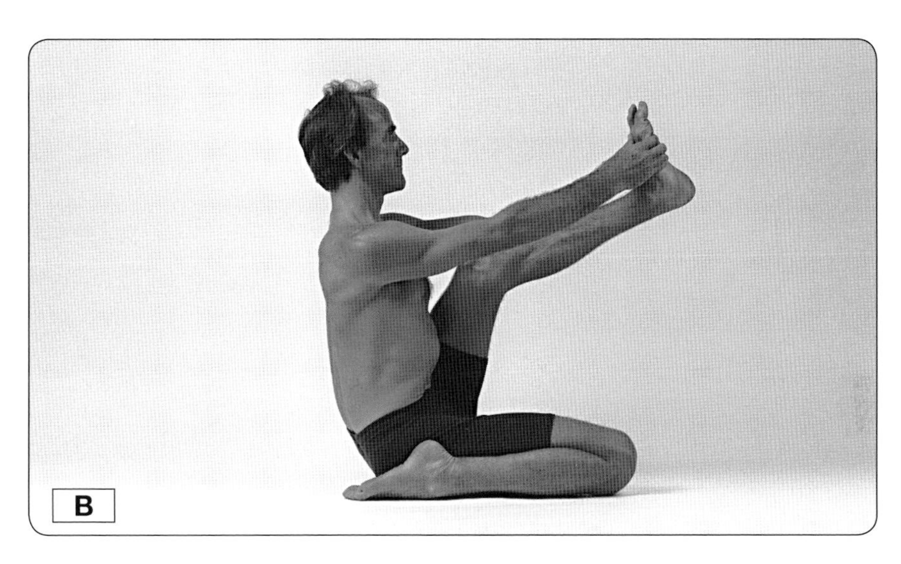

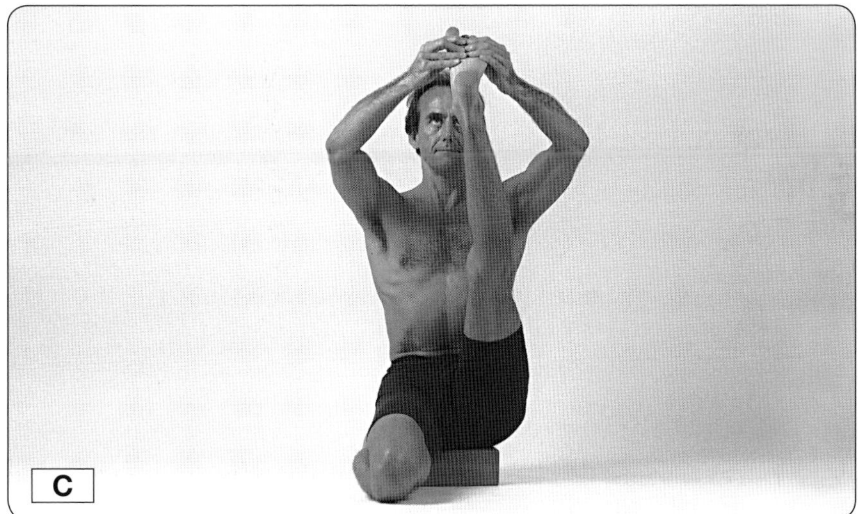

Comments - There is a tendency for the lower back to sag in this posture. To avoid this you may bring full awareness to your bandhas. By engagement of the lower abdominal area the lower back will remain supported. This supportive action may be further enhanced by using the hands to pull against the lifted foot as the foot pushes back against the hands. Lift the chest and shine your heart at your toes. Eventually you may enter **Krounchasana** directly from **Downward Dog** by jumping through with the right leg curled back.

Shalabhasana A

Shalabha = Locust

"Locust Posture"

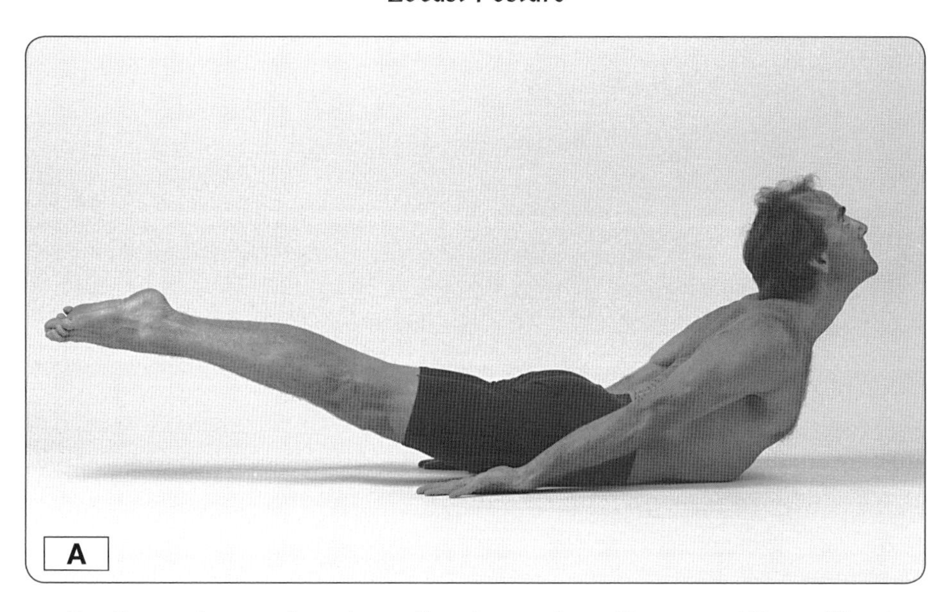

A

For the next several postures the vinyasa from Downward Dog will *not* bring you all of the way through to sitting to enter the next asana. The particular entry will be described for each.

1) **Exhale** and lie down on your belly from **Downward Dog**.

2) **Inhale** lift your chest and feet. Place the back of the hands on the floor. Keep the feet together **(A)**. If it is too difficult to raise the chest and feet simultaneously, you may leave the feet on the floor and raise only the chest **(B)** or raise only one foot at a time as in **(C)**. If you choose option **(C)** you may raise each foot for a five breath count.

Remain Here for 5 Deep Breaths

Enter the Next Asana from Here

Drishti ~ **Nose**

Shalabhasana A

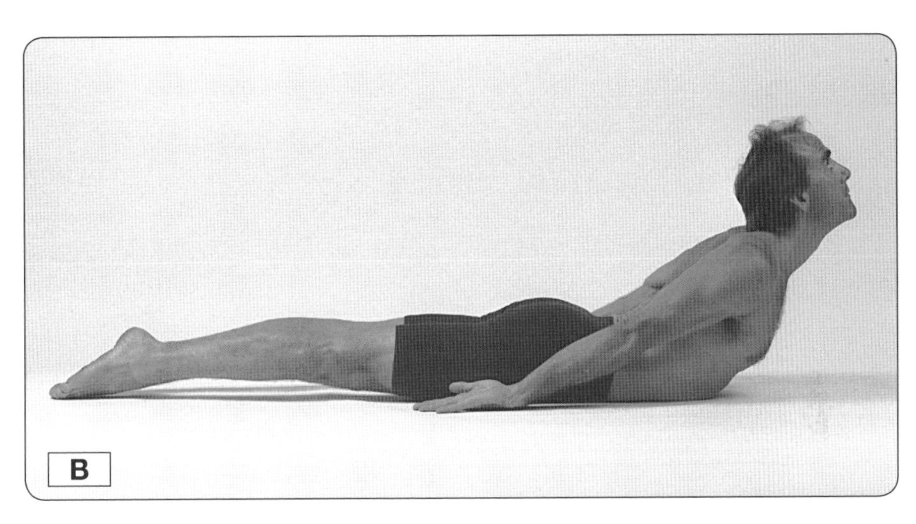

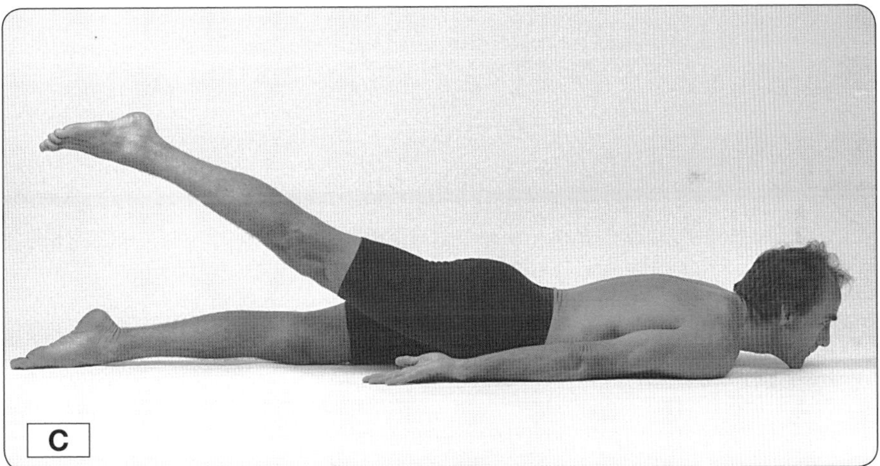

Comments - This asana is excellent for strengthening the lower back. Many physical therapists use a similar approach to treat people with lower back complaints. If you find discomfort from your pelvis pressing into the floor you may place a thin cushion or towel under the area and that will relieve it. Use the action of pressing the back of your hands into the floor to gain greater lift in the chest. This will also distribute the action into the shoulders. Pull the shoulders back in order to keep the heart open wide. One of the great challenges of this asana is to keep the feet together. They generally want to separate. Engage the adductor muscles of the inner legs to keep the feet touching.

Shalabhasana B

Shalabha = Locust

"Locust Posture"

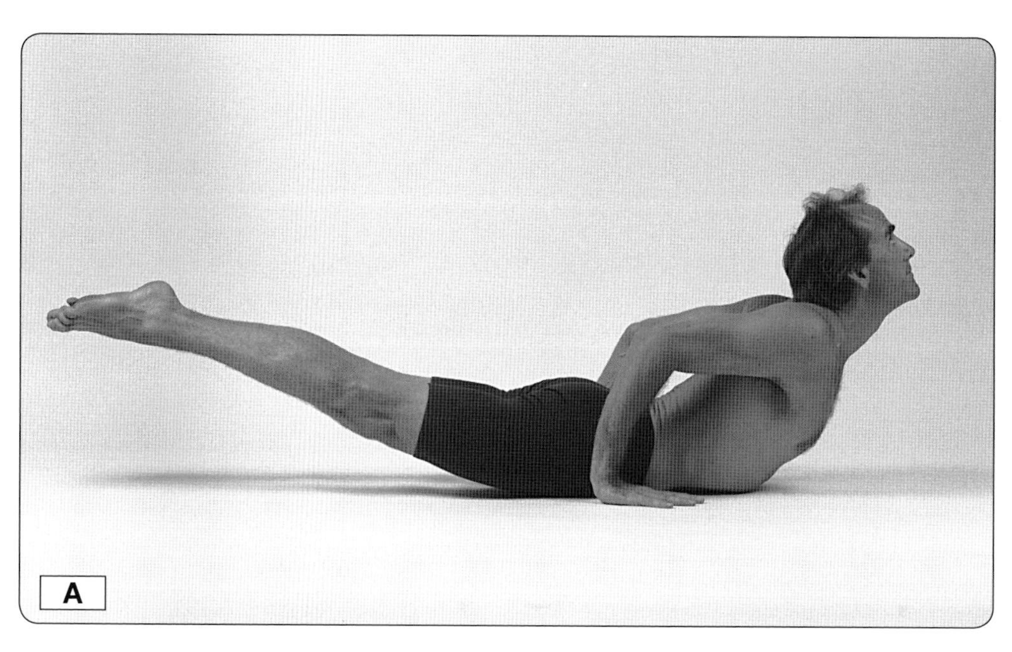

1) **Inhale** bring the hands forward toward the waist with the elbows bent. Place the palms on the floor with the fingers pointing straight ahead. Lift the chest a bit higher than in the previous asana **(A)**. If it is too difficult to take the hands beside the waist you may outstretch your arms and take the hands to the floor in front of you as in **(B)**. You may also choose to place the forearms and palms on the floor in front for additional support while leaving the legs on the floor **(C)**.

Remain Here for 5 Deep Breaths

2) **Exhale** release the asana by lowering the chest and feet and take the hands under the shoulders.

~VINYASA~

Enter the Next Asana from Downward Dog

Drishti ~ **Nose**

Shalabhasana B

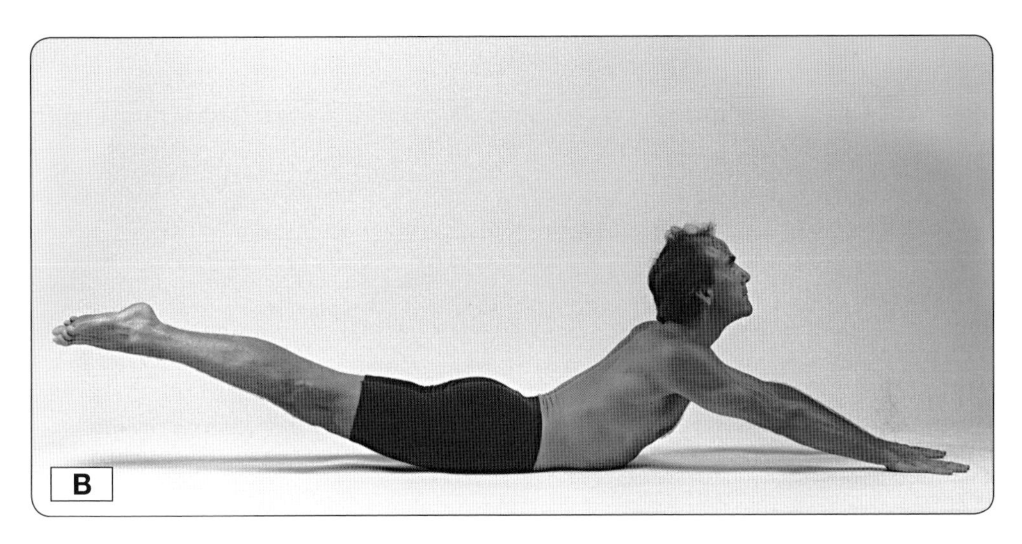

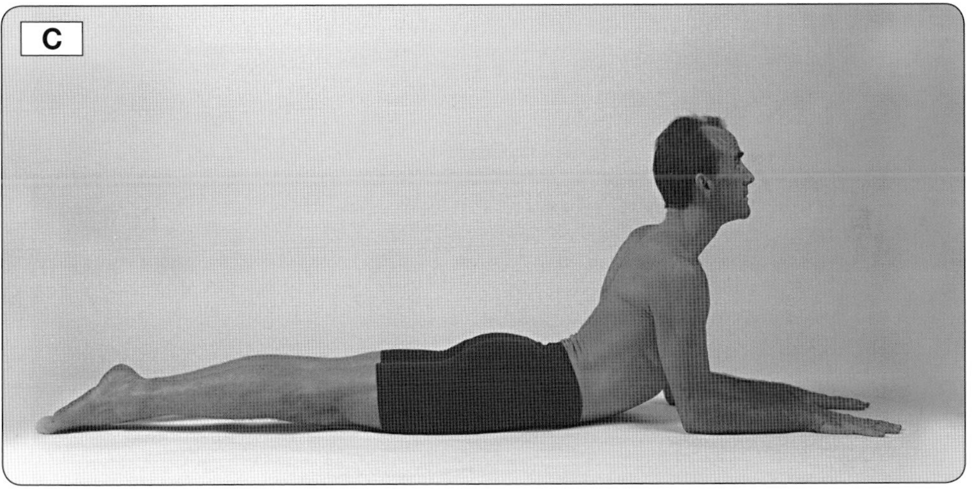

Comments - In this version of **Shalabhasana** the object is to create greater lift in the chest by the action of the palms pressing into the floor beside the hips. Keep the feet lifting as you raise the chest. It is tempting to push with the arms so much that the upper body begins to lift into an **Upward Dog**. It is not necessary to lift that high. That is the reason for the hands remaining near the waist rather than under the shoulders. Use the muscles of the back for the main support unless you feel discomfort; in which case, it is best to back off. Create an equality of effort between the right and left side of your body so that you are not lifting higher on one side than the other. If you need to come down in between **Shalabhasana A** and **B** that is fine.

Bhekasana

Bheka = Frog

"Frog Posture"

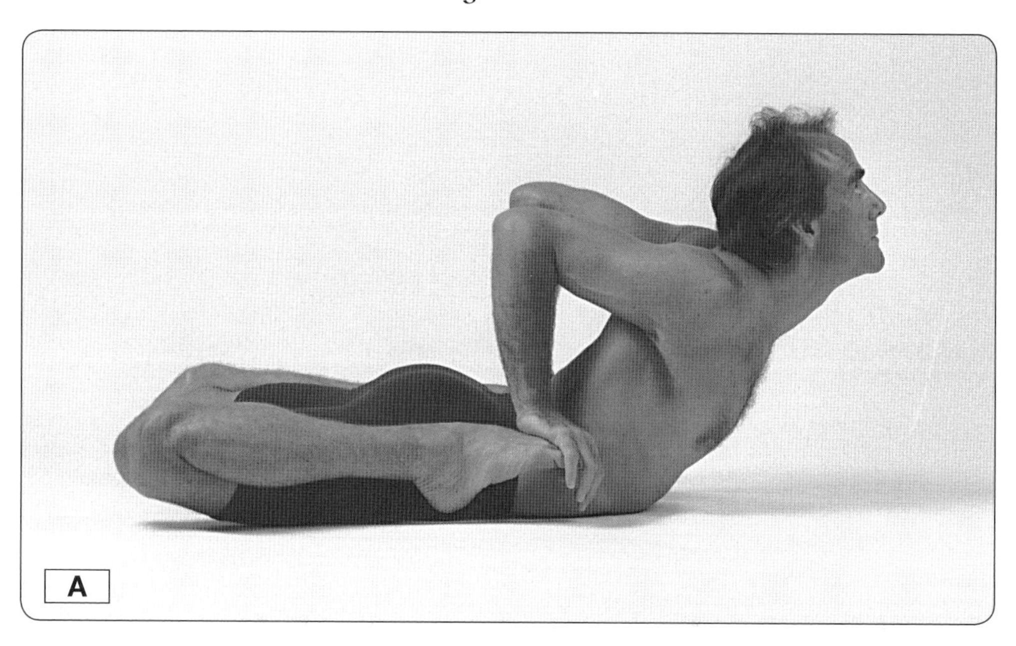

1) **Exhale** and lie down on your belly from **Downward Dog**. Bend your knees and pull the feet toward the floor outside of the hips. The hands should grab the feet so that the fingers and toes run in the same direction. Point the elbows toward the sky and lift the chest as you press the feet toward the floor **(A)**. It may be too intense in the beginning to press both feet down as described in **(A)**, so you may practice with one foot at a time as shown in **(B)**. Another option is to take both feet at the same time but point the fingers toward the knees instead of toward the toes and take the feet only partway toward the floor **(C)**.

Remain Here for 5 Deep Breaths

2) **Exhale** release the asana.

~VINYASA~

Enter the next asana from downward dog

Drishti ~ **Nose**

Bhekasana

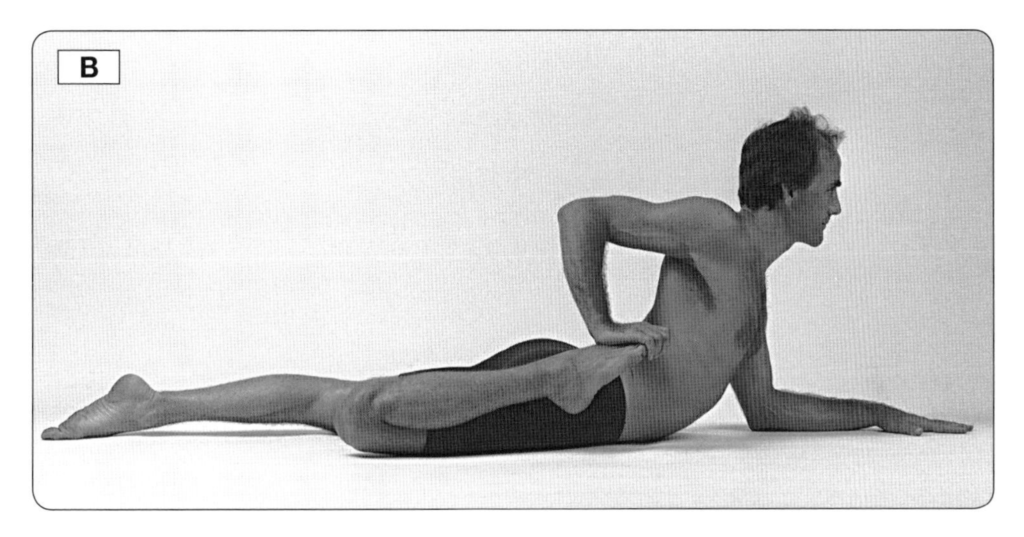

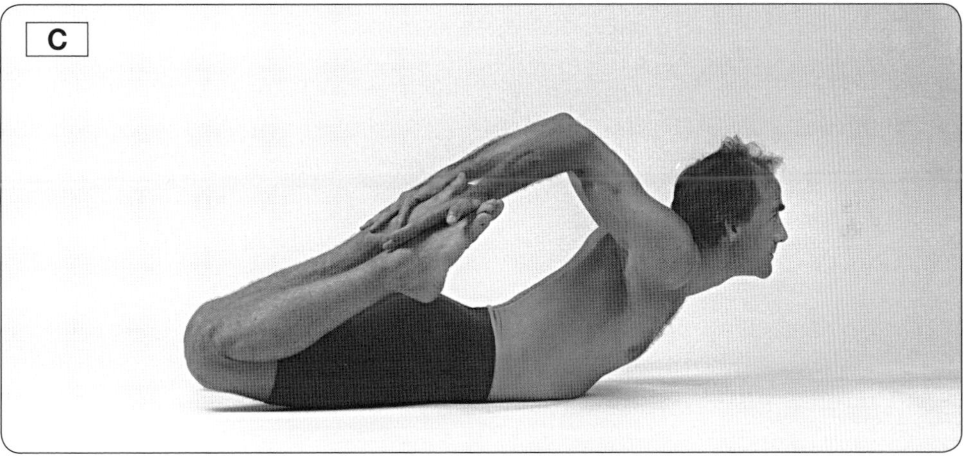

Comments - Take precautions with your knees in this asana. You must keep the top of the feet pointing straight up toward the sky with the heels moving toward the floor. ***DO NOT*** **roll the toes out so that they are pointing away from the hips**. Turning out of the toes will put undue strain on the inner knee and you will risk injury. The stretch is meant to be directed at the quadriceps and the front of the knee. If you feel pain or discomfort release the asana without delay. Choose the most suitable approach for your body. Another action of this asana is the lifting of the chest and opening of the heart. Use the downward motion of the hands against the feet to gain lift in the chest. Keep the shoulders rolling down the back.

Dhanurasana

Dhanura = Bow

"Bow Posture"

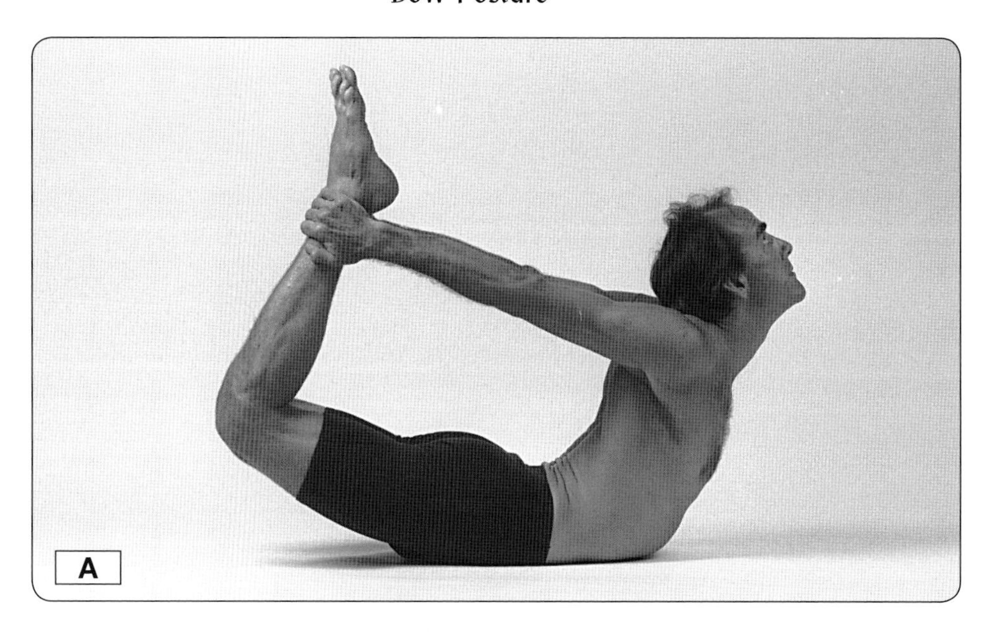

1) **Exhale** and lie down on your belly from **Downward Dog**. Bend your knees and grab the ankles with your hands.

2) **Inhale** push the ankles against the hands as you pull with the arms and lift the chest high while keeping the knees touching and the feet together **(A)**. If it is too intense to keep the legs together then you may open them until you find a comfort zone while keeping the chest and knees away from the floor **(B)**. Another option is to leave the knees on the floor and lift only the chest **(C)**.

Remain Here for 5 Deep Breaths

Enter the Next Asana from Here

Drishti ~ **Nose**

Comments - This is another excellent asana for strengthening the back as well as opening the chest. The key to the lift here is the dynamic of opposition which is created between the hands and ankles. By pushing away with the feet while simultaneously lifting with the arms the heart automatically begins to open. It is a wonderful feeling to experience the energy expansion which occurs while holding **Dhanurasana**. The arms are like the string of a bow and the body is the bow itself. The energy being propelled through the spine and up to the crown of the head is the arrow. If you feel tension in your neck then drop your chin toward your chest and that should relieve it. The drishti will also aid in keeping the neck from bending back too far.

Dhanurasana

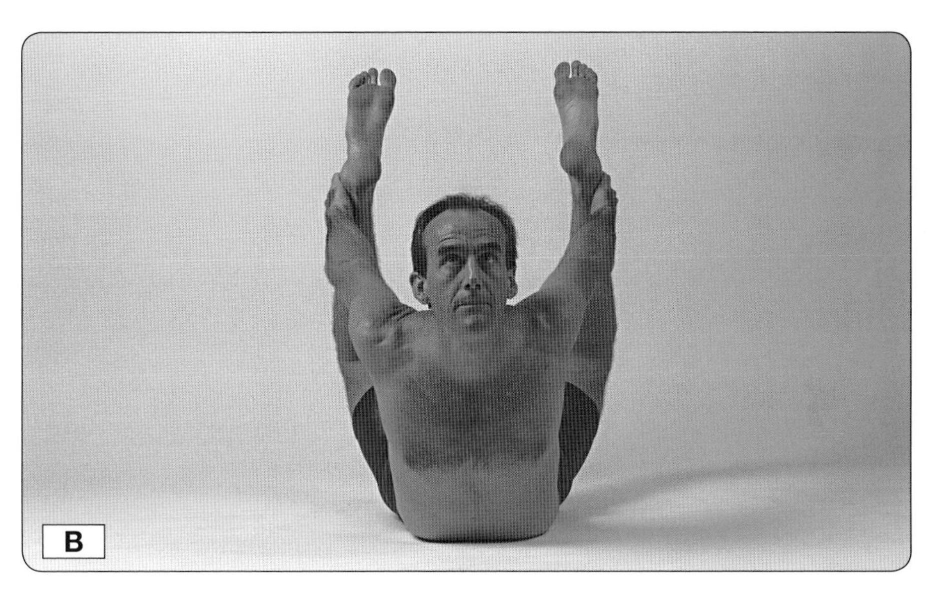
B

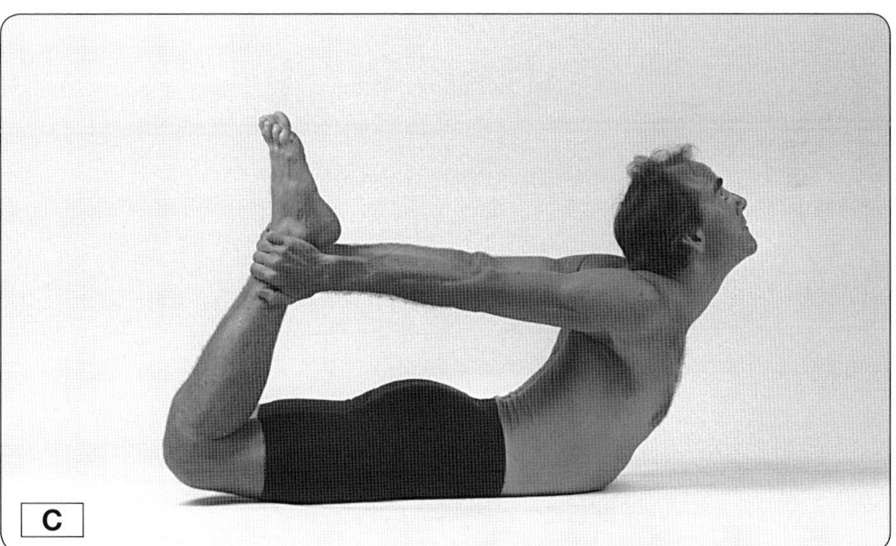
C

Parsva Dhanurasana

Parsva = Side   Dhanura = Bow

"Sideways Bow Posture"

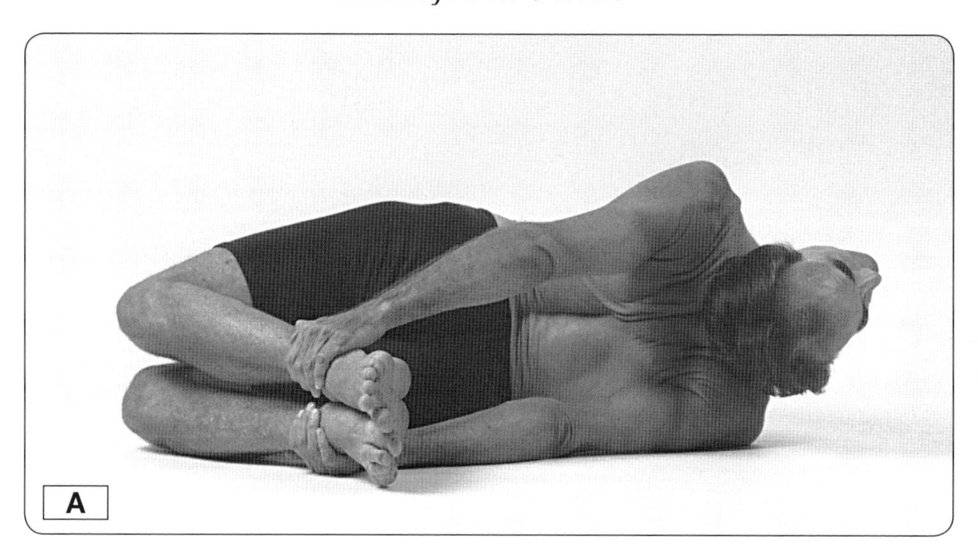

A

1) **Exhale** roll over onto your right shoulder while continuing to hold the ankles. Keep the knees together and the heart open fully as you arch the back like a bow with a full extension of the chest **(A)** or you may separate the knees and keep the feet touching as in **(B)**. A third option is to rest the left leg on top of the right so that the ankles are touching and the knees are together as in **(A)**, yet create some slack in the bowstring by releasing the opposition of force between the ankles and hands **(C)**.

Remain Here for 5 Deep Breaths

2) **Inhale** roll up to the center.

3) **Exhale** roll onto the left shoulder.

Remain Here for 5 Deep Breaths

4) **Inhale** return to the center and hold **Dhanurasana**.

Remain Here for 5 Deep Breaths

Repeat one of the options from Dhanurasana. Hold it for 5 Breaths before releasing.

5) **Exhale** release the asana.

~VINYASA~

Enter the Next Asana from Downward Dog

Drishti ~ **Nose**

Parsva Dhanurasana

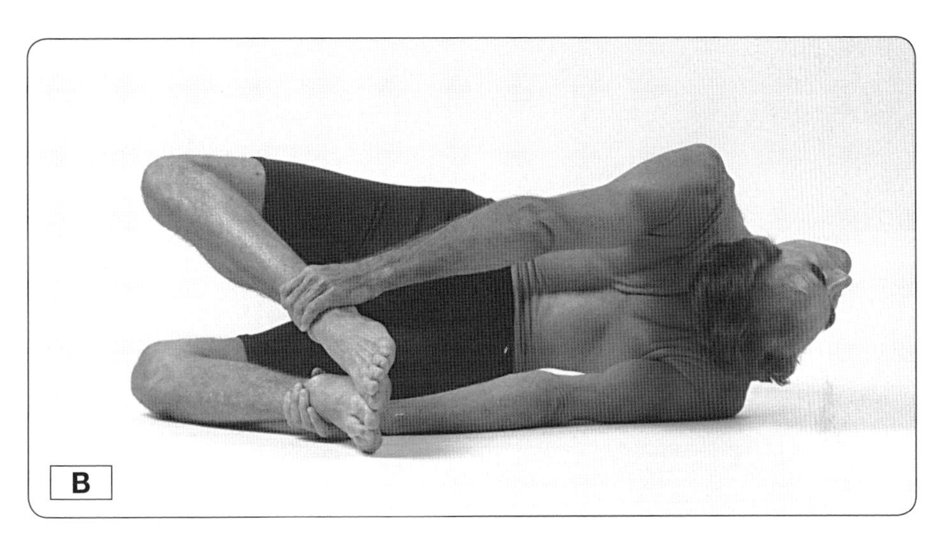
B

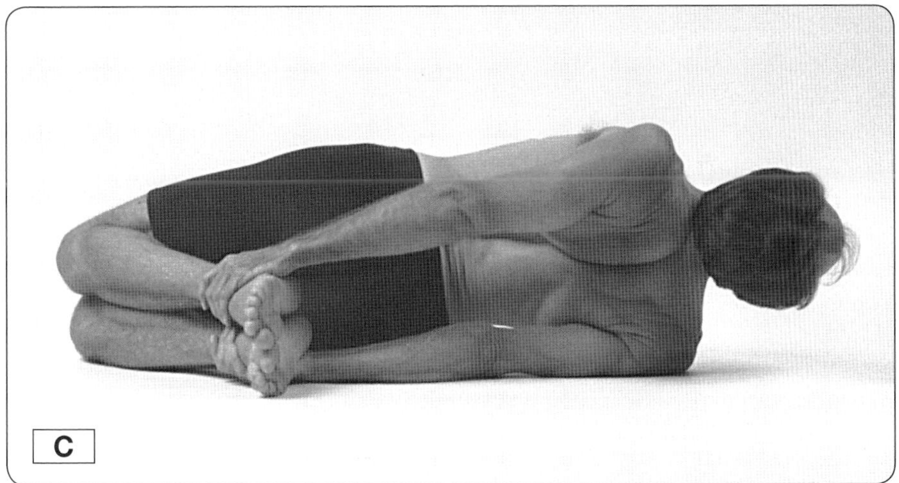
C

Comments - It is a great challenge, in **Parsva Dhanurasana,** to maintain the openness in the chest which was achieved in **Dhanurasana**. When rolling to the side it will be necessary to release some of the lift in the chest. After rolling over it may be regained by reinitiating the opposing forces. If your neck becomes tired rest your head on the floor. If you feel discomfort in the lower back then loosen the "bowstring".

Ushtrasana

Ushtra = Camel

"Camel Posture"

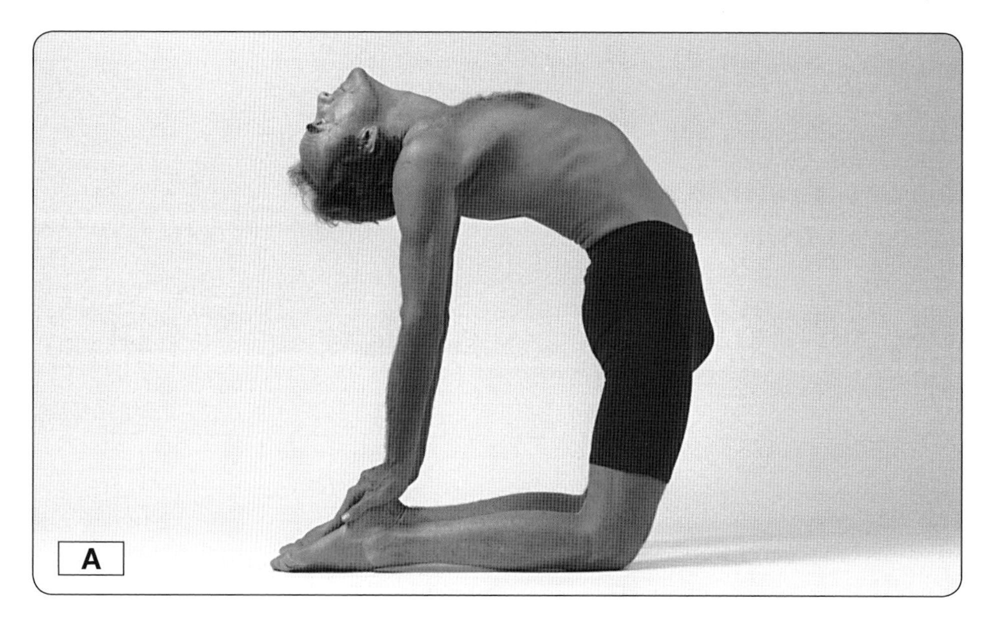
A

1) **Inhale** and come forward into a kneeling position from **Downward Dog**. Keep the tops of the feet on the floor with the toes pointing back.

2) **Exhale** lean back and place your heels in the palms of your hands with the fingers running down the soles of the feet. Drop the head back and lift the chest **(A)**. If it is too intense to place the hands on the heels with the tops of the feet on the floor you may curl the toes under and elevate the heels as in **(B)** or leave the hands on the back of the thighs for support **(C)**.

Remain Here for 5 Deep Breaths

3) **Inhale** release the asana by coming up and placing the hands on the floor and sit on the heels.

~VINYASA~

Enter the Next Asana from Downward Dog

Drishti ~ **Nose**

Comments - When entering a backbend there is a tendency to use the lower back like a hinge, instead of distributing the movement throughout the spine from bottom to top. One way to avoid "hinging" in this asana is to keep the legs fully engaged as you are extending the hands toward the feet. Even after the hands have made contact it is important to keep the legs working. This will add extra structural support for the lower back. Another assistance is to be aware of the front of the body, particularly the chest and heart area. Keep the heart open fully. Roll the shoulders back. Use the hands for additional support by pressing them against the feet to create more lift in the chest.

Ushtrasana

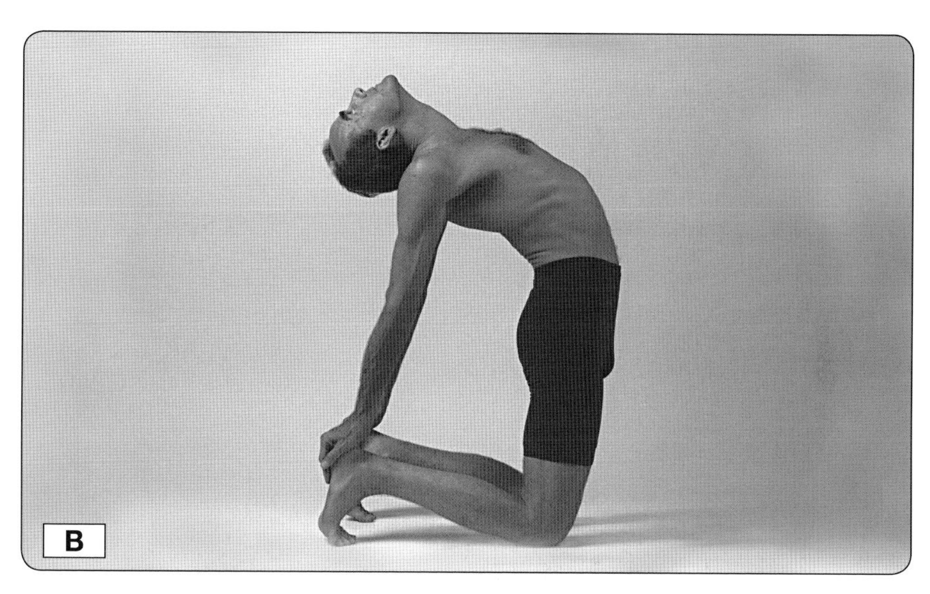

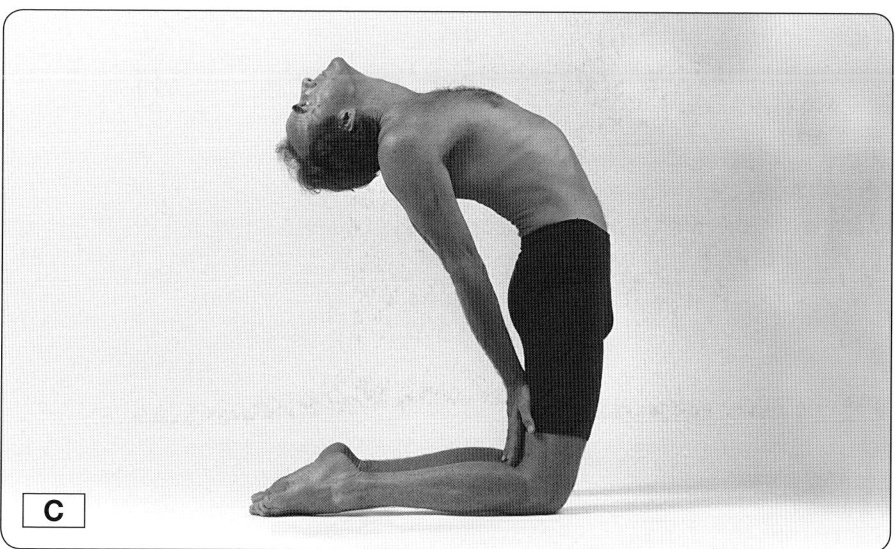

Laghuvajrasana

Laghu = Little or Small   Vajra = Thunderbolt

"Little Thunderbolt Posture"

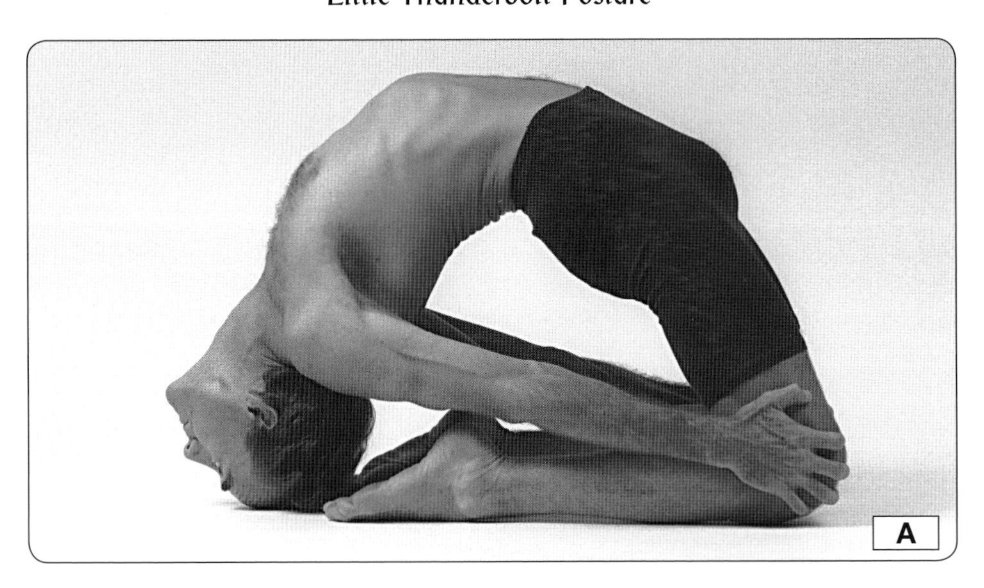

1) **Inhale** and come into a kneeling position from **Downward Dog**.
2) **Exhale** hold the knees with the hands and lower the head toward the feet **(A)**. If holding the knees is not possible at this time then you may hold your thighs as in **(B)** or leave the hands on the back of the calves for support **(C)**. Another option is to hold the thighs as in **(B)** but take the head only part of the way down toward the floor and remain in that position **(D)**. **You may also choose to either omit this asana for now or repeat one of the options from Ushtrasana**.

Remain Here for 5 Deep Breaths

3) **Inhale** release the asana by coming up and placing the hands on the floor and sit on the heels.

~VINYASA~

Enter the Next Asana from Downward Dog

Drishti ~ **Third Eye**

Comments - The back-bending asanas are moving progressively deeper as we travel from **Ushtrasana** to **Laghuvajrasana** and next on to **Kapotasana**. Listen to your body and move at your own pace and depth. Do not hurry. If you choose to move into this asana you must keep the legs working fully just as in **Ushtrasana**. It is even more imperative that the legs remain engaged here. Without the hands on the feet, as in **Ushtrasana** for support, the quadriceps must do even more work to keep the stretch distributed evenly throughout the spine. One consolation of the hands holding the thighs is that it will enable you to pull the shoulders back more fully and evenly which will enhance the opening of the heart area. When exiting use the legs to lift you up.

Laghuvajrasana

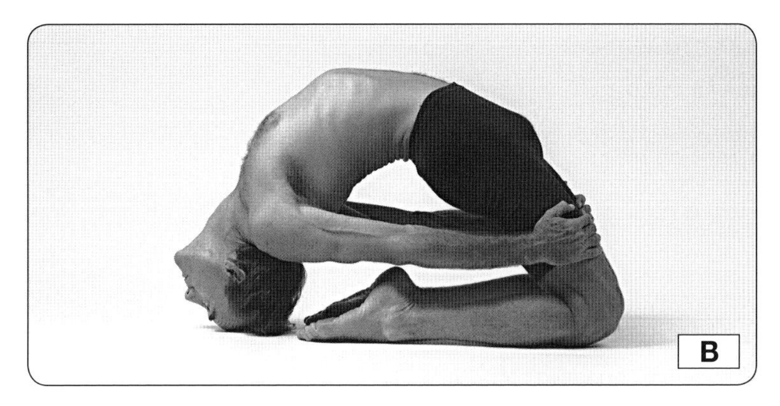

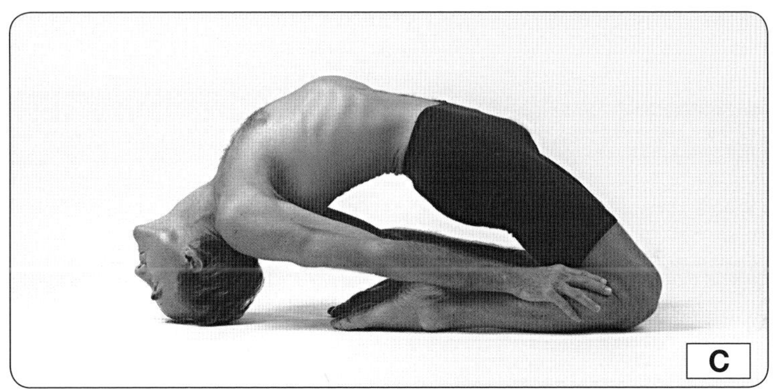

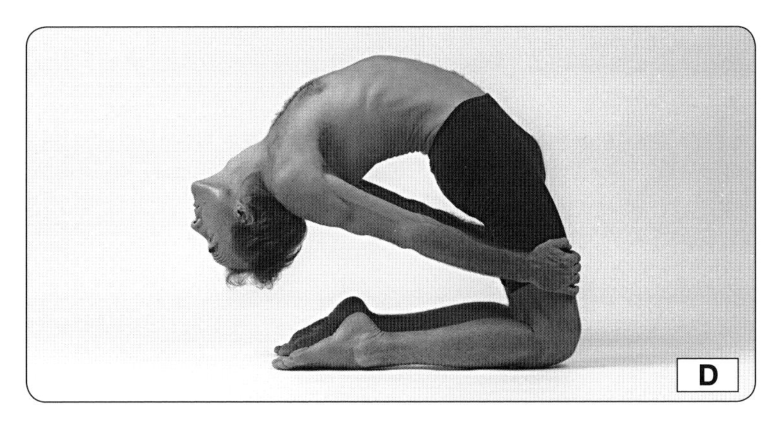

Kapotasana

Kapota = Pigeon

"Pigeon Posture"

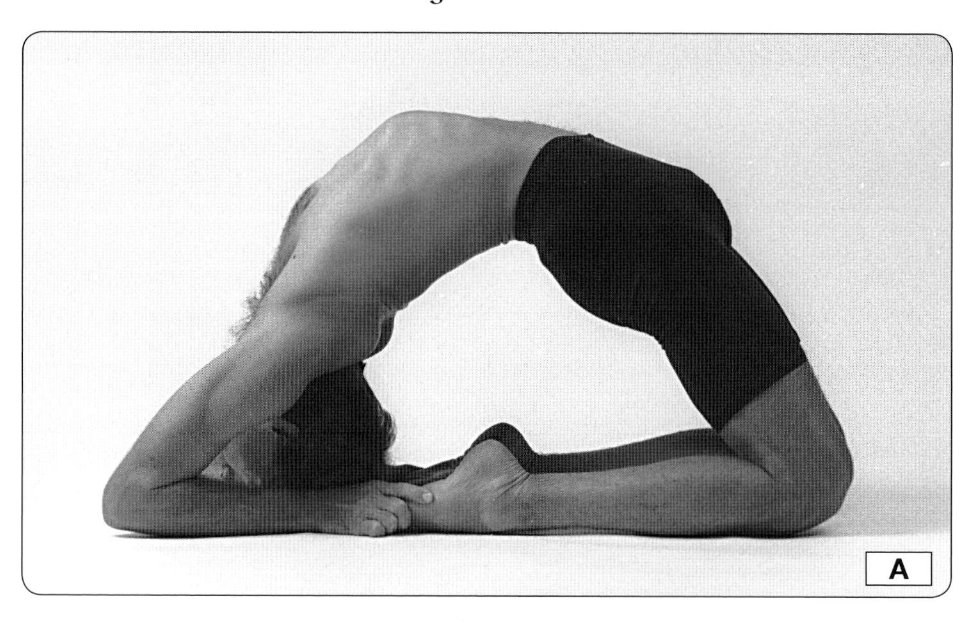

1) **Inhale** and come into a kneeling position from **Downward Dog**.

2) **Exhale** extend the arms over head and bend back until the hands reach the floor behind you. Clasp the feet or heels as in **(A)** or if you are unable to reach the feet you may leave the hands on the floor as close to the feet as is comfortable **(B)**. If taking the hands to the floor is too intense then you may raise the arms overhead with the palms together and lean back only part of the way toward the floor and remain there **(C)**. Another option is to position yourself near a wall. Lean back against the wall for support at whatever depth of stretch feels most appropriate, as seen in **(D)**. **You may also choose to either omit this asana for now or repeat one of the options from Ushtrasana or Laghuvajrasana**.

Remain Here for 5 Deep Breaths

3) **Inhale** release the asana by coming up and placing the hands on the floor and sit on the heels.

~VINYASA~

Drishti ~ **Nose**

Comments - Of the three asanas in this back-bending sequence (**Ushtrasana, Laghuvajrasana and Kapotasana**), **Kapotasana** requires the greatest flexibility as well as the greatest action in the legs. The opening of the chest and upper back should be initiated before you engage the lower back. This is done by taking the arms overhead and contracting the quadriceps muscles. Lift the heart before actually travelling backwards toward the floor. The legs continue to act as supports as the arms press against the floor.

Kapotasana

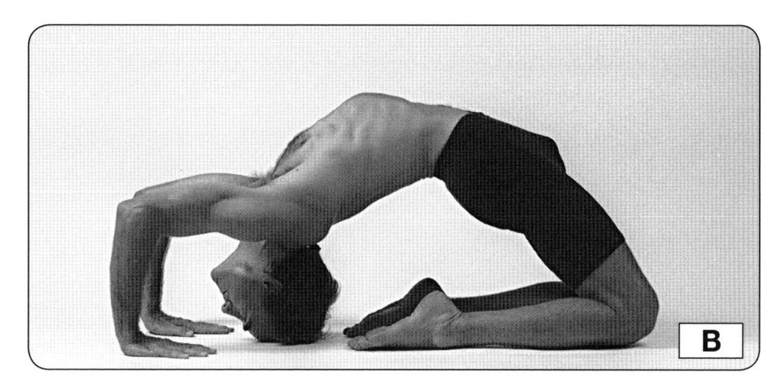

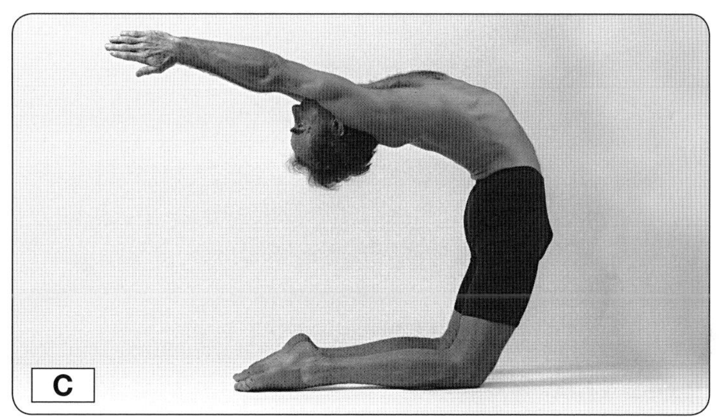

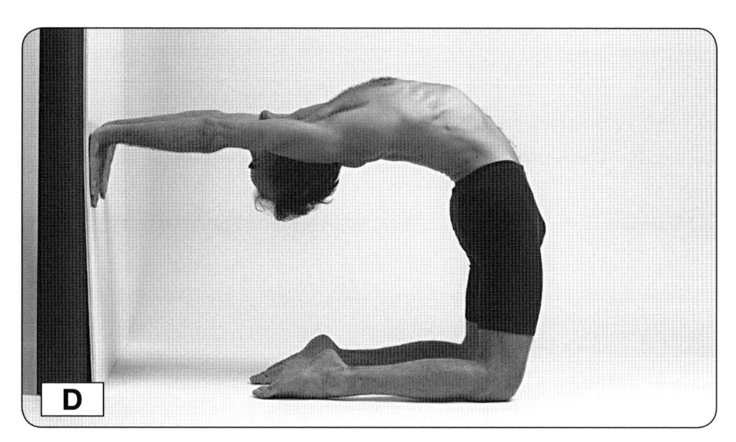

Supta Vajrasana

Supta = Lying Down or Sleeping   Vajra = Thunderbolt

"Lying Down Thunderbolt Posture"

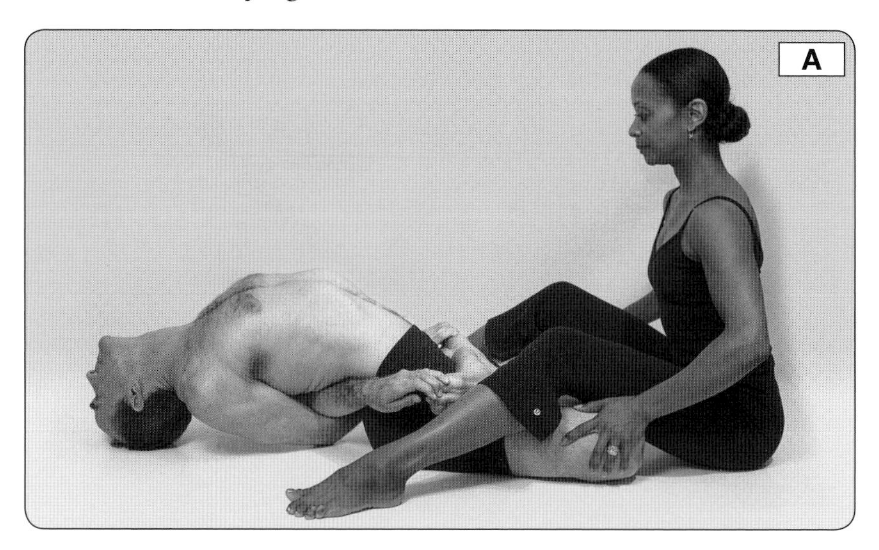

You will need an assistant to practice this asana fully, otherwise you may practice it partially

1) **Exhale** and place your legs in full-lotus or in "no-lotus" with the ankles crossed.

2) **Inhale** reach the arms behind the back. If sitting in lotus grab the feet. Clasp the foot that is on top first. Your assistant may sit in front of you with their legs on top of yours. If you are unable to clasp your feet then clasp hands with your assistant instead. If lotus is too much then sit with legs crossed. Another option is to keep the legs straight and have your assistant place their legs over yours.

3) **Exhale** lean back from one of the methods described above. Take your head to the floor while in full lotus, with an assistant to hold your knees down **(A)** or full lotus with an assistant holding your hands and supporting the knees **(B)**. Another option is crossed legs with an assistant **(C)** or with straight legs and an assistant **(D)**. Without an assistant, remain sitting and lift the chest without dropping back **(E)**.

Remain Here for 5 Deep Breaths

4) **Inhale** sit up. **Exhale** drop back. **Repeat this Up and Back motion 5 Times if you have assistance.**

5) **Exhale** take your head back to the floor again after the five repetitions of step 4.

Remain Here for 5 Deep Breaths

6) **Inhale** sit up.

7) **Exhale** release the asana and straighten your legs.

~VINYASA~

Enter the Next Asana from Downward Dog

Drishti ~ **Nose**

Supta Vajrasana

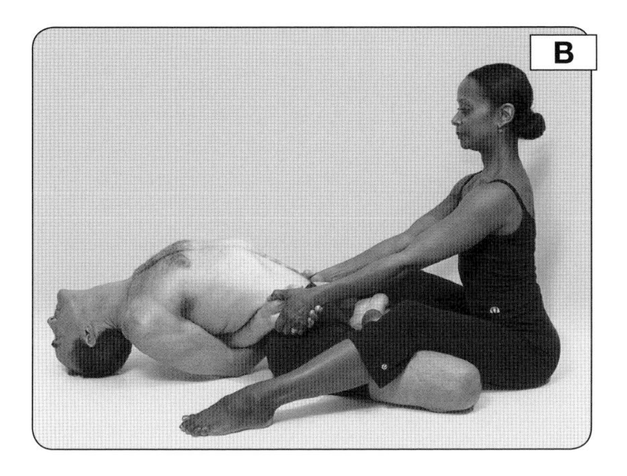

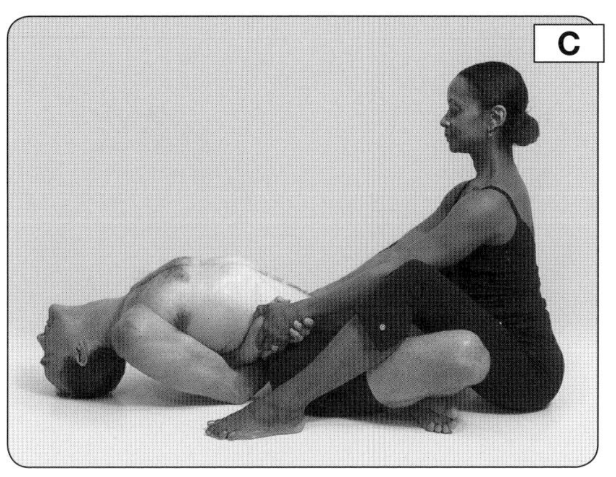

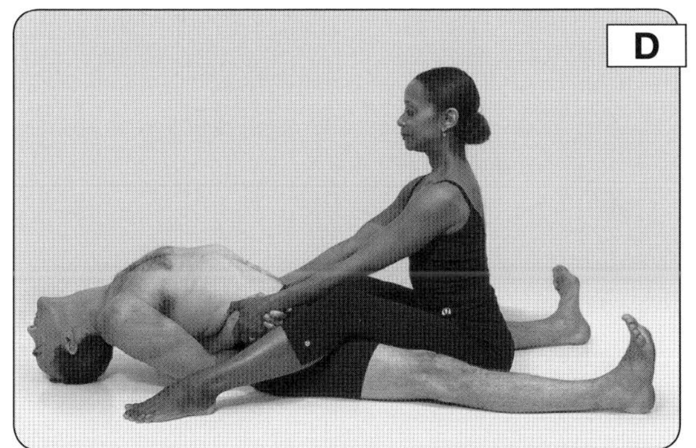

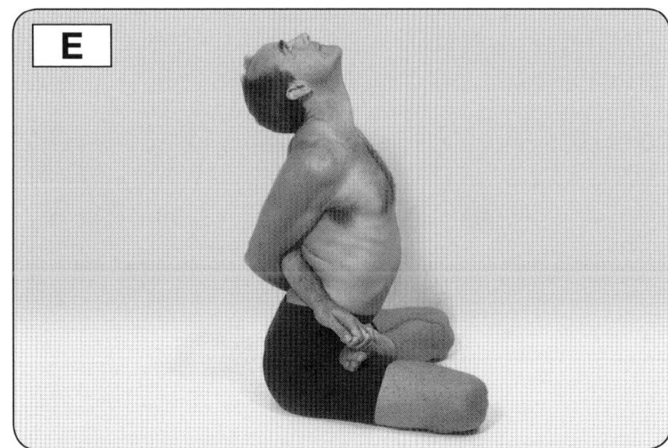

Comments - Communicate with your assistant so that they do not place too much pressure on your knees. The weight should be just enough to keep your legs from lifting. ***If you feel discomfort, back off or come out***. Keep the chest open. Lead with your sternum when coming up and not with your chin. Use the inhales to lift you and the exhales to lower. You may omit this asana for now and move on if it is too intense.

Bakasana A & B

Baka = Crane

"Crane Posture"

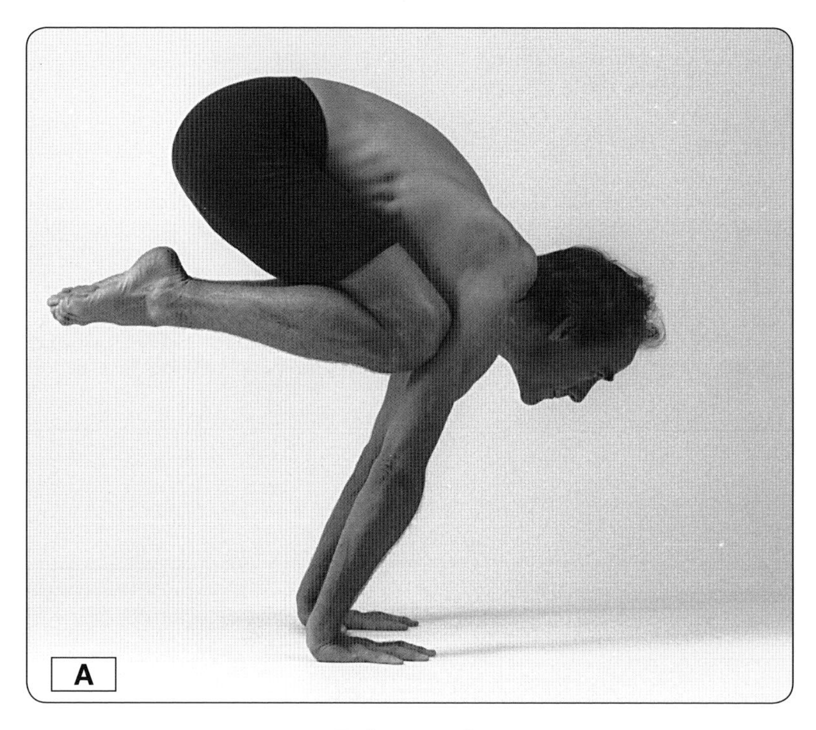

Bakasana A

1) **Inhale** from **Downward Dog** and bring the feet forward near the hands.

2) **Exhale** place the knees in the armpits **(A)** or put the knees on top of the elbows with bent arms **(B)**. Another option is to place the inner thighs on top of the elbows **(C)**.

3) **Inhale** from one of the options in **Step 2** and lift the feet away from the floor. If it is too much to lift the feet you may leave them on the floor as in **(D)**.

Remain Here for 5 Deep Breaths

~VINYASA~

Bakasana B

4) **Inhale** jump forward and land the legs in one of the Bakasana positions from options **(A)**, **(B)**, **(C)** or **(D)**.

Remain Here for 5 Deep Breaths

~VINYASA~

Drishti ~ **Nose**

Bakasana

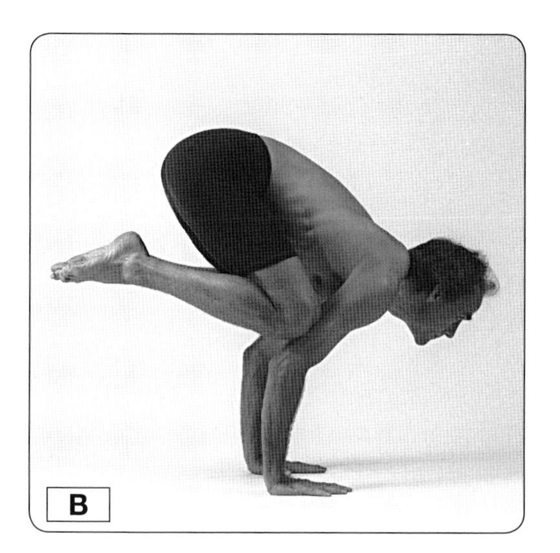

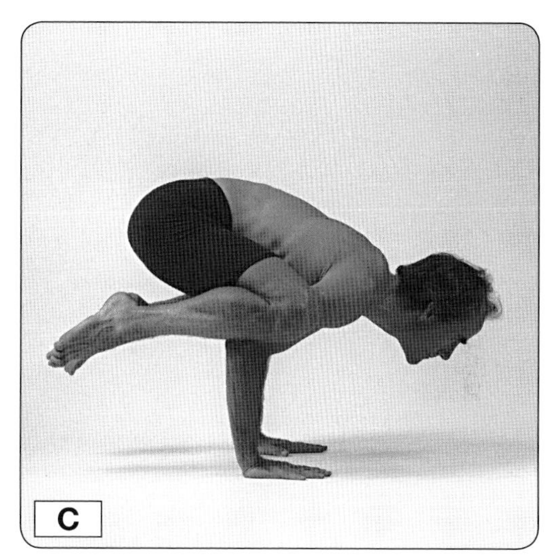

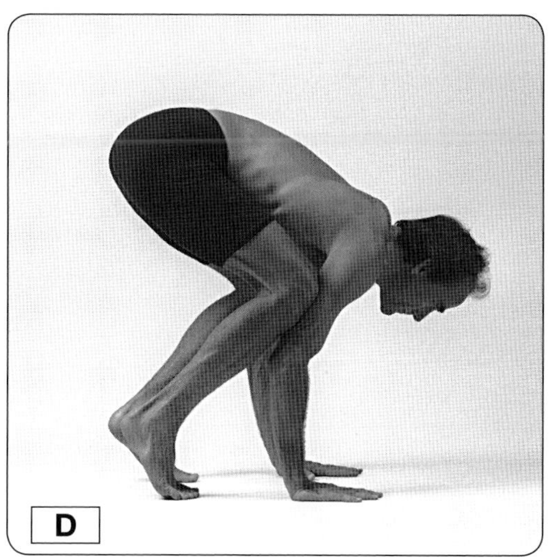

Comments - Bakasana is repeated twice. The first time is more supported than the second. It is initiated with the feet still on the ground. **Bakasana B** is meant to be jumped into from **Downward Dog**. This will require a great amount of control. The bandhas play a crucial role in creating the lightness required to land softly. Maintain a lifting action in the hips when the knees are resting on the arms, otherwise gravity will overpower and it will become increasingly difficult to maintain the asana. It is best to learn the second version under direct supervision. You may choose to eliminate **Bakasana B** for now and repeat **A** twice.

Bharadvajasana

Bharadvaja was a great warrior described in the Mahabharata

This Posture Is Dedicated To Bharadvaja

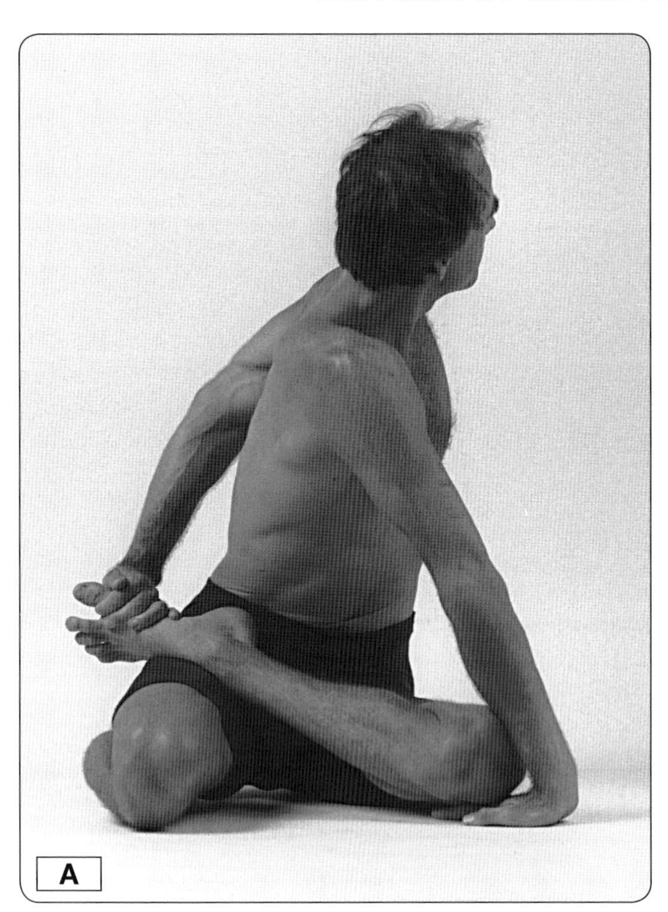
A

1) **Exhale** from a seated position and bend your right leg back so that the top of the foot is on the floor with the toes pointing back and the knees far apart. Place the left leg in half-lotus on top of the right. Reach around your back with your left hand and clasp the left foot. Place the right hand under the left knee so that the palm is pressing down with the fingers pointing back under the knee. Twist the upper body **(A)**. If you are unable to clasp the left foot you may use a strap to hold it and place the right hand on top of the left knee instead of under it as in **(B)**. If the first two options are too intense you may elevate your hips with a block and leave the left foot on the floor instead of in half-lotus **(C)**.

Remain Here for 5 Deep Breaths

2) **Inhale** gaze to the front.

3) **Exhale** release that side and straighten your legs.

~VINYASA~

Repeat Steps 1-3 on the Left Side

~VINYASA~

Drishti ~ **Over the Shoulder**

Bharadvajasana

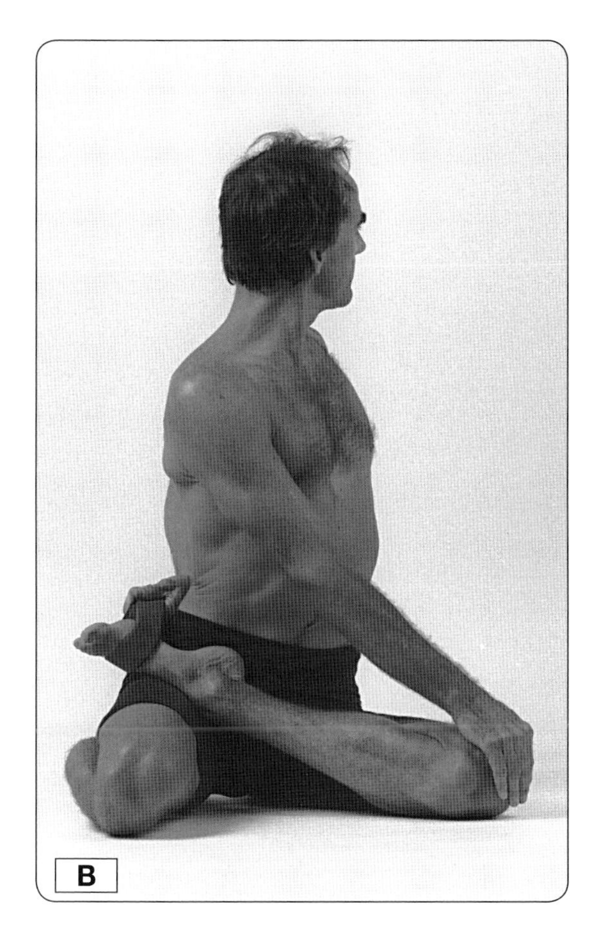

B

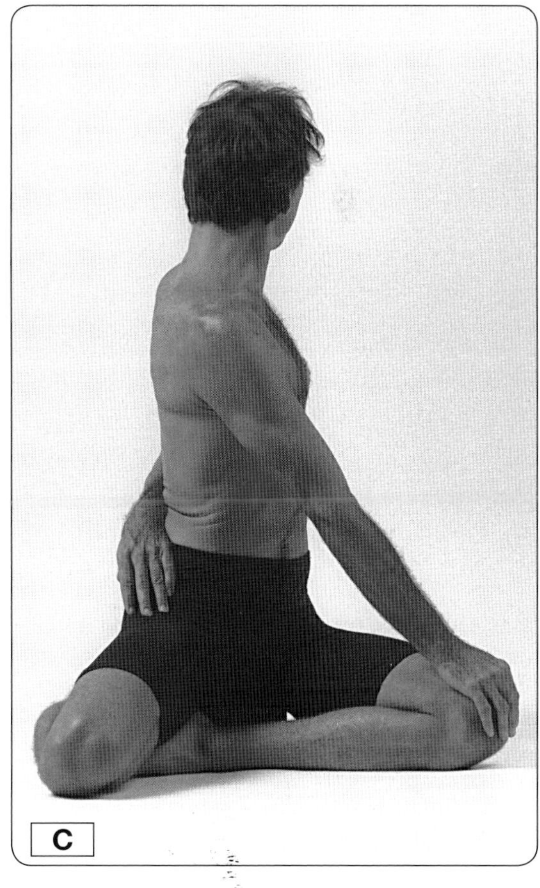

C

Comments - There are numerous asanas present within **Bharadvajasana**. There is a spinal twist, the half-lotus position of one leg and the drawing back of the other. The main emphasis is the twisting. This is meant to bring the spine back to a neutral point after the deep back bending. Create length by engaging opposing forces. Pull with the hand that is behind the back and also push away with the other. Sit up tall. Extend from the base of the spine through the top of your head. Work with the appropriate option and breathe.

Ardha Matsyendrasana

Ardha = Half   Matsyendra = Lord of the Fishes

"Half Lord of the Fishes Posture"

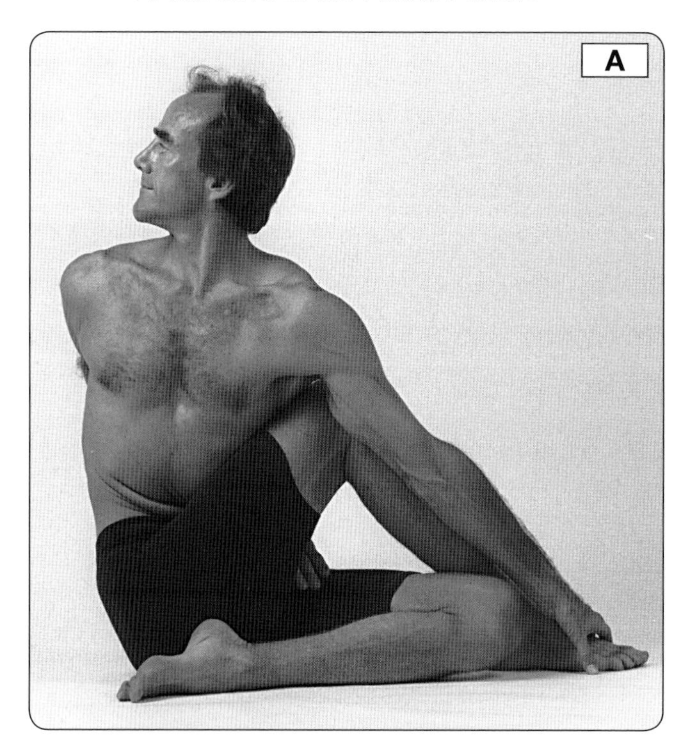

1) **Exhale** place the left foot near the right buttock. Bring the right foot outside the left knee. Take the left arm outside the right knee and run the arm down the outside of the right lower leg. Clasp the right foot with the left hand. Take the right arm behind the back. Grab the left thigh as you twist **(A)**. Instead of taking the left hand to the foot, you may keep the left elbow outside the right knee and place the right hand on the floor behind you **(B)** or if reaching the elbow outside of the knee is too much you may hold the right knee with two hands and lift the chest in a spiraling motion **(C)**. Another option is to keep the right foot on the inside of the left knee instead of taking it all of the way to the outside **(D)**.

Remain Here for 5 Deep Breaths

2) **Inhale** gaze to the front.

3) **Exhale** release that side and straighten your legs.

~VINYASA~

Repeat Steps 1-3 on the Left Side

~VINYASA~

Drishti ~ **Over the Shoulder**

Ardha Matsyendrasana

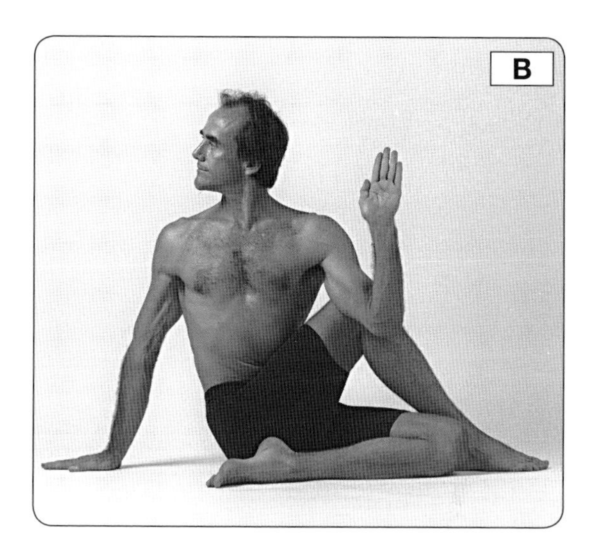

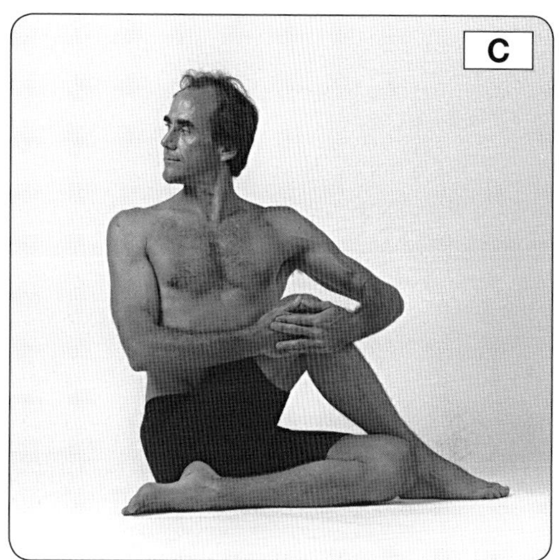

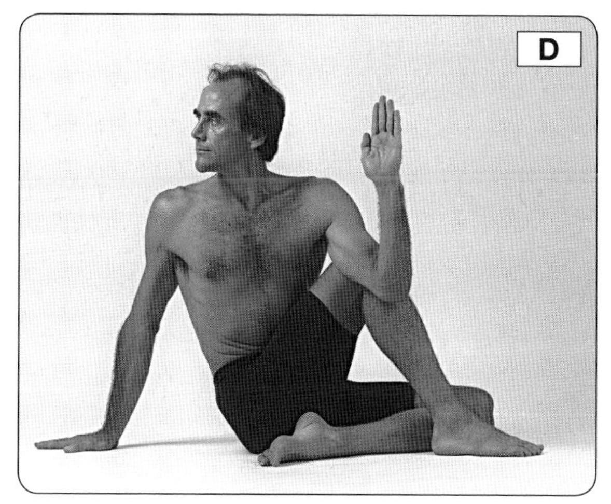

Comments - The same rules of opposition apply here as in **Bharadvajasana**. Use the outer elbow and the knee to push against each other to enhance depth in the asana. Keep the shoulders rolling down the back away from the ears. The upper body acts like a spiral. Use the arm that is behind to further open the chest and heart. Create space for the lungs by bringing the ribs outside of the upper leg. Depth in twisting asanas is achieved by creating length. Drop the sit-bones and draw energy up your spine to the top of your head.

Eka Pada Sirsasana A

Eka = One Pada = Foot or Leg Sirsa = Head

"One Foot To Head Posture"

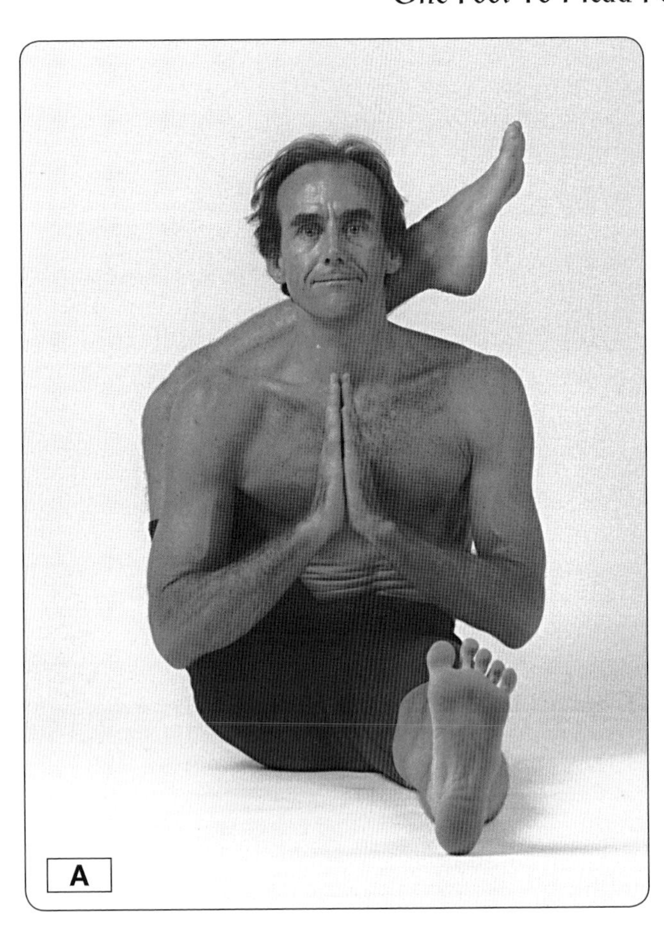
A

1) **Exhale** take the right leg behind the head by lifting the foot with both hands and rotating the hip as you bend the knee and take the foot across toward the back of the neck. Place the palms in a prayer fashion in front of the chest. Sit up straight and keep the left leg straight, toes pulled back **(A)**. If you are able to get the leg behind the head but it will not stay there when you release your hands you may place your chin in your palms for support to release pressure from the neck as in **(B)**. Taking the leg fully behind the head may be too extreme. Another option is to take the right leg behind the shoulder and then straighten it with the foot pointing toward the sky. Grab the right foot with the left hand and lift it. Keep the right shoulder pressing against the right leg for support as in **(C)** or you may take the right knee behind the shoulder and leave the leg bent **(D)**. A great preparation for **Eka Pada Sirsasana** is to stand with the back leg straight and the front leg bent at a ninety-degree angle. Then take the right arm under the right knee and clasp the ankle from the outside. Leave the left hand on the floor inside the right foot and take the head toward the ankle until you feel a nice stretch in the right hip. Hold that position **(E)** or sit up straight and take the right foot into the inner left elbow and the right knee into the right elbow **(F)**.

Remain Here for 5 Deep Breaths

Enter the Next Asana from Here Before Changing Sides

Drishti ~ **Nose**

Eka Pada Sirsasana A

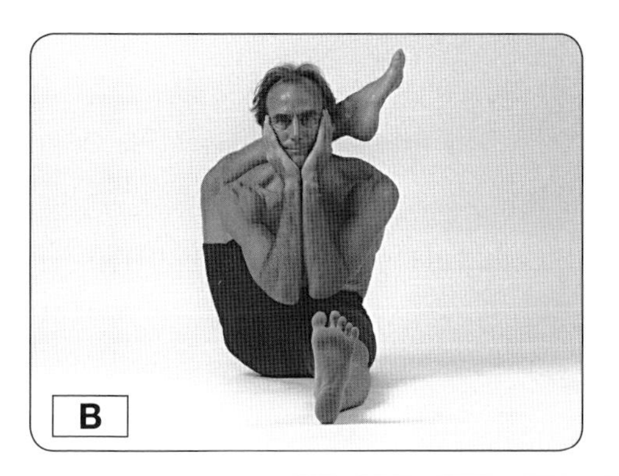

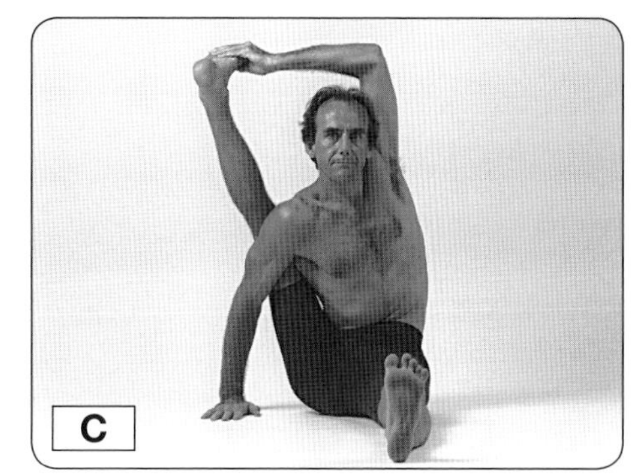

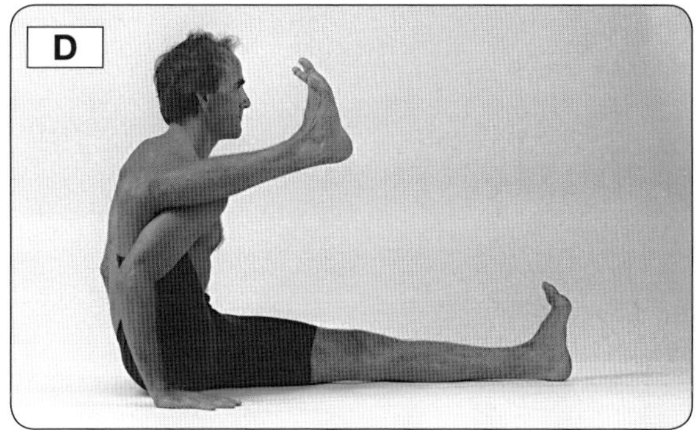

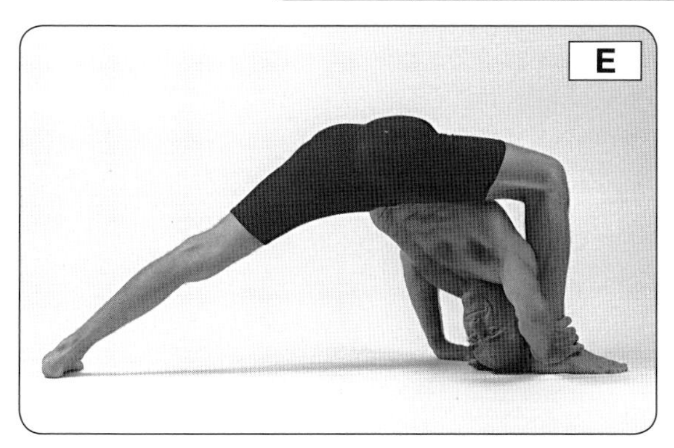

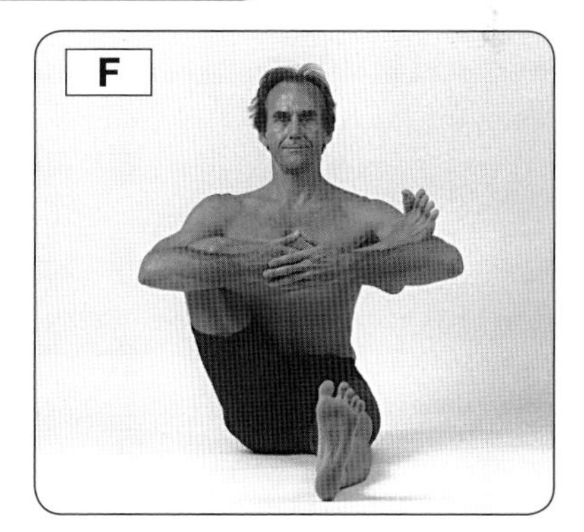

Comments - This asana is one of the greatest challenges in the Intermediate Series. Be patient and choose one of the options offered above and you will find a steady increase in flexibility in the hips and hamstrings. Opening must occur in these areas first so that the knee does not take too much of the stretch. Use the shoulder to assist in holding the leg in place. Avoid collapsing in the lower back by lifting the chest and heart.

Eka Pada Sirsasana B

Eka = One Pada = Foot or Leg Sirsa = Head

"One Foot To Head Posture"

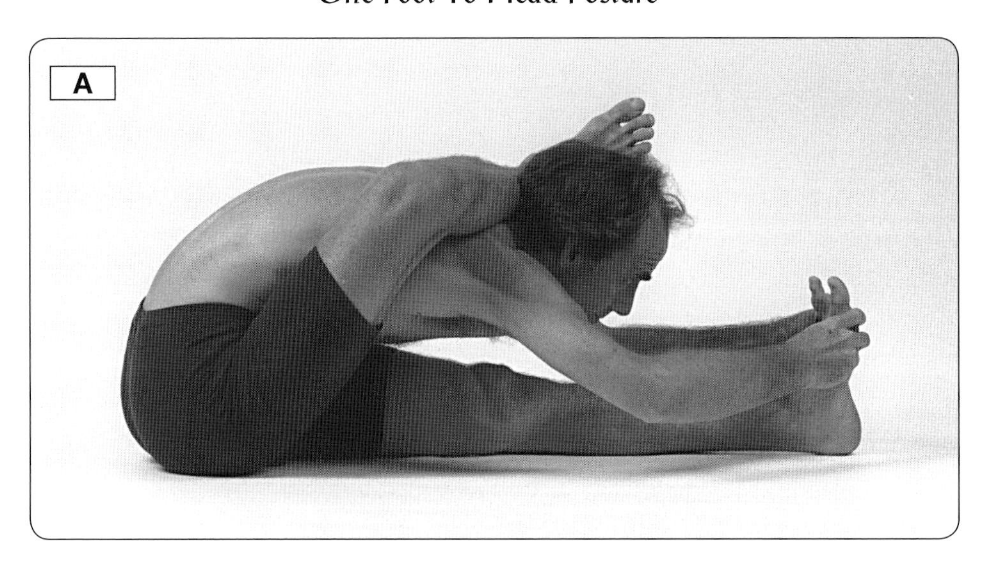

1) **Exhale** fold forward. Grab the left foot with both hands. Keep the right leg fully behind the head with the elbows lifted **(A)**. If it is too much to keep the leg behind the head you may leave it resting on the shoulder and lean forward. Take the hands to the floor with the elbows bent and keep the foot lifting as in **(B)** or leave the right knee behind the shoulder and when you lean forward take the right foot to the floor instead of keeping it in the air **(C)**. You may also approach it from **Option (F)** in **Eka Pada Sirsasana A** by holding the right leg across the chest and then lean forward as far as feels appropriate for you as in **(D)**.

2) **Inhale** lift the head while maintaining one of the options from above.

3) **Exhale** fold forward into **Eka Pada Sirsasana B**.

Remain Here for 5 Deep Breaths

Enter the Next Asana from Here Before Changing Sides

Drishti ~ **Nose**

Comments - The second and third versions of **Eka Pada Sirsasana** require a greater amount of control than the first. You may find it to be more effective to wait until you are comfortable with **Eka Pada Sirsasana A** before moving into B and C. If you find yourself straining, back off until you regain your composure, then continue. **If you omit Eka Pada Sirsasana B, take a vinyasa after A and repeat it on the left side**. The breath is your barometer. If your breathing becomes constricted or forced then you are trying too hard. Do not force your way into an asana. Take the slower more steady route of following your breath. Create depth over time. If you choose to approach **Eka Pada Sirsasana B**, maintain full control of your bandhas. Use the shoulders as a stabilizer rather than the lower back. Keep the left leg extended and engaged.

Eka Pada Sirsasana B

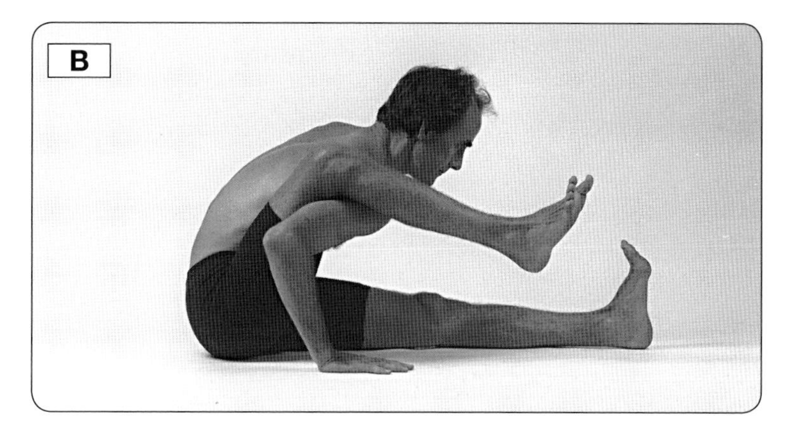

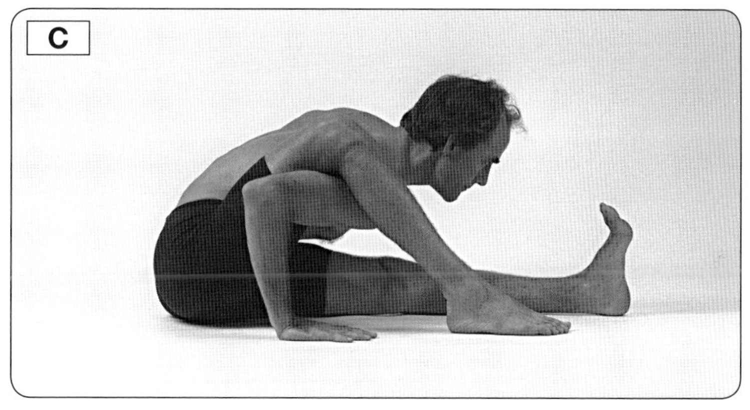

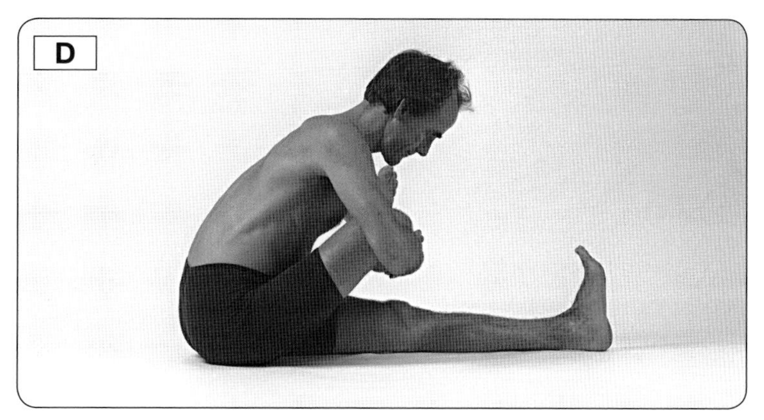

Eka Pada Sirsasana C

Eka = One Pada = Foot or Leg Sirsa = Head

"One Foot To Head Posture"

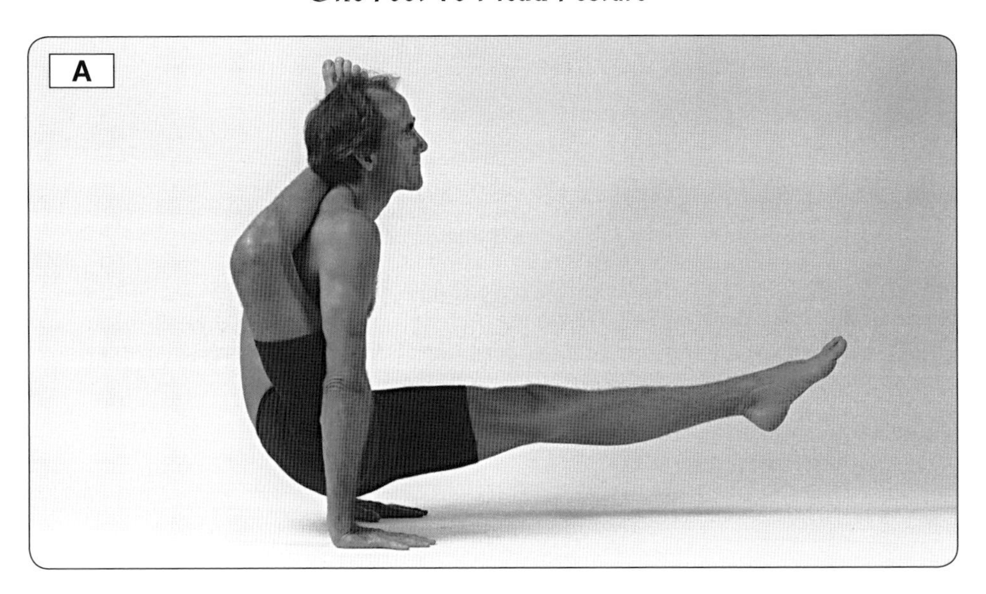

1) **Inhale** sit up.

2) **Exhale** place your hands on the floor.

3) **Inhale** lift your body away from the floor with the right leg behind the head and the left leg lifted parallel to the floor with the toes pointed **(A)**. Another option is to leave the right knee behind the shoulder with the leg bent and the left leg lifted parallel to the floor as in **(B)** or leave the right leg bent over the shoulder and raise only the hips leaving the left leg straight with the foot on the floor when you lift **(C)**.

Remain Here for 5 Deep Breaths

~VINYASA~

Repeat All Stages of Eka Pada Sirsasana A, B and C On the Left Side

~VINYASA~

Drishti ~ **Toes**

Eka Pada Sirsasana C

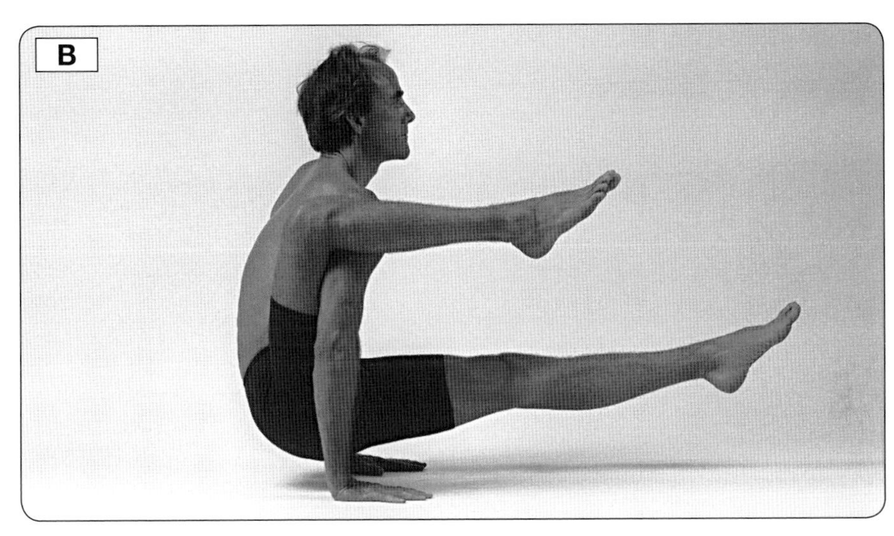

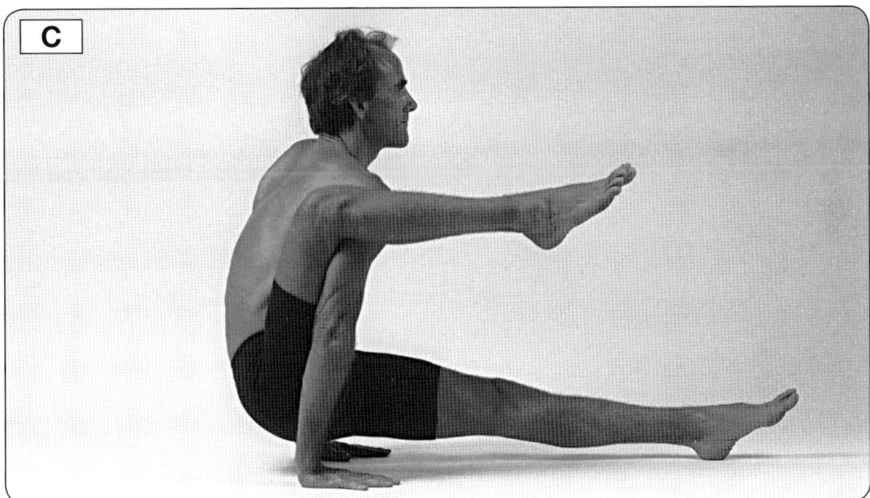

Comments - If you find **Eka Pada Sirsasana C** to be too intense, you may leave it out for now. **If you omit Eka Pada Sirsasana C, take a vinyasa and repeat A and B on the left side**. Keep your arms absolutely straight in the lifting phase of **Eka Pada Sirsasana C**. Straight arms will support much more weight with less effort than if you have your arms bent. The lifting comes from the bandhas and a contraction of the lower abdominal muscles rather than from upper body strength. It also helps to keep the extended leg fully engaged with the quadriceps muscles lifting above the knee. As you push your hands against the earth you may also lift the chest and open the heart. If you are lifting the extended leg away from the floor, keep it parallel to the earth, not pointed up. Pointing it up is an asana from Advanced A.

Dwi Pada Sirsasana A

Dwi = Two Pada = Foot or Leg Sirsa = Head

"Two Feet To Head Posture"

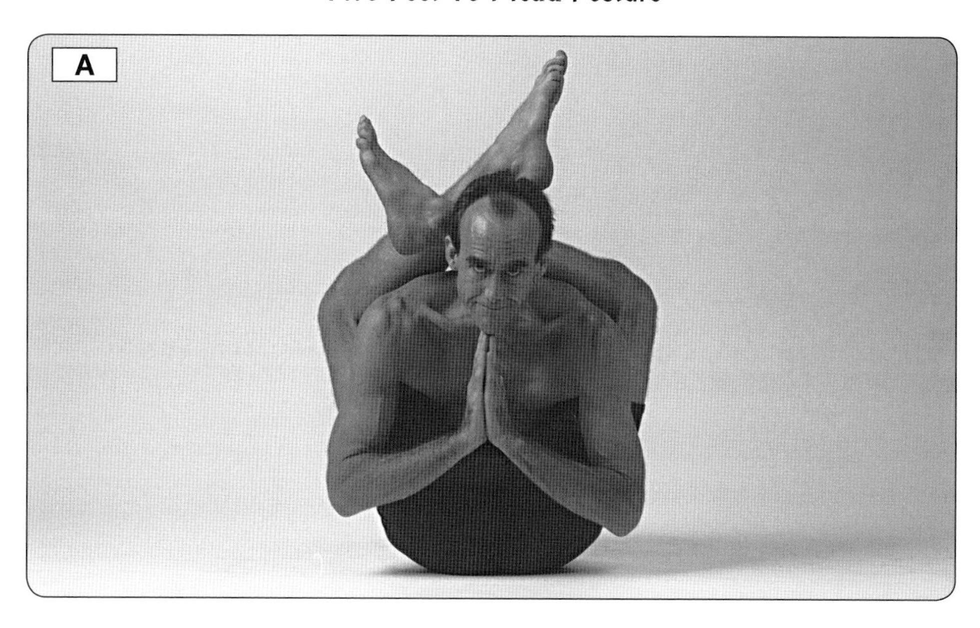

1) **Exhale** take both legs behind the head by first taking one back and then hooking the second one behind the ankle of the first. Place the palms in prayer fashion and balance in that position as seen in **(A)**. If it is too much to take the legs behind the head then you may leave them behind the elbows with the ankles crossed in front of the chest with the palms in prayer fashion behind the feet **(B)** or keep the knees behind the elbows but instead of crossing the ankles you may leave the feet hovering in the air while the hands are praying as in **(C)**.

Remain Here for 5 Deep Breaths

Enter the Next Asana from Here

Drishti ~ **Nose**

Comments - Dwi Pada Sirsasana doubles the challenge which was experienced in **Eka Pada Sirsasana A, B** and **C**. One of the difficulties in this asana is to keep the heart area open when both legs are brought toward the head. There is a tendency to round the shoulders in order to make room for the legs. A little of that action is alright but too much rounding and the clavicle bones become compressed and the torso loses its capacity to house a full **inhale**. If you find your breath becoming constricted or the chest collapsing, come out of the asana and either re-approach it with less intensity or leave it out for now. The elbows and shoulders play an important role in keeping the chest open. By pressing the shoulders back you may lift the chest and spine. Another point of challenge here is the balance. Once you have the legs up it is necessary to balance precariously on your sit bones. Use the lifting of the chest and the opposing forces between the shoulders and legs to find your still point of least resistance.

Dwi Pada Sirsasana A

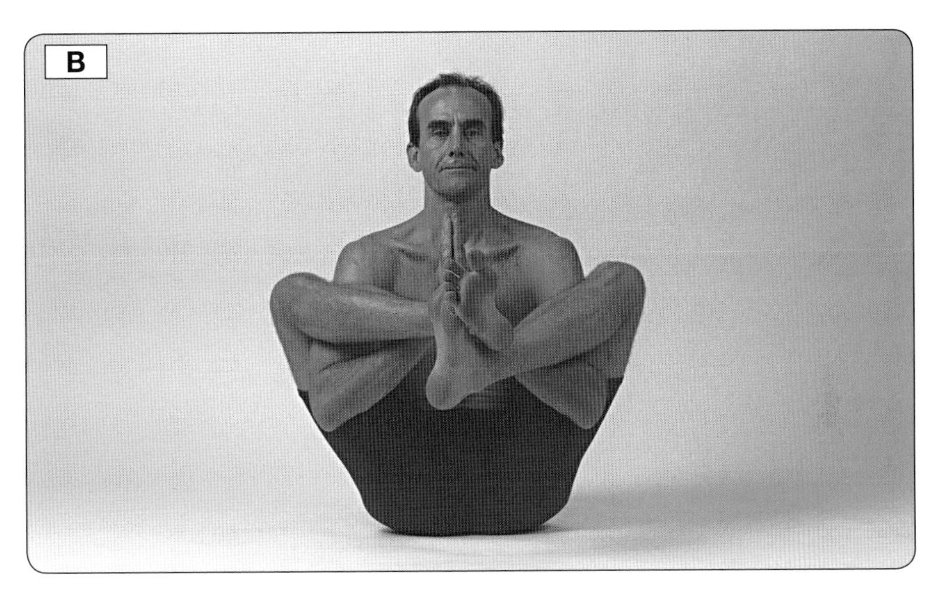

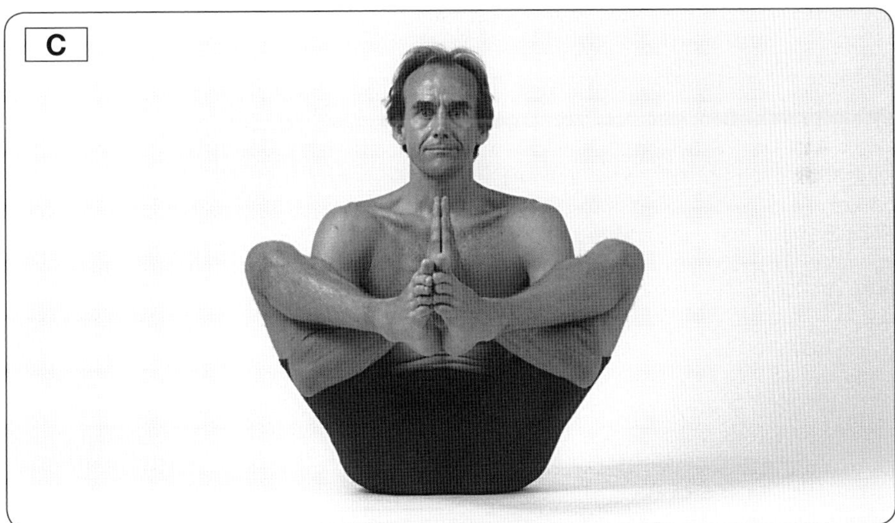

Dwi Pada Sirsasana B

Dwi = Two Pada = Foot or Leg Sirsa = Head

"Two Feet To Head Posture"

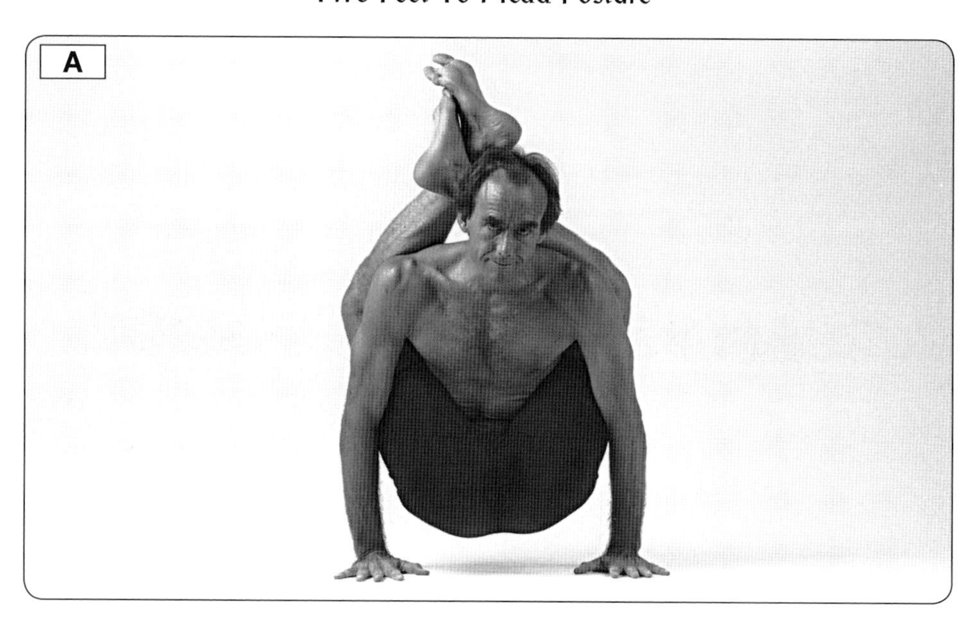

1) **Inhale** place your hands on the floor and lift the body up while keeping both legs behind the head **(A)**. If it is too much to take the legs behind the head then you may take the knees behind the shoulders and and straighten the legs as much as possible so that the toes point up to the sky with the hips dropping toward the floor **(B)**. A third choice is to bend the legs over the upper arms with the elbows bent. Keep the lower leg parallel to the floor and the hips dropped **(C)**.

Remain Here for 5 Deep Breaths

~VINYASA~

Drishti ~ **Nose**

Comments - Use the opposition of forces to aid in your "lift-off". Pressing the hands down is the first stage of creating lift. That downward action must then be countered by the upward movement of the mid-section coupled with engagement of the bandhas. The arms are the foundation from which a stable flight may grow. Just as in **Eka Pada Sirsasana C** the dynamic action between the shoulders and legs are an additional point of opposition which may be utilized to your benefit. Press the shoulders back to create a greater opening in the chest and it will also assist the lift. Eventually the Vinyasa out of **Dwi Pada Sirsasana B** is initiated directly from the lifted position. First the feet are released and the legs straightened, parallel to the floor **(D)**. Next, the feet curl back as in **(E)** to give the momentum to shoot the legs behind. This method of jumping out is quite difficult and is more easily learned under direct supervision so you may choose to sit down on the floor and then untie your legs and take your favorite method of Vinyasa to move into the next asana.

Dwi Pada Sirsasana B

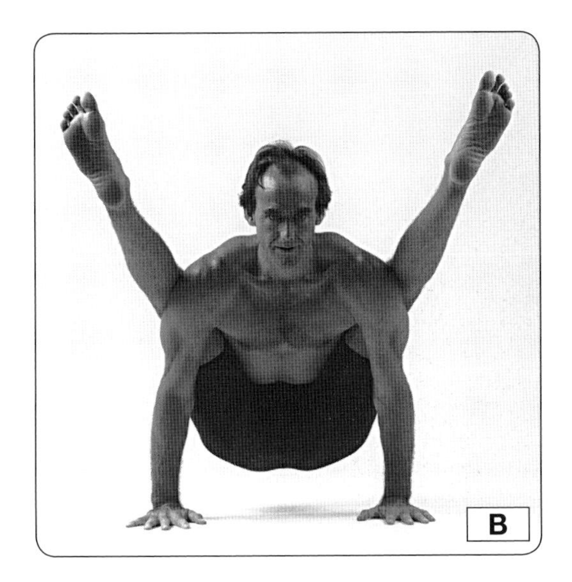

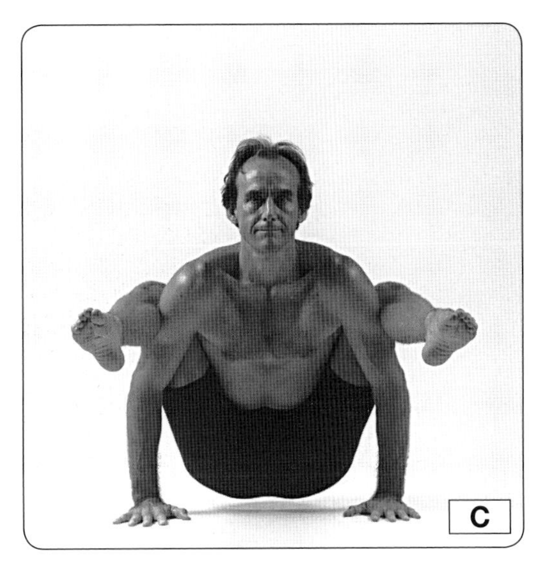

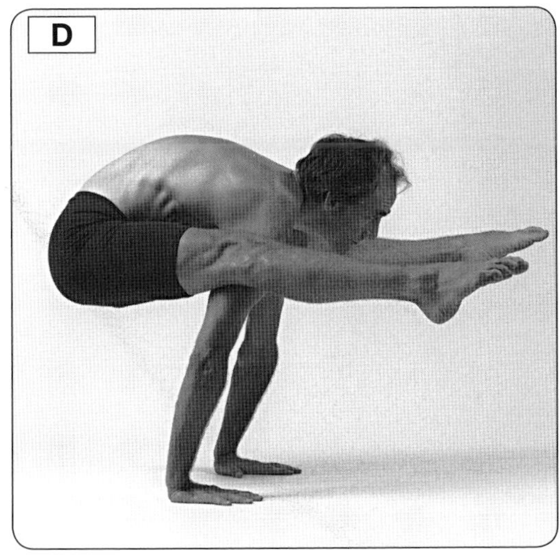

Transition. Do Not Hold.

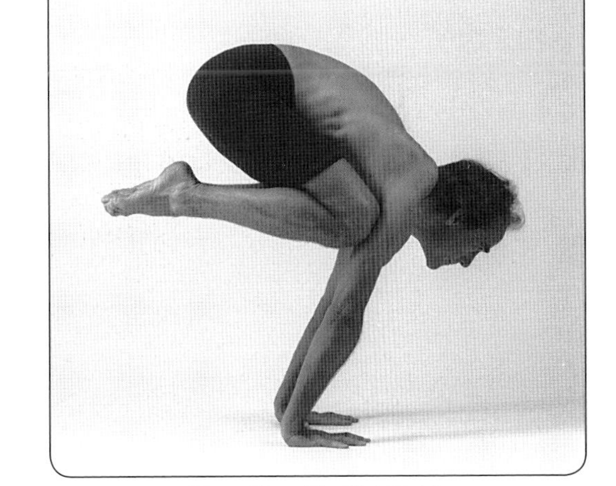

Transition. Do Not Hold.

Yoganidrasana

Nidra = Sleep

"Yogi's Sleep Posture"

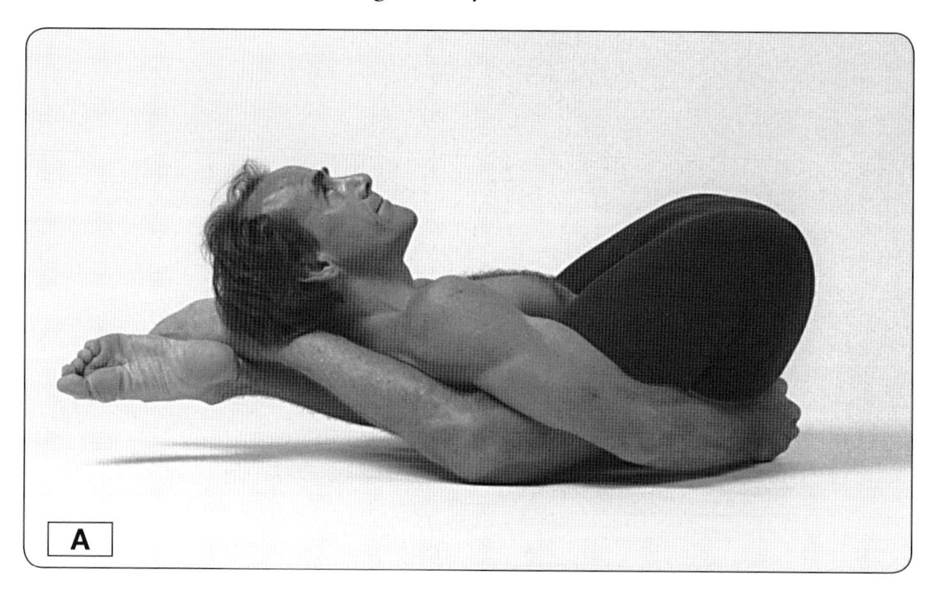

A

1) **Exhale** lie down on your back.
2) **Inhale** lift your feet and bend your knees in preparation to enter the asana.
3) **Exhale** take both legs behind the head and rest the head against them. Extend the arms over the thighs and clasp the hands behind the back **(A)**. If it is too extreme to take the legs behind the head you may bend the knees and take the arms over the thighs and clasp the hands behind the back. Leave the feet in the air without crossing them and let the head rest on the floor **(B)**. Another option is to bend the knees with the feet pointing up toward the sky. Grab the feet with both hands and pull them down in order to draw the knees closer to the floor **(C)**.

Remain Here for 5 Deep Breaths

~CHAKRASANA~

Remember your options from pages 120-121 or apply your favorite jumping Vinyasa

Drishti ~ **Third Eye**

Comments - This asana is called "Yogi's Sleep" due to its reclining appearance. K. Pattabhi Jois is fond of saying: "Where is your pillow?", when he is assisting a student in this asana. The "pillow" is the leg closest to the neck. It should act as a support upon which the head may rest as the hands clasp behind the back. Use these points to create opposing forces in the posture's full expression. For the variations offered you may still use equality of opposition by using the arms against the thighs or the hands against the feet. In all of the options you should work toward pulling the shoulders through the legs in order to open the chest. Keep the face relaxed as though you are dreaming.

Yoganidrasana

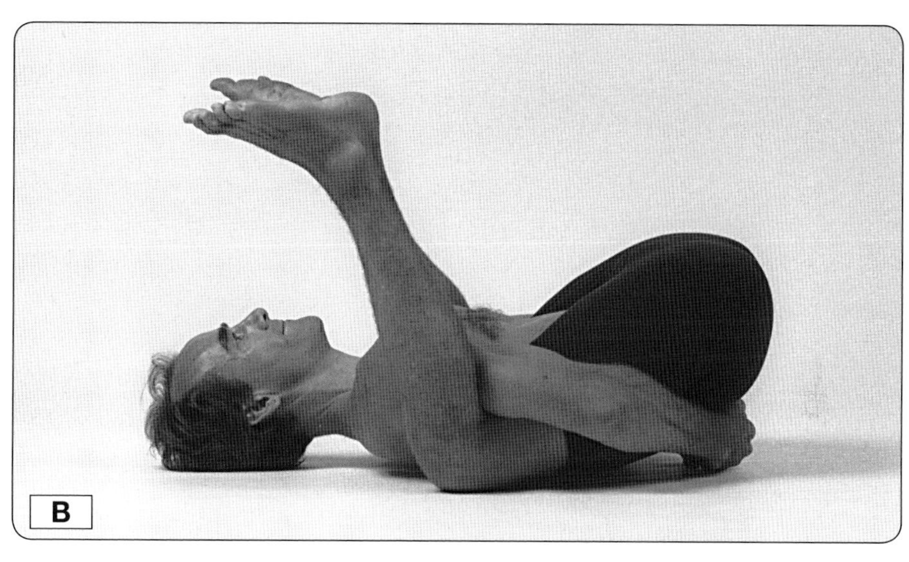

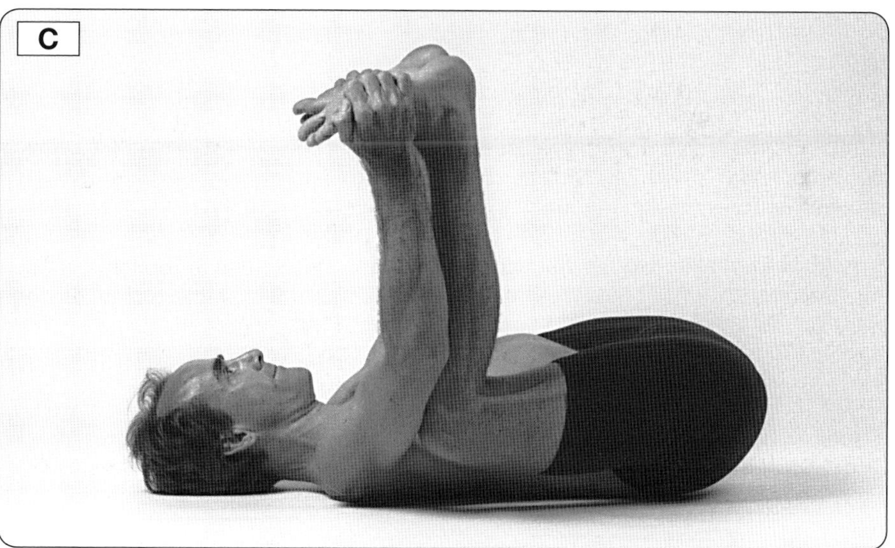

Tittibhasana A

Tittibha = Insect

"Insect Posture"

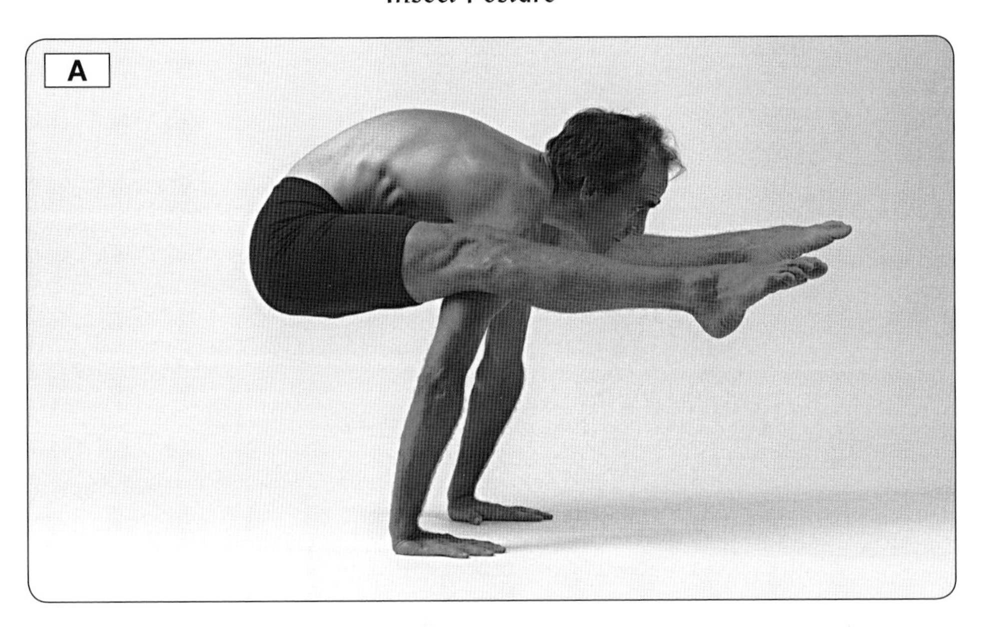

1) **Inhale** jump your legs onto the arms from **Downward Dog**. Keep the legs straight and the toes pointed with the hips lifting and the arms straight **(A)**. This method of entry requires a great amount of control. It should be learned under direct supervision of a qualified instructor. A safe approach to gain the necessary control is to jump the feet outside of the hands before entry as seen in **(B)**. From this position drop the hips and bend the elbows until the back of the thighs are able to rest on them. Next, wriggle the feet forward and lift them away from the floor. Straighten the legs with the toes pointed and the arms straight **(A)**. If it is not possible to keep the arms straight you may bend them slightly and rest the back of the thighs on the elbows as in **(C)**. If it is too much to straighten the legs, leave them bent as in **(D)**.

Remain Here for 5 Deep Breaths

Enter the Next Asana from Here

Drishti ~ **Nose**

Tittibhasana A

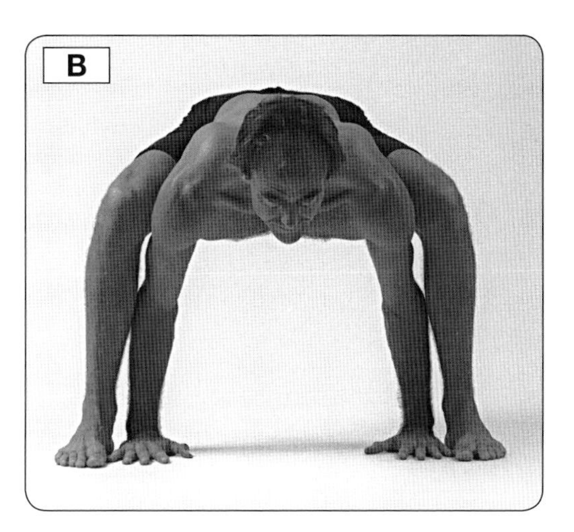

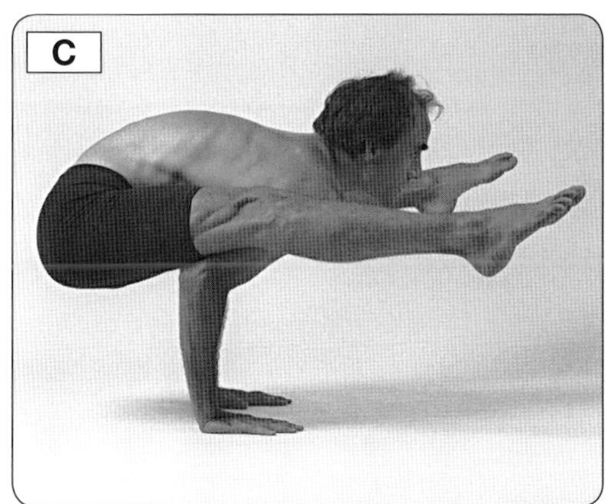

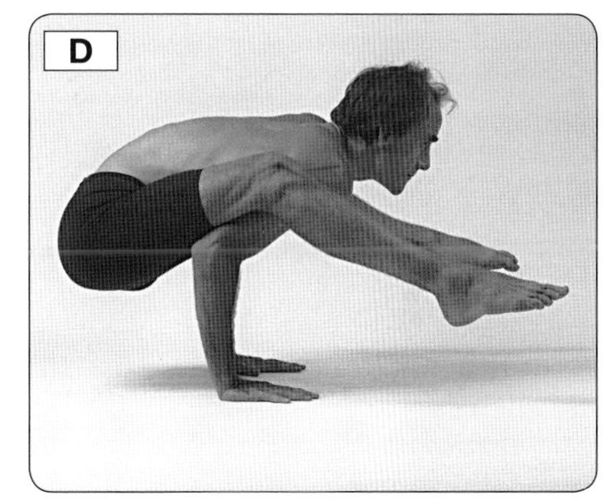

Comments - The official method of entry here is to jump directly into the asana from **Downward Dog**. It is best to practice it by walking or jumping the feet onto the floor outside the hands first to develop control. Once you have the legs on top of the arms, whether jumping them or walking and slowly wrapping them, the next phase is the same. The quadriceps must engage fully in order to lift the feet away from the floor. At the same time the hips need to rise at an equal rate to create the desired opposition of force. The arms are the fulcrum for this asana. If you create an equality of weight distribution between the rising of the feet and hips you will find the least amount of energy required from the arms to maintain the asana.

Tittibhasana B

Tittibha = Insect

"Insect Posture"

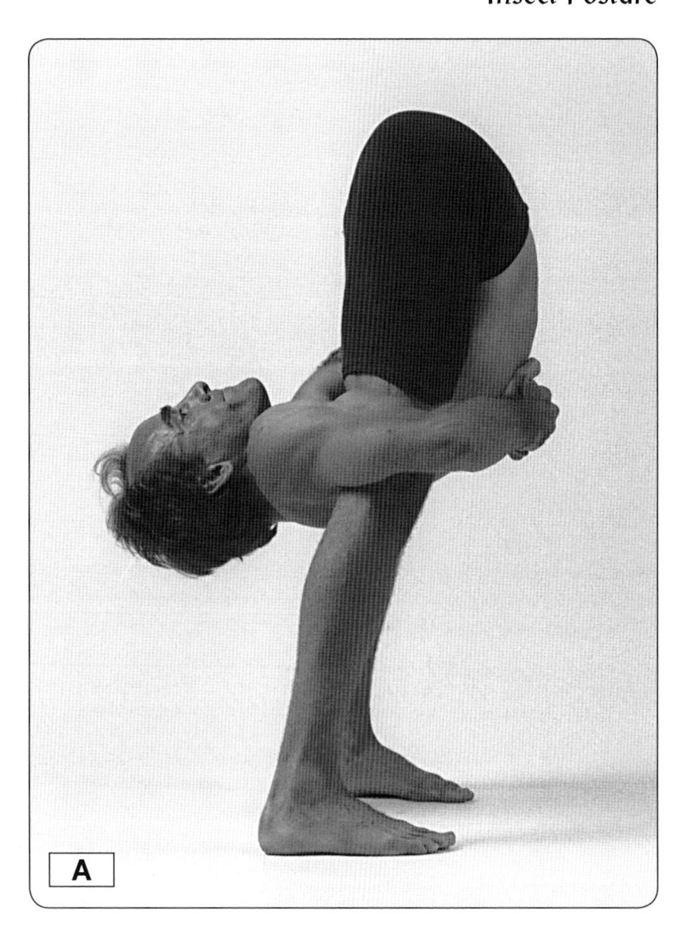

1) **Exhale** from **Tittibhasana A** position and lower the feet to the floor outside the hands.

2) **Inhale** reach the arms through the legs and around the thighs. Clasp the hands behind the back and straighten the legs **(A)**. If you are able to clasp the hands but it is too much to straighten the legs then keep them slightly bent as in **(B)**. If your hands do not reach then you may use a strap to connect them as in **(C)** or instead of taking both arms through the legs at the same time you may take one arm through while the other reaches behind the back without wrapping around the other leg. You would then hold this position for five breaths on each side as seen in **(D)**. Another option is to grab the ankles with both hands and pull the chest through while keeping the legs bent instead of taking the hands behind the back **(E)**.

Remain Here for 5 Deep Breaths

Enter the Next Asana from Here

Drishti ~ **Nose**

Comments - The full expression of this asana, as shown in option **A,** requires a great amount of flexibility in the hamstrings. It is best to take it slowly and work with the alternative options so as not to over-stretch the back of the legs. The quadriceps must engage fully in order to maintain stability and to assist in bringing the chest through the legs. At the same time that the legs are working the shoulders should press back against them to create a balance of opposition. If you feel discomfort in the lower back or too much stretch in the hamstrings then bend the legs a bit. This will induce a slackening of the hamstrings which will reduce the intensity. Find a point of even distribution of weight across the bottom of the feet. Listen to your breath.

Tittibhasana B

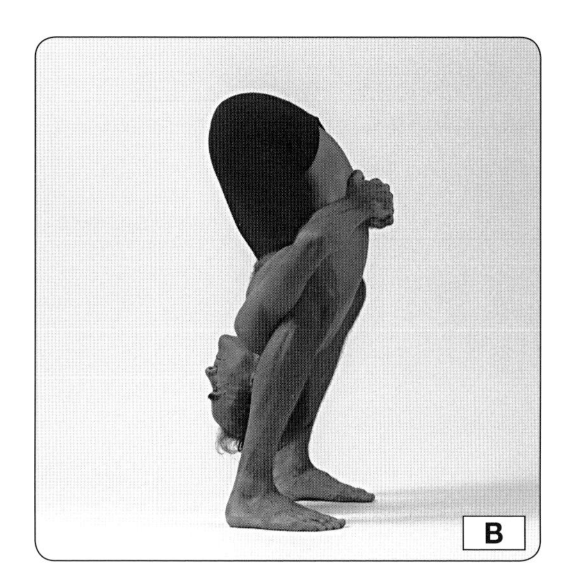

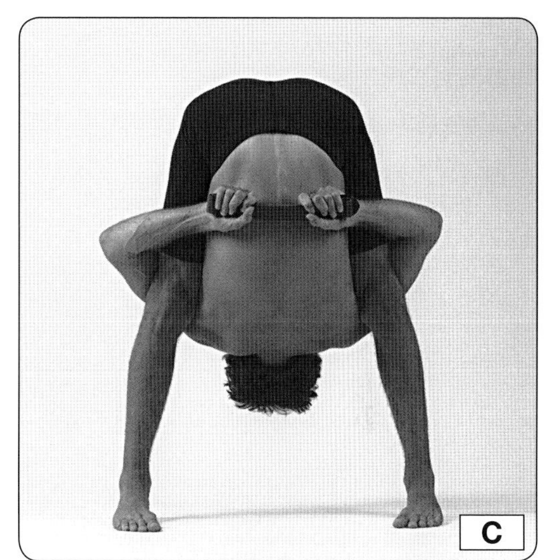

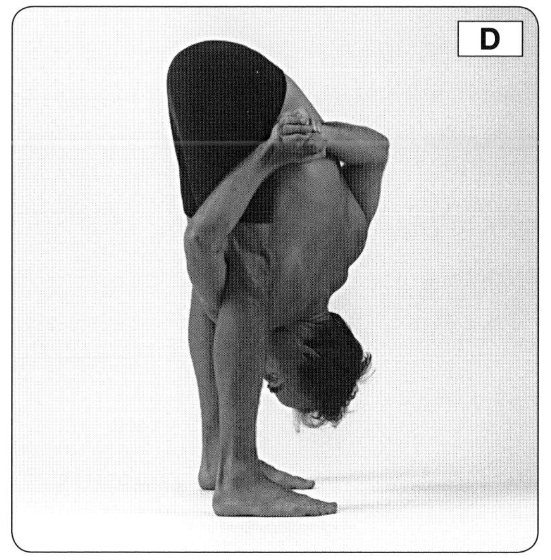

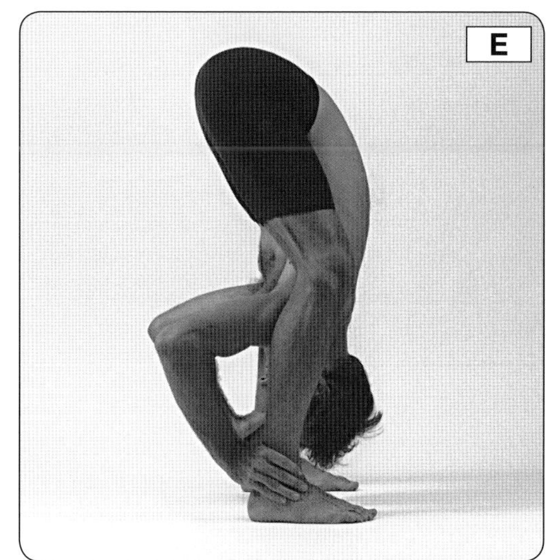

Tittibhasana C

Tittibha = Insect

"Insect Posture"

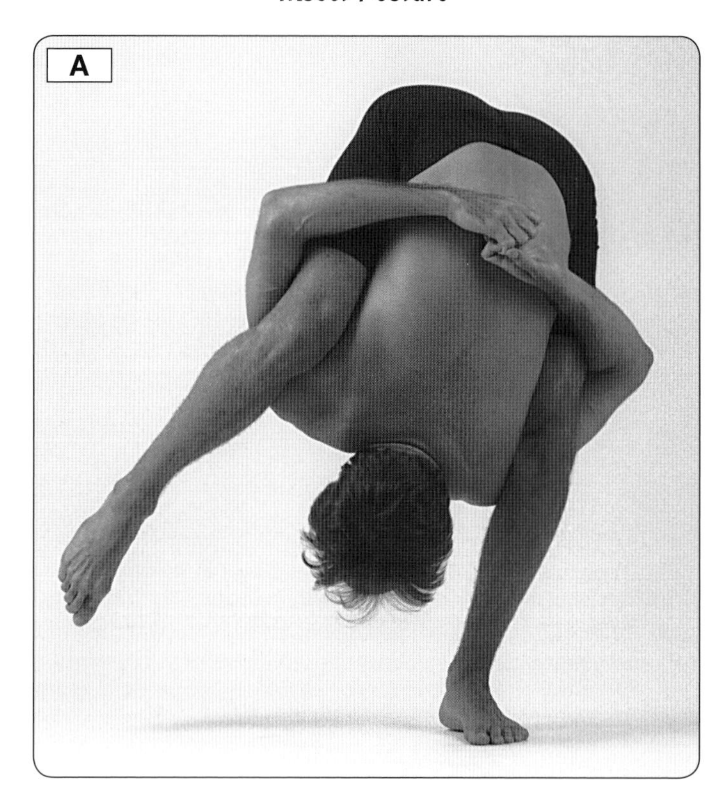
A

1) **Inhale** lift the right foot and take a step forward while keeping both hands clasped behind the back.

2) **Exhale** as you lower the right foot.

3) **Inhale** lift the left foot. Take another step forward while keeping the hands clasped.

4) **Exhale** as you lower the left foot . . . .

Continue walking forward in this fashion for five complete steps.
Then repeat the process in reverse so that you end in the same place that you started

Eventually as you raise and lower the feet the hands should remain fully clasped behind the back as seen in **(A)**. If you were using a strap in Tittibhasana B then maintain your grip on it as you walk forward and back **(B)**. If you were holding your ankles you may continue on your stroll from that position as seen in **(C)**.

Enter the Next Asana from Here

Drishti ~ **Nose**

Tittibhasana C

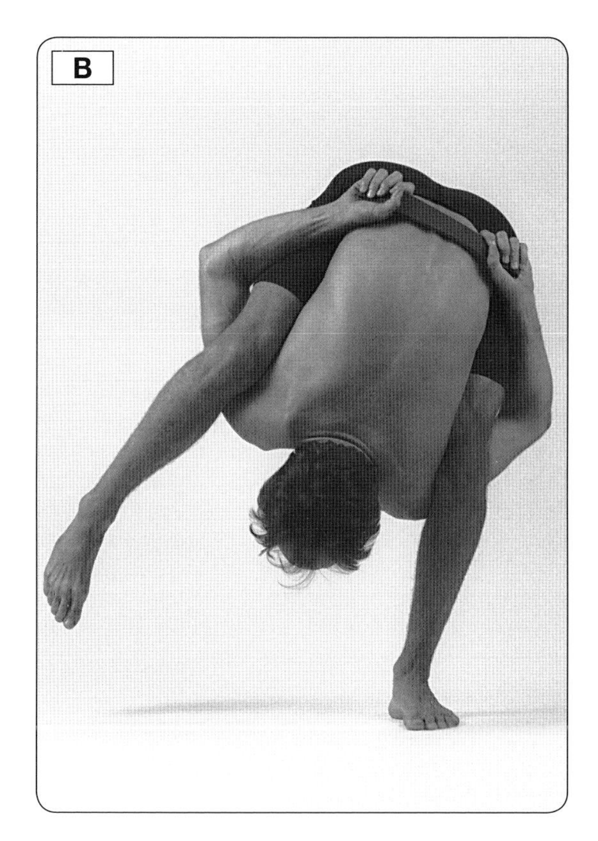

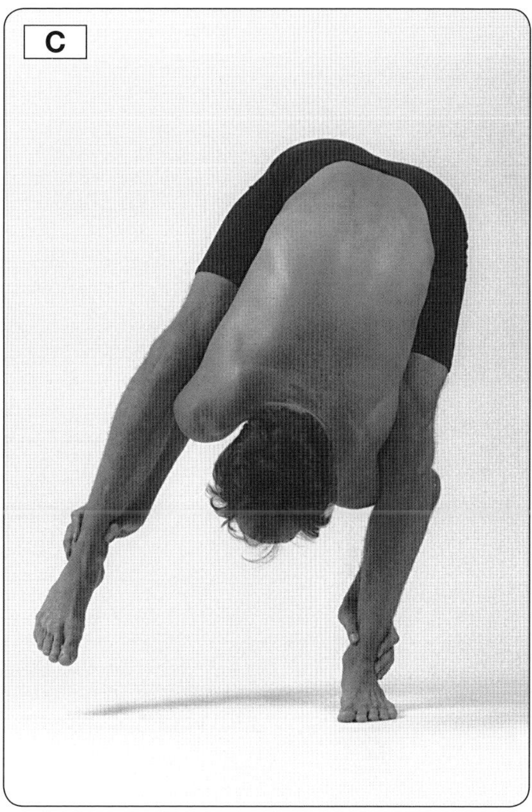

Comments - This asana is unique in that the actual holding of it is in motion. One of the keys to walking is to utilize the breath to initiate each movement. The inhales lift the foot and the exhales lower the foot. Give a little rotation in the body each time that you raise a foot to create the forward or backward progression. In the beginning do not attempt to lift the foot too high. Just take it high enough to bring it forward or back. If this asana is too intense or strange, you may always omit it for now and work toward it over time. It is quite a fun and silly asana. It will develop balance, control and confidence once you get the hang of it. The prescribed Drishti is the nose. You may find it best to look between the feet at first.

Tittibhasana D

Tittibha = Insect

"Insect Posture"

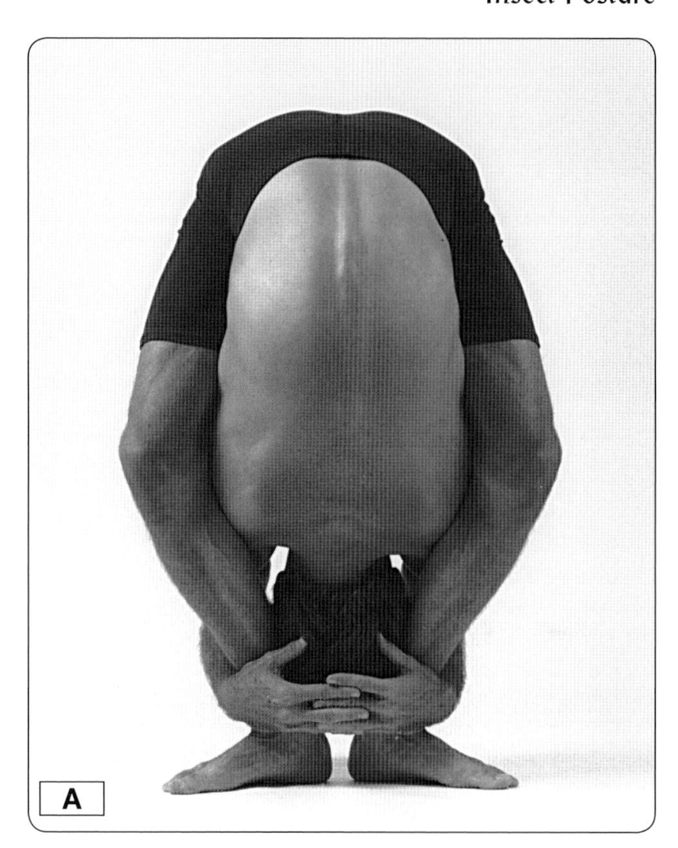

1) **Inhale** release the hands from behind the back. Bend the knees. Bring the heels toward each other with the toes pointing out.

2) **Exhale** grab the ankles. Pull the shoulders through the legs and tuck the chin into the chest. Release the ankles. Take the hands around the outside of the ankles. Interlace the fingers behind the back of the head as in **(A)**. If it is too much to keep the heels together or to clasp the hands together behind the head you may separate the heels to an appropriate distance and use the wrists to assist in pulling the shoulders through while gradually moving the fingers toward each other **(B)** or take the arms through the legs and grab the ankles **(C)**.

Remain Here for 5 Deep Breaths

3) **Inhale** lift the head and look forward.

4) **Exhale** hands to the floor. Lower the hips and bend the elbows.

5) **Inhale** lift the feet into Tittibhasana A, as seen in **(D)**. Bend the knees as you curl the feet back into Bakasana **(E)**.

6) **Exhale** jump back.

If Steps 5 & 6 are too much then take your Vinyasa after Step 4

~VINYASA~

Enter the next asana from Downward Dog

Drishti ~ **Nose**

Tittibhasana D

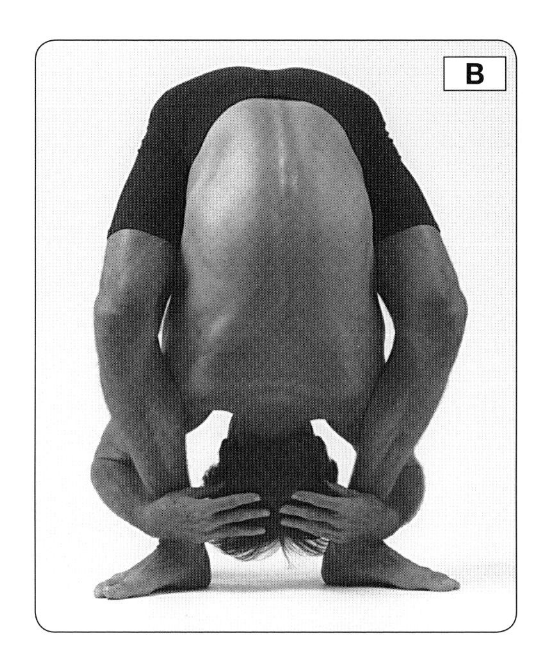

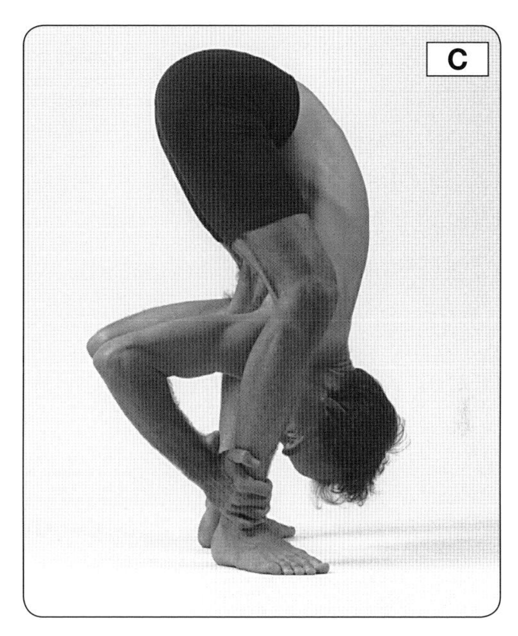

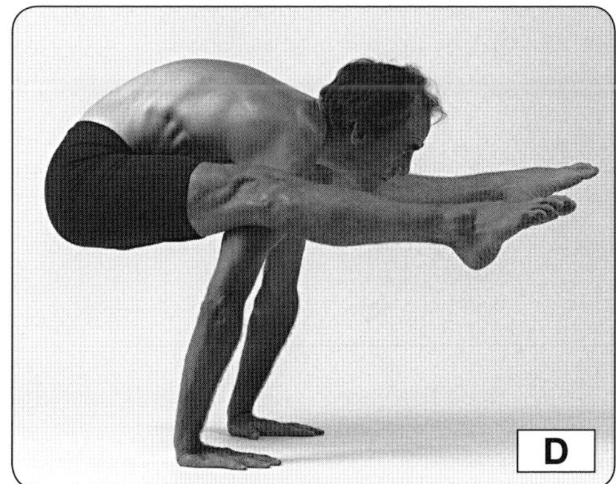

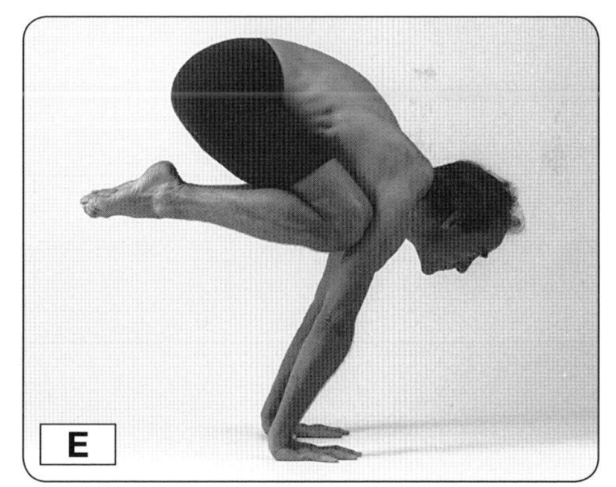

Comments - The feet need to be turned so that they point out at a forty-five degree angle like Charlie Chaplin. When the knees are bent they also should point out in the direction of the toes. This will protect the knees and it will also create space between the legs for your shoulders to fit. Feel the weight distribution on the feet. It should be distributed evenly so that you are not leaning too far forward or back. Once the legs are in place then the arms may assist in bringing the upper body through. You will find that the quadriceps are engaged immensely in this asana. Breathe deeply. If you find the breath constricted then back off until it is flowing smoothly again. Do not hold steps 5 & 6. They are transition stages of the Vinyasa.

Pincha Mayurasana

Pincha = Feather   Mayura = Peacock

"Feather of the Peacock Posture"

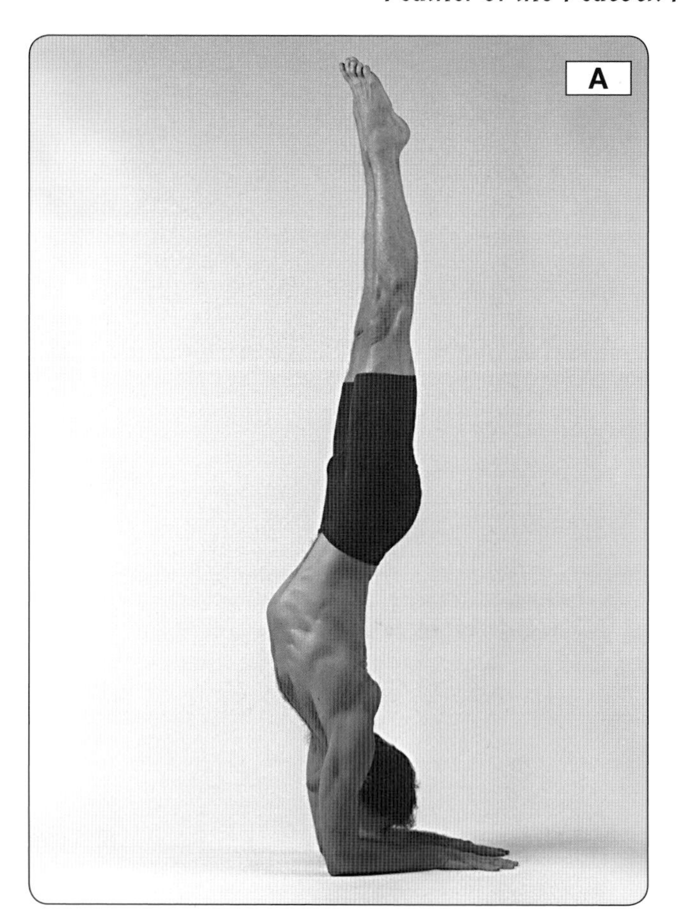

1) **Inhale** forward into a kneeling position.

2) **Exhale** forearms on the floor, palms down.

3) **Inhale** jump up with both feet. Straighten the legs, keeping the feet together with the toes pointed as in **(A)**. If it is too difficult to balance in the middle of the room you may place your mat near a wall. **Be sure that there are no pictures, nails or other obstructions on the wall above you**. Position your forearms on the floor as described in **#2** with the fingertips about one foot away from the wall. Kick the feet up one at a time and bring them together. Use control so that you do not crash into the wall with too much force. Find your balance and hold that position **(B)** or place a chair on top of your mat with the back legs of it touching the wall so that it will not slip. Position yourself so that you are facing away from the chair after putting your forearms on the floor. Place your feet on the seat of the chair and straighten your legs **(C)**. A method to build strength and confidence before moving on to the more challenging approaches is to leave the feet on the floor and lift only the hips **(D)**.

Remain Here for 5 Deep Breaths

4) **Exhale** return the feet to the floor.

~VINYASA~

Enter the next asana from Downward Dog

Drishti ~ **Nose**

Pincha Mayurasana

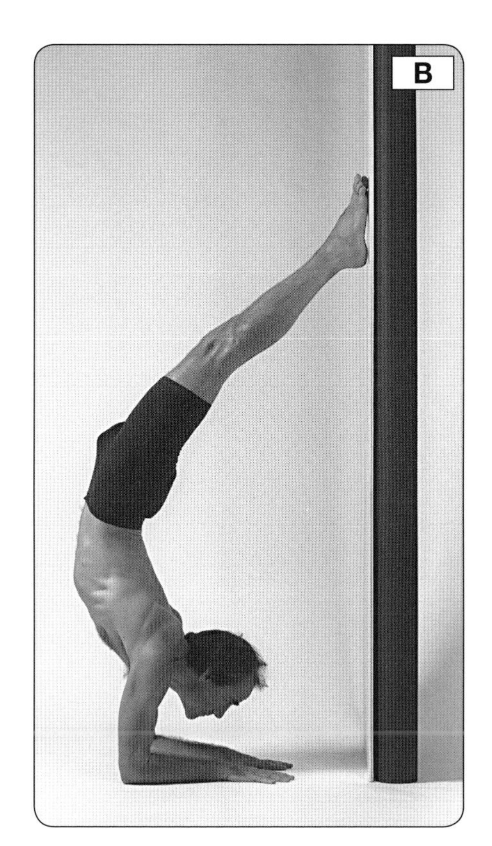

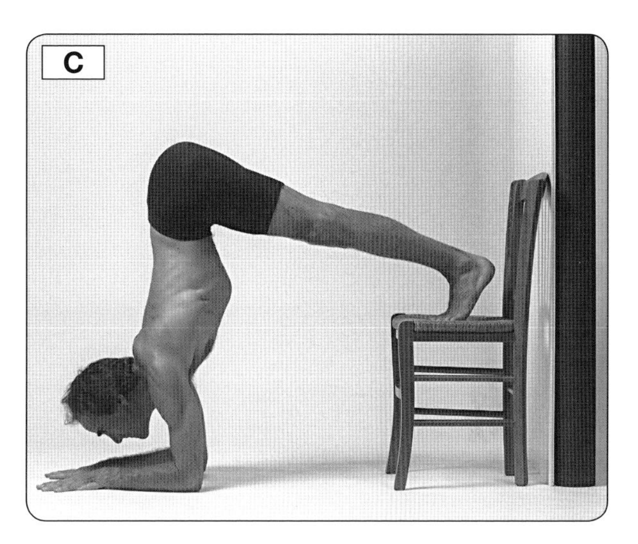

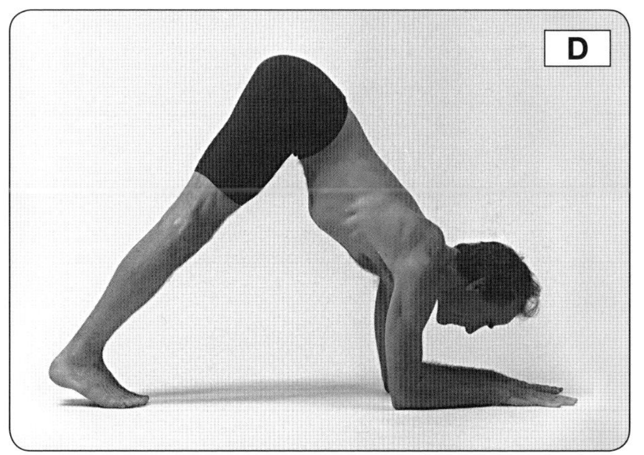

Comments - This asana is dynamic and challenging yet once you have the confidence to support your weight on your forearms it is not as difficult as it first appears. There is a natural fear-factor inherent in this type of inversion when our weight is supported solely on the arms. Use the more supported versions offered in options **(C)** & **(D)** before approaching **(A)** or **(B)**. It is best to learn this posture under the guidance of a qualified yoga instructor before attempting options **(A)** or **(B)** on your own. Feel the weight distribution running along the forearms and across the palms. Use the fingertips for fine-tuning your balance. Keep the legs working with the feet together. Point the toes toward the sky. Fully engage your bandhas. Lift the chest away from the floor.

Karandavasana

Karandava = A Sort of Duck

"Duck Posture"

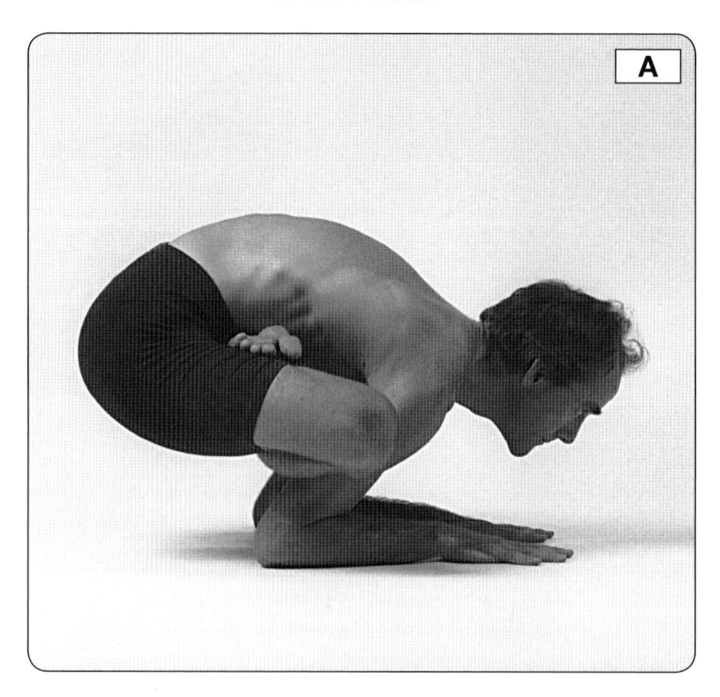

1) **Inhale** to your knees from **Downward Dog**.

2) **Exhale** place your forearms on the floor with the palms down.

3) **Inhale** jump up with both feet. Straighten the legs. Feet together and the toes pointed.

4) **Exhale** place your legs in full-lotus and lower them onto your forearms while keeping the head and chest lifted **(A)**. If you are able to place the legs in lotus while balancing in **Pincha Mayurasana** but it is too difficult to lower them to the arms then lower only partway and hold that position **(B)**. If it is too difficult to build your lotus while inverted you may cross the legs and lower only part of the way toward the arms **(C)** or sit on the floor in full-lotus and then lean forward with the forearms on the floor and slide the legs up onto the arms from the seated position until they are lifted fully into option **(A)** or on top of the elbows as seen in **(D)**.

Remain Here for 5 Deep Breaths

5) **Inhale** lift the legs up and release the lotus.

6) **Exhale** and lower the feet to the floor.

~VINYASA~

Enter the next asana from Downward Dog

Drishti ~ **Nose**

Karandavasana

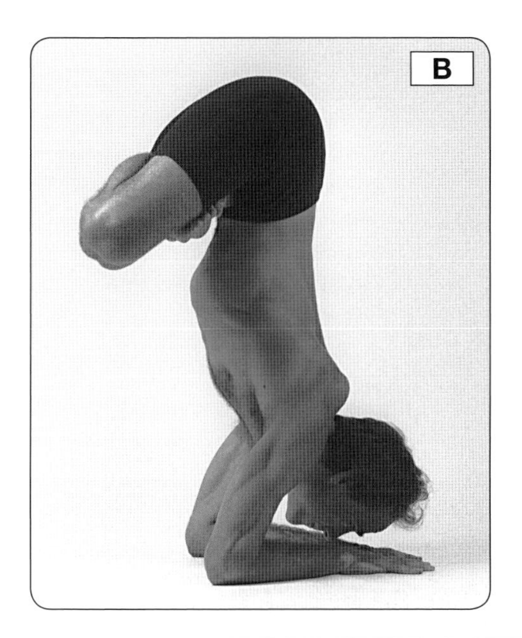

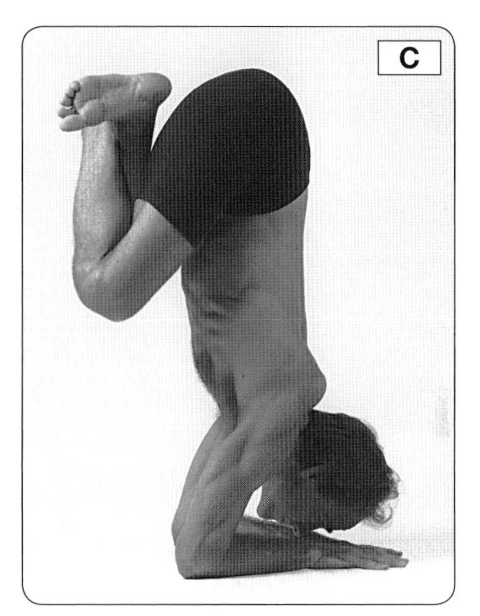

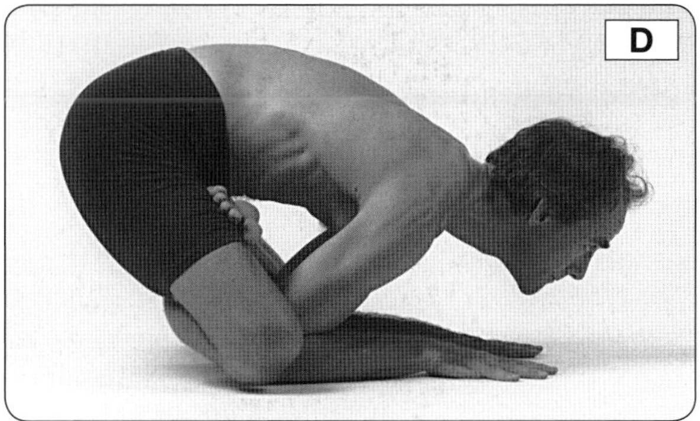

Comments - In order to build the lotus while in an inverted position you may drop the left leg back a bit and then place the right foot on the upper left thigh. Next, bend the left leg slightly so that the right foot may push against it and wriggle its way deeper. You may then open the right hip and move the right knee back to create space for the left foot to move on top and wriggle it into place. Once in lotus the next challenge is lowering. It is imperative that you maintain opposing forces of lifting and lowering at the same time. This means that as you are going down you are simultaneously lifting up yet with slightly less effort. This will control your descent. The bandhas are your support line. Once the legs touch the arms you must maintain an equality of both lifting and lowering. If you allow your weight to sink at this point it will not be possible to climb back up. To come up, add energy to the lifting mode and decrease the sinking force.

Vrishchikasana

Vrishchika = Scorpion

"Scorpion Posture"

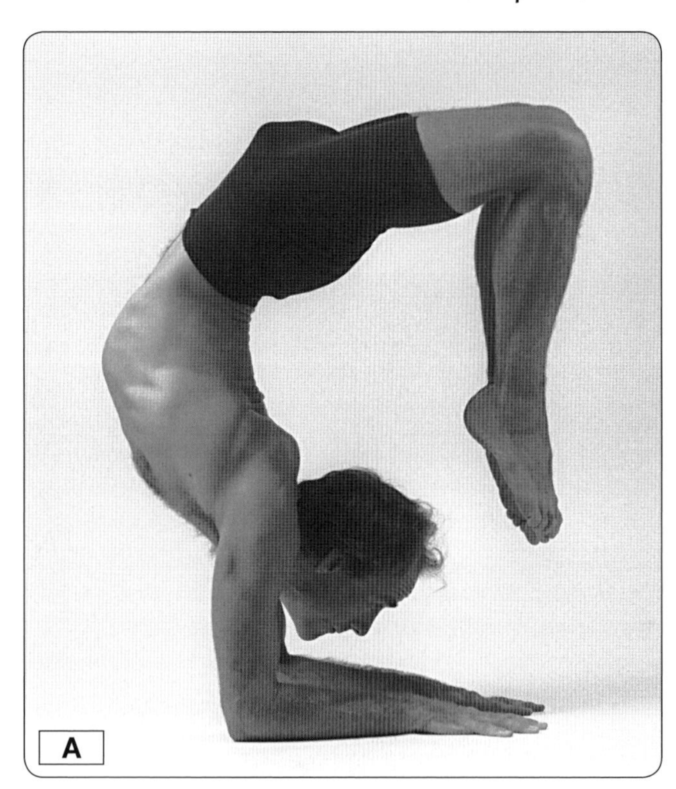
A

1) **Inhale** from **Downward Dog** to your knees.

2) **Exhale** place your forearms on the floor.

3) **Inhale** jump up with both feet as in **Pincha Mayurasana**. Feet together and toes pointed.

4) **Exhale** bend your knees and lower your feet toward the head with the toes pointing toward the floor. Let your hips follow the feet as you arch your back and open the chest **(A)**. If it is too intense to take the feet all of the way down you may bend the knees without dropping the hips or arching the back **(B)**. If it is too difficult to maintain your balance you may practice near a wall as in **Pincha Mayurasana. Remember to make sure that the wall is clear of obstructions**. This time begin with the fingertips about one-and-half to two feet away from the wall. Jump up and bend your knees until the feet find the wall. Walk them down slowly until you reach your maximum stretch and hold it **(C)**.

Remain Here for 5 Deep Breaths

4) **Inhale** lift the feet.

5) **Exhale** lower into **Chaturanga Dandasana**.

~VINYASA~

Take this vinyasa to standing as though finishing Surya Namaskara A

Drishti ~ **Nose**

Vrishchikasana

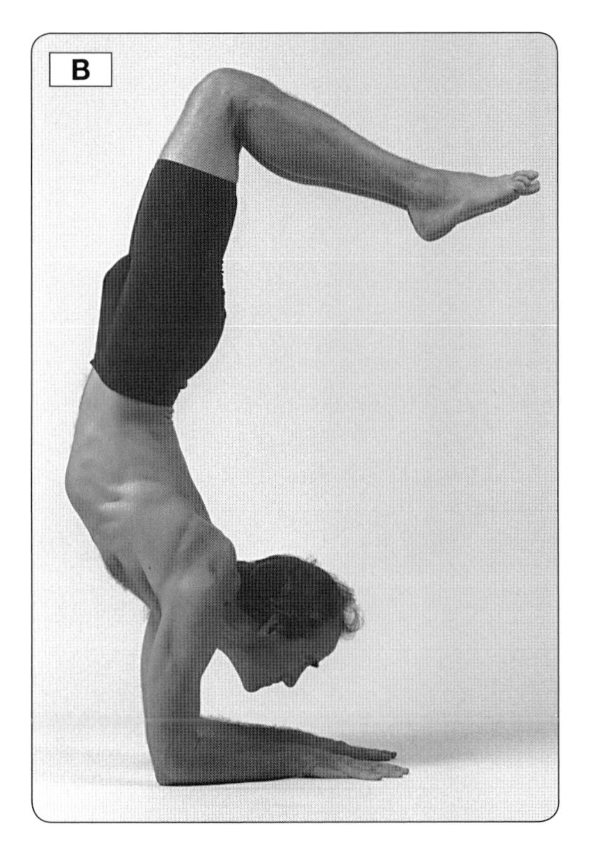

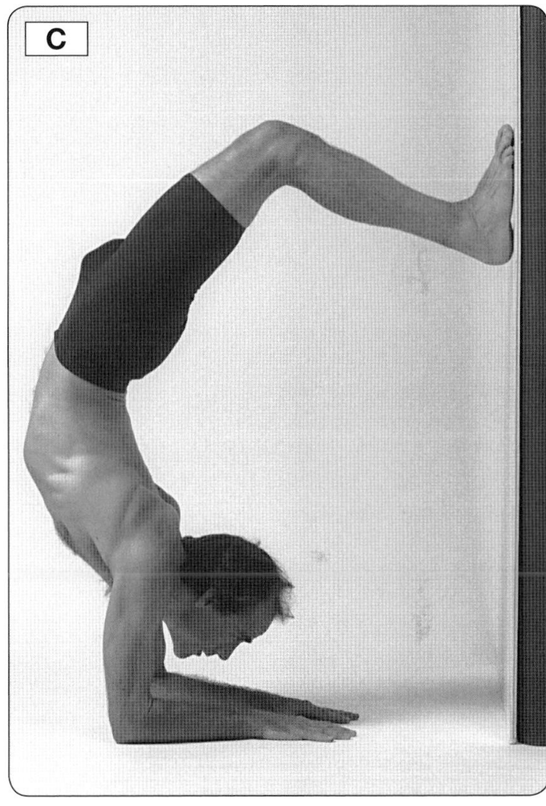

Comments - The key to finding balance when taking the feet over is to utilize the equalizing effects of opposing forces. In this asana you will find the oppositions in the opening of the chest and the lowering of the feet. This action will create an even distribution of weight so that you may have greater control. Without the compensation of extending the chest your weight will begin to pull you over as the feet drop. The same resistance must be engaged here as you utilized in **Karandavasana**. As the feet lower you must continue to lift them simultaneously. Keep the head lifted so that it does not start to sink toward the floor. When you lift your head it will assist in opening the chest and upper back. Distribute the weight from the elbows along the forearms and out to the fingertips. The major source of balance is achieved from the movement of the chest, hips and feet but the fingertips may be used for subtle adjustments.

Mayurasana

Mayura = Peacock / "Peacock Posture"

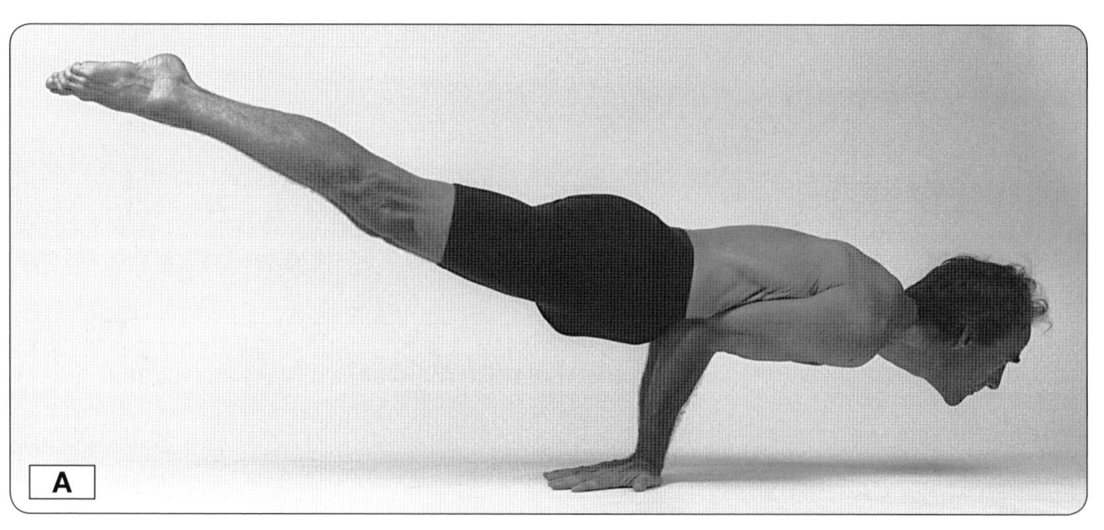

Come to standing from Downward Dog as though you are finishing Surya Namaskara A

1) **Inhale** beginning from a standing position take your arms overhead and separate the feet slightly.
2) **Exhale** forward, palms facing up **(D)**. Place the hands between the feet palms down, fingers back **(E)**.
3) **Inhale** look up.
4) **Exhale** jump back leaving the hands pointing backwards.
5) **Inhale** Upward-Facing Dog.
6) **Exhale** Downward Dog.
7) **Inhale** jump to a kneeling position with the knees outside the hands.
8) **Exhale** pull the elbows in toward the lower belly. Take the head toward the floor. Knees bent.
9) **Inhale** walk the feet back. Lift the head and arch your back. Take both feet from the floor **(A)** or raise only one leg and leave the other grounded **(B)**. You may also leave both feet on the floor as in **(C)**.

Remain Here for 5 Deep Breaths

10) **Exhale** lower the feet to the floor.
11) **Inhale** lift into Upward Dog keeping the hands reversed.
12) **Exhale** Downward Dog with the hands still reversed.
13) **Inhale** jump forward. Land the feet outside the hands. Hands still reversed. Lift your gaze.
14) **Exhale** fold forward with the hands in the same position.
15) **Inhale** up to standing, arms overhead until the palms touch.
16) **Exhale** lower your arms to your sides and take the feet together in preparation for the next asana.

Drishti ~ **Nose**

Mayurasana

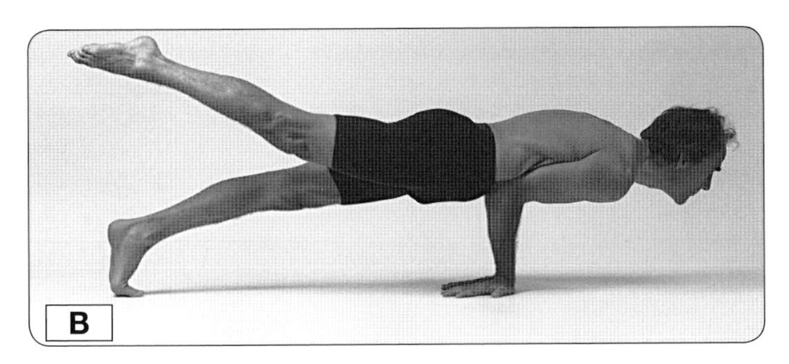
B

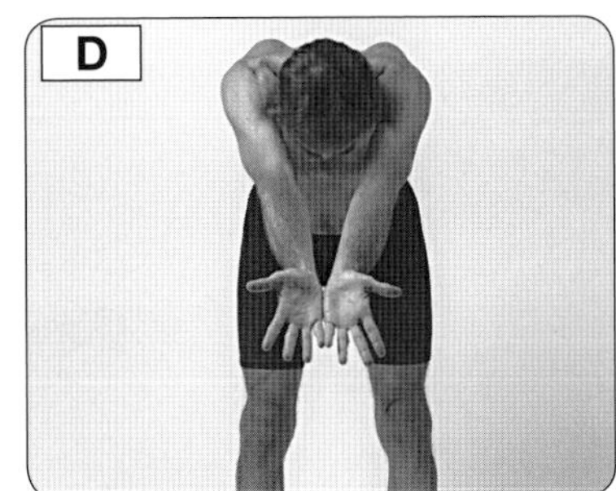
D

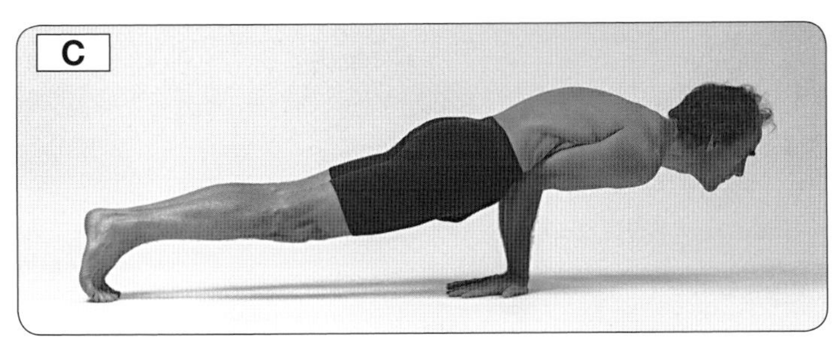
C

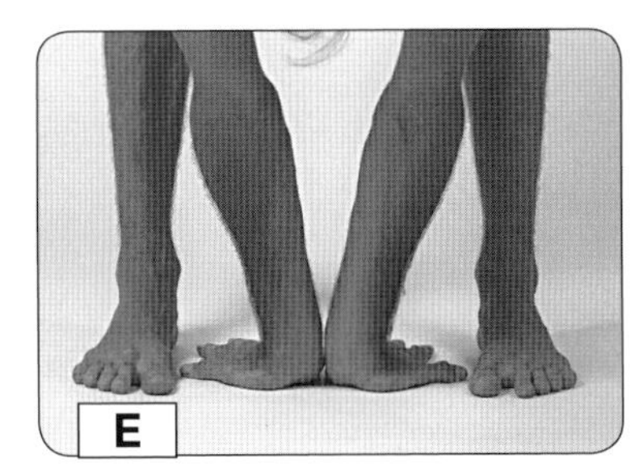
E

Comments - Mayurasana and the next three postures are all entered from a standing position. The Vinyasa begins exactly as though you are practicing **Surya Namaskara A**. After the hands are raised over the head and the palms touch, the first changes begin. As soon as the exhale forward is initiated, the feet should be separated slightly. At the same time the hands are turned so that the palms are facing up with the outer edges of the little fingers touching and the thumbs pointing out to the sides as shown in **(D)**. As the hands reach the floor the heels of the hands point to the front and the fingers point back **(E)**. The hands then remain in this position for the duration of the Vinyasa sequence as well as during the asana. The hand position is only released after coming back to standing. This is the prescribed method of Vinyasa for **Mayurasana**. It is quite difficult to move through the entire set of movements with the hands in this reversed position. It requires a great amount of strength and flexibility in the wrists. If it feels too intense, you should enter this as though you are practicing **Surya Namaskara** without the hand reversal.

The key to lifting the feet and head away from the floor is the proper placement of the elbows. The closer you can arrange your elbows to the center of your body the easier it will be to raise the feet. The pubic bone is the landmark to aim for. If you can reach the elbows just in front of this area then your body will have the ideal fulcrum upon which to balance. There is a tendency for the elbows to want to separate. You must remain focused on keeping them as close together as possible. The engagement of the lower abdominal region also plays a crucial role in finding stability in this asana. This may be achieved by working the bandhas fully. Once the legs are straight and the feet are still on the floor you may gently begin to push the floor away with the toes and simultaneously lift the chest and the head. Keep the legs active with the toes pointed and the feet together. If all of this seems like too much you may always choose to omit it for now and work toward it over time.

Nakrasana

Nakra = Crocodile / "Crocodile Posture"

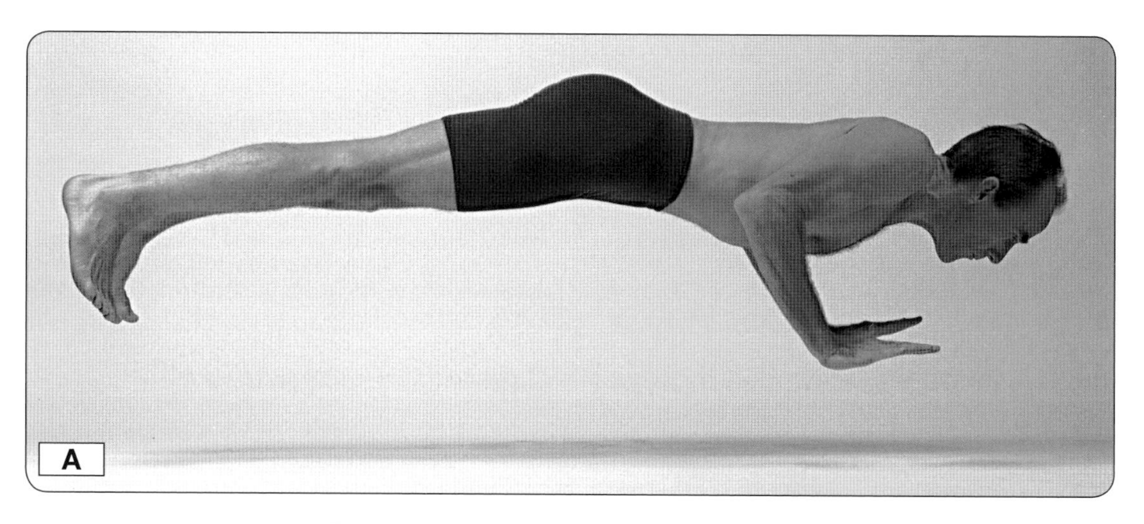
A

Enter this asana from a standing postion.

1) **Inhale** take your arms up over your head.

2) **Exhale** fold forward. Hands to the floor outside the feet. Lower your head.

3) **Inhale** look up.

4) **Exhale** jump back into Chaturanga Dandasana.

5) **Inhale** push with your hands and feet. Jump the body into the air with a slight forward motion **(A)**. If it is too much to propel the full body into the air then jump only the feet up without any forward motion and leave the hands in place **(B)** or leave the hands and feet on the floor and lift only the hips **(C)**.

6) **Exhale** as you land and lower into Chaturanga Dandasana.

Repeat Steps 5 and 6 four more times for a total of five hops forward. Then repeat the process in reverse. Hop five times back so that you return to the place from which you started.

11) **Inhale** lift into Upward Dog.

12) **Exhale** Downward Dog.

13) **Inhale** jump forward. Lift your gaze and lengthen the spine.

14) **Exhale** fold forward.

15) **Inhale** up to standing. Raise the arms overhead.

16) **Exhale** lower your arms to your sides in preparation for the next asana.

Drishti ~ **Nose**

Nakrasana

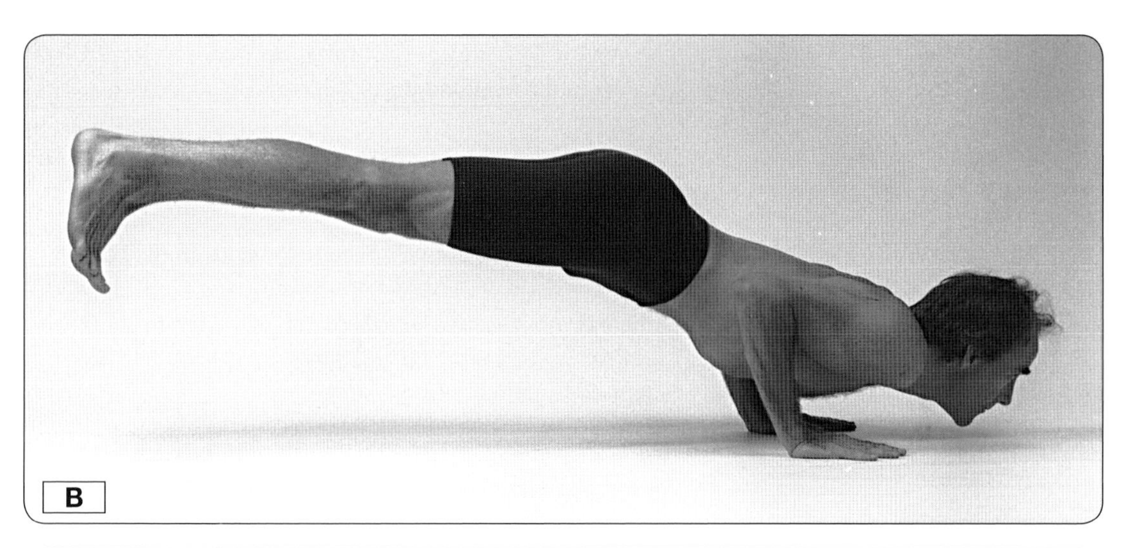

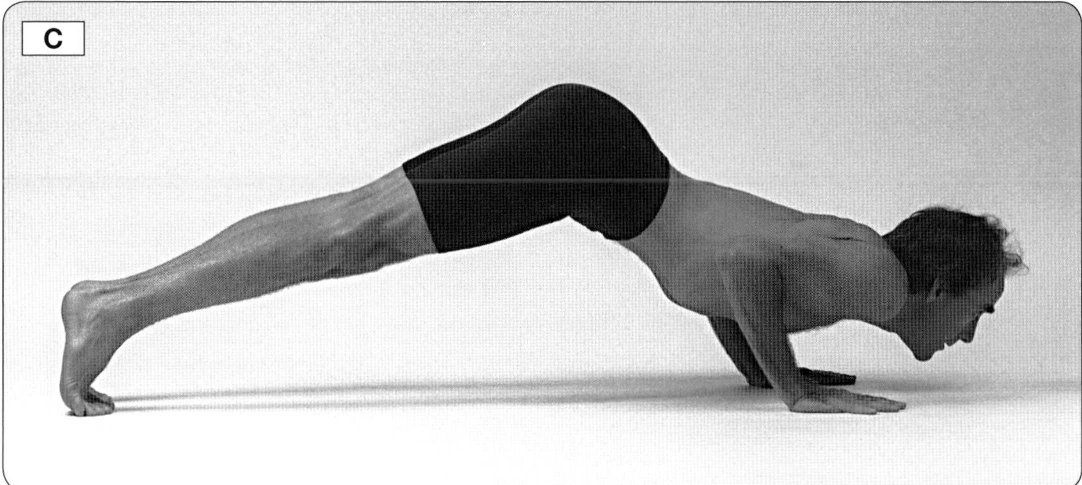

Comments - This asana requires a cooperative orchestration of movement. Every finger and toe acts as a spring to bounce the body. The hips lead the projection of motion. The arms, feet and legs give the extra push to rise. In **option (B)** you may focus on the hips and toes while leaving the hands stationary. **Option (C)** is a great approach to develop the strength required to eventually bounce the body away from the floor. If practicing **option (B)** or **(C)** you may repeat the action five times. Then take a Vinyasa back to standing.

Vatayanasana

Vatayana = Horse / "Horse Posture"

Enter this asana from standing.

1) **Inhale** lift the right foot into half-lotus. Remain standing.

2) **Exhale** reach behind the back and clasp the right foot with the right hand as in **Ardha Baddha Padmottanasana**.

3) **Inhale** raise the left arm overhead.

4) **Exhale** fold forward. Release the right foot but keep it in half-lotus. Take both hands to the floor.

5) **Inhale** lift your gaze to the horizon and lengthen the spine.

6) **Exhale** jump back into **Chaturanga Dandasana** with the right leg still on top of the left thigh.

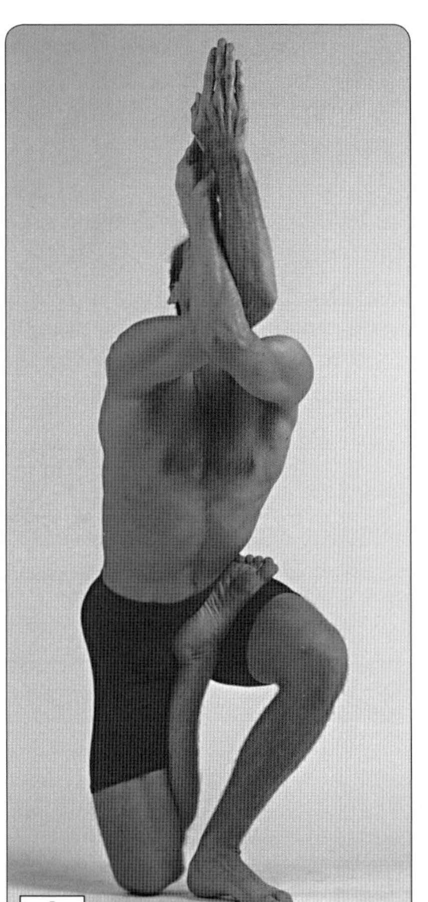
A

7) **Inhale** into **Upward Dog**, right knee away from the floor.

8) **Exhale Downward Dog**.

9) **Inhale** jump the left foot forward between the hands. Lift your gaze and lengthen the spine.

10) **Exhale** lower the right knee to the floor near the left heel.

11) **Inhale** lift the hands from the floor. Intertwine the arms with the right arm on top. Bend the elbows with the palms together and the fingers pointing toward the sky **(A)**. If it is too intense to keep the right knee close to the left heel then take the left foot further away until it is more comfortable **(B)** or instead of placing the right foot in half-lotus you may leave it on the floor for easier balance and less intensity **(C)**.

Remain Here for 5 Deep Breaths

12) **Exhale** lower your hands to the floor.

13) **Inhale** straighten the left leg and gaze to the horizon with the right leg still in half-lotus.

14) **Exhale** jump back, still keeping the right leg in half-lotus.

15) **Inhale Upward Dog**, right knee away from the floor.

16) **Exhale Downward Dog**. Release the right foot. Lower it to the floor.

17) **Inhale** place the left foot in half-lotus.

18) **Exhale** lower to **Chaturanga Dandasana**.

19) **Inhale Upward Dog**. Keep the knee away from the floor.

20) **Exhale Downward Dog** with leg still in half-lotus.

21) **Inhale** jump the right foot forward while keeping the left foot in half-lotus.

22) **Exhale** lower the left knee to the floor.

23) **Inhale** lift the hands from the floor. Move into whichever option is most appropriate from **step 11**.

Vatayanasana

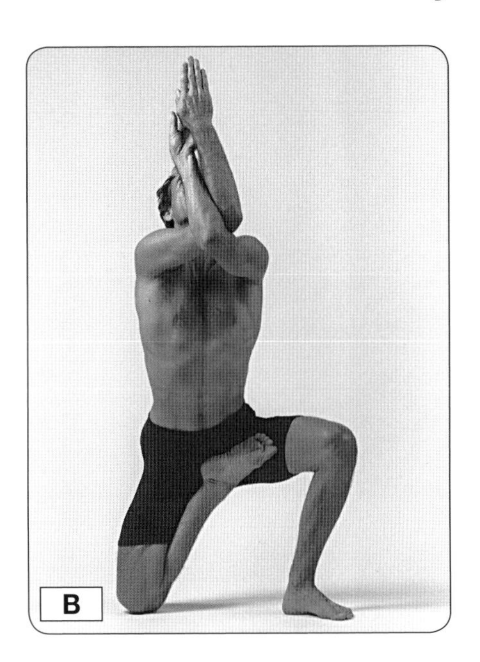

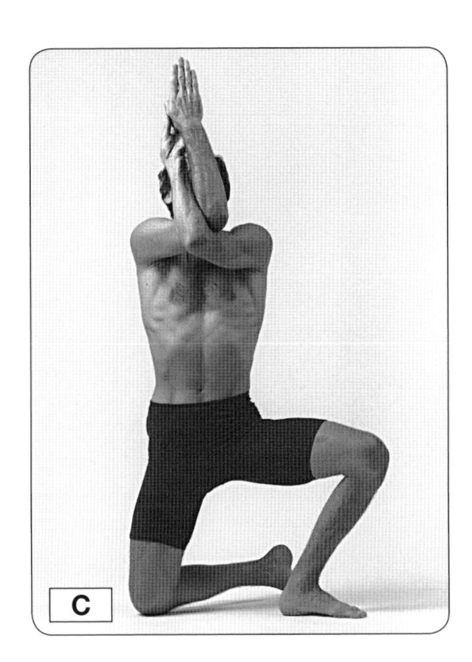

Remain Here for 5 Deep Breaths

24) **Exhale** lower your hands to the floor.
25) **Inhale** straighten the right leg and gaze to the horizon while keeping the left leg in half-lotus.
26) **Exhale** jump back, still keeping the left leg in half-lotus.
27) **Inhale** Upward Dog keeping the left knee away from the floor.
28) **Exhale** downward dog.
29) **Inhale** jump forward with the right foot. Lift your gaze to the horizon and lengthen the spine.
30) **Exhale** fold forward. Reach around the back with the left hand and grab the left foot.
31) **Inhale** stand up as you continue to hold the left foot in half-lotus. Raise the right arm over the head.
32) **Exhale** release the left foot and lower it to the floor as you take both arms to your sides.

Drishti ~ **To the Sky**

Comments - *Be Careful With Your Knees!* Choose the most appropriate option. If it is too intense to practice this Vinyasa with the foot in half-lotus you may practice a standard Vinyasa and jump forward with both feet. From there you may then place one foot in half-lotus and proceed. The closer you take the knee to the foot the more intense is the stretch. Proceed with caution and listen to your body. An additional challenge is the balance required when lifting the hands. It is a fine line. You must create an equality of weight distribution by drawing the hips forward as the hands and torso lift. There is a tendency to fall back due to an imbalance of weight transferal. This occurs when the hips are left behind as the chest and arms lift.

Parighasana

Parigha = Cross of a Gate

"Cross Beam of a Gate Posture"

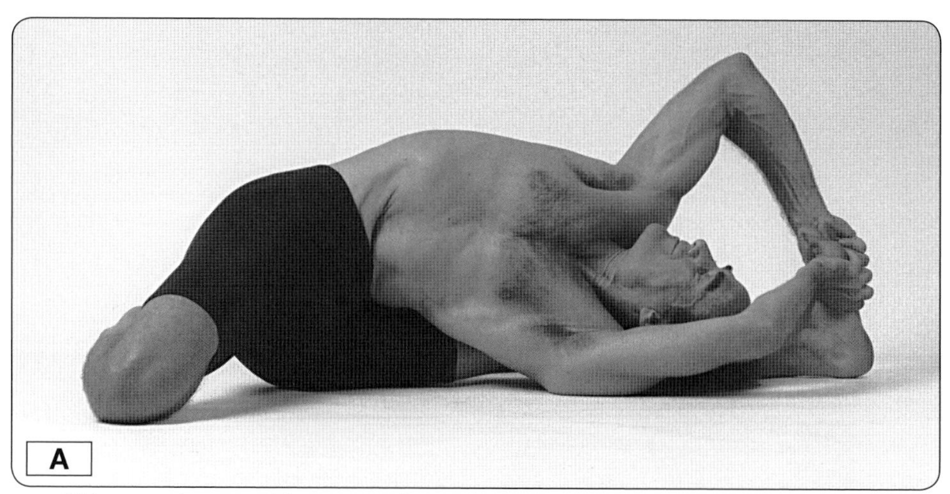

This asana is entered from a standing sequence due to the exit from Vatayanasana

1) **Inhale** raise both arms overhead and look at the thumbs.
2) **Exhale** fold forward and lower the head.
3) **Inhale** look to the horizon. Lengthen the spine.
4) **Exhale** jump back into **Chaturanga Dandasana**.
5) **Inhale** lift into Upward Dog.
6) **Exhale** Downward Dog.
7) **Inhale** jump forward and land with the right leg bent back with the right foot behind the right hip. Straighten the left leg with the hands on the floor between the thighs.
8) **Exhale** lower the left shoulder toward the inner left knee. Roll the chest open toward the sky. Take the right hand toward the left foot first, then the left hand toward the foot until you are able to clasp it with both hands **(A)**. If you cannot reach both hands to the foot you may clasp it with the right hand only and leave the left arm on the floor perpendicular to the left leg **(B)**. Another option is to roll the chest open and lean out over the left leg. Leave the left arm on the floor parallel to the left leg and take the right arm beside the right ear with the palm facing down and extend out through the fingertips as seen in **(C)**.

Remain Here for 5 Deep Breaths

9) **Inhale** release the foot and come out of the posture.

~VINYASA~

This is a standard Vinyasa. Do not take it to standing. Repeat Steps 7 & 8 On the Left Side

~VINYASA~

Enter the next asana from downward dog

Drishti ~ **To The Sky**

Parighasana

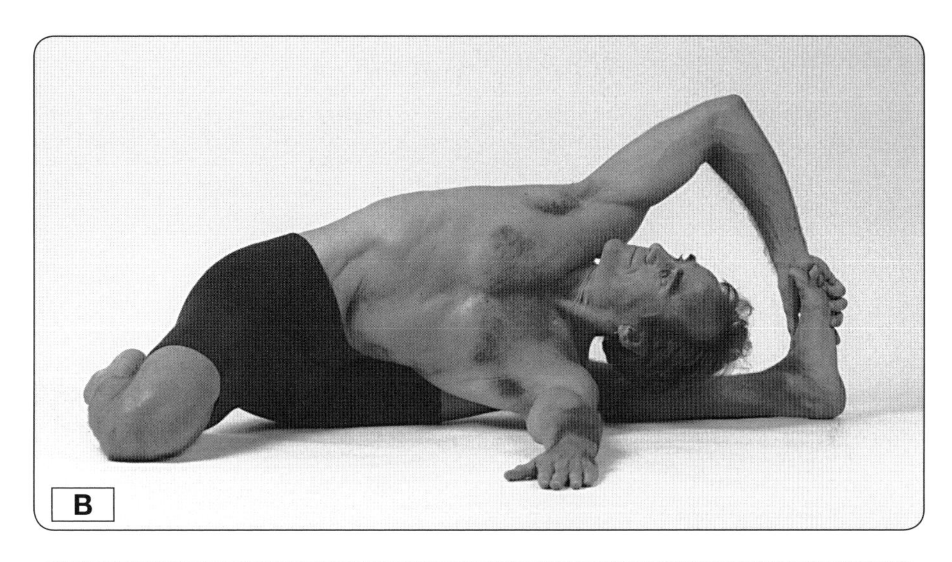

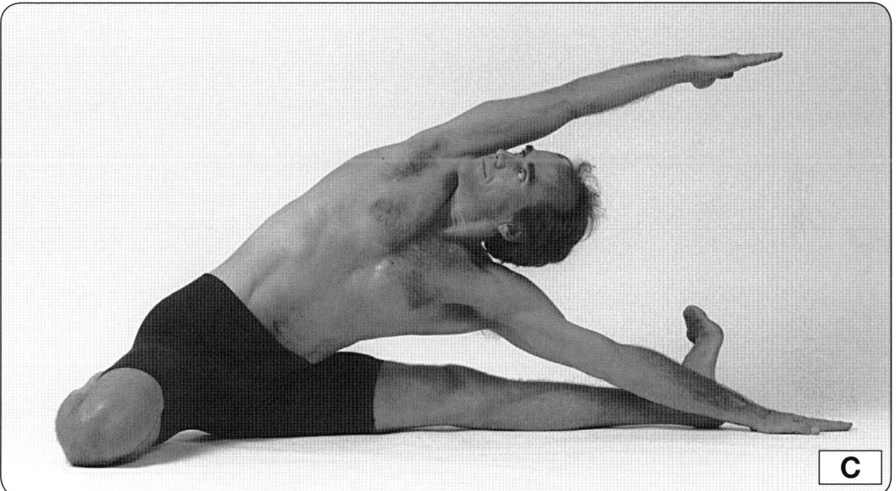

Comments - Lengthen the spine and rotate the torso. Take the shoulder to the inner knee. Press them against each other to enhance the spiraling action. If taking the shoulder to the knee is too much, then use the elbow instead. Keep the extended leg active. The back foot should be close to the thigh with the heel pointing up.

Gomukhasana A

Gomukha = Cow Face

"Cow Face Posture"

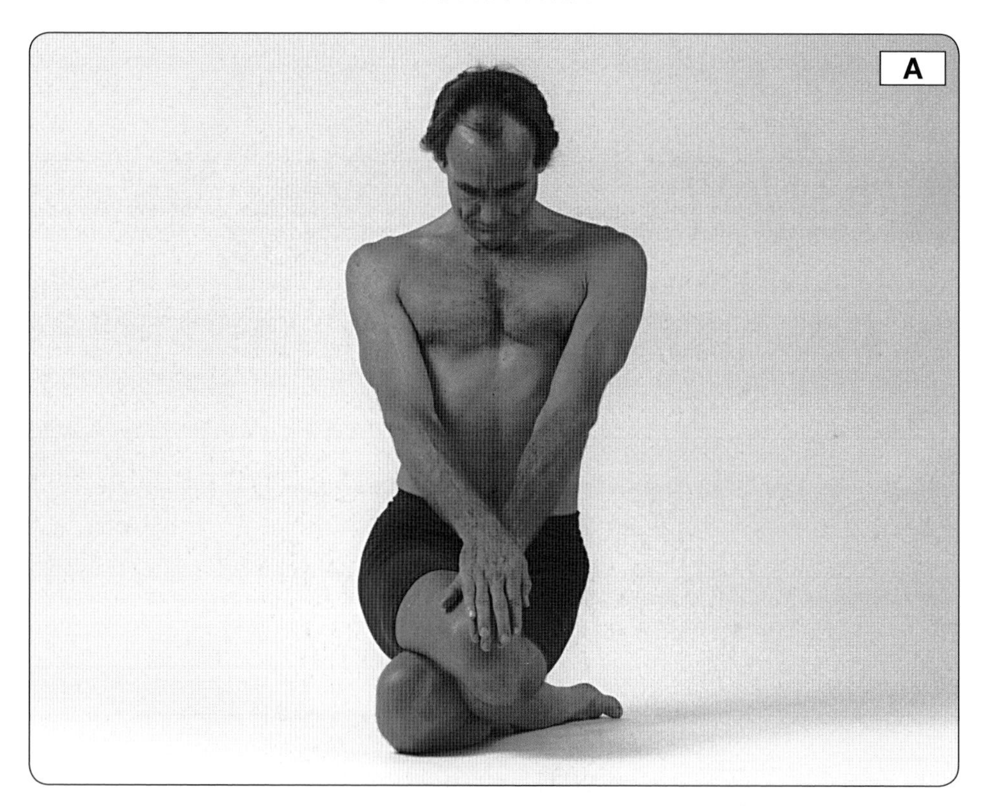

1) **Inhale** jump from **Downward Dog**. Land with the right leg crossed over the left. Toes pointing back.
2) **Exhale** bring the heels close together with the toes pointed back and the tops of the feet on the floor. Sit on top of the heels. Place the hands on the knees with the right hand on top of the left with the fingers pointing at the floor. Drop the chin to the chest **(A)**. If it is too much to bring the heels so close together you may sit on the left heel and let the right foot move slightly to the side as in **(B)** or leave the feet separated and sit on the floor between them **(C)**.

Remain Here for 5 Deep Breaths

Enter the Next Asana from Here

Drishti ~ **Nose**

Comments - Press the hands against the knees. Roll the shoulders down the back. Open the chest and heart. Avoid collapsing in the lower back by engaging the bandhas and slightly tilting your pelvis forward. When you draw your chin into your chest be aware that you do not slump forward at the same time.

Gomukhasana A

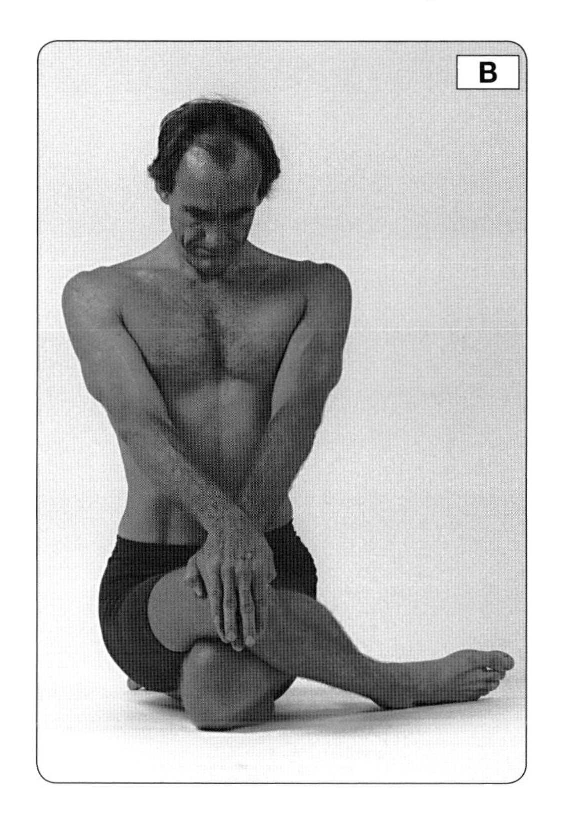

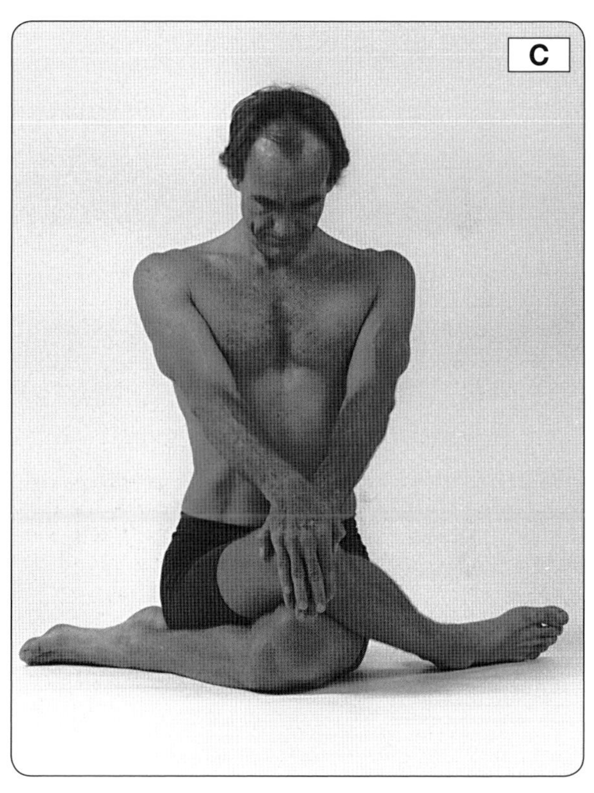

"Yoga is the Cessation of the Fluctuation of the Mind."

Patanjali

Gomukhasana B

Gomukha = Cow Face

"Cow Face Posture"

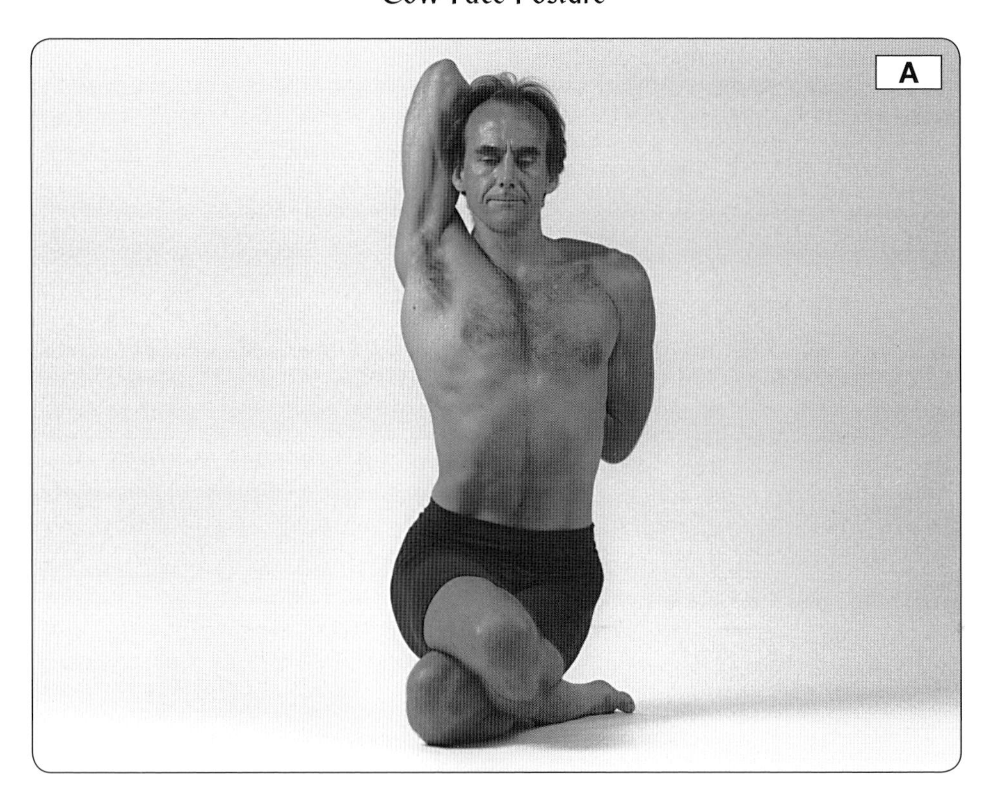

1) **Inhale** lift the hands from the top of the knees. Maintain your seated posture from **Gomukhasana A**. Take the right hand and reach over the top of the right shoulder. Wrap the left arm behind the back until both hands meet and clasp **(A)**. If you are seated with the ankles together yet are unable to reach the hands you may use a strap to connect them **(B)** or use the strap while seated between the heels **(C)**.

Remain Here for 5 Deep Breaths

2) **Exhale** release the hands and take them to the floor.

Repeat Gomukhasana A and B On The Left Side

~VINYASA~

Drishti ~ **Nose**

Comments - The shoulder of the upper arm should be rotated externally with the elbow pointing toward the sky. Keep your neck long. Use opposing forces between the hands to create an equal stretch on both arms. If you feel too much strain it is best to back off for now and come back to this version another day.

Gomukhasana B

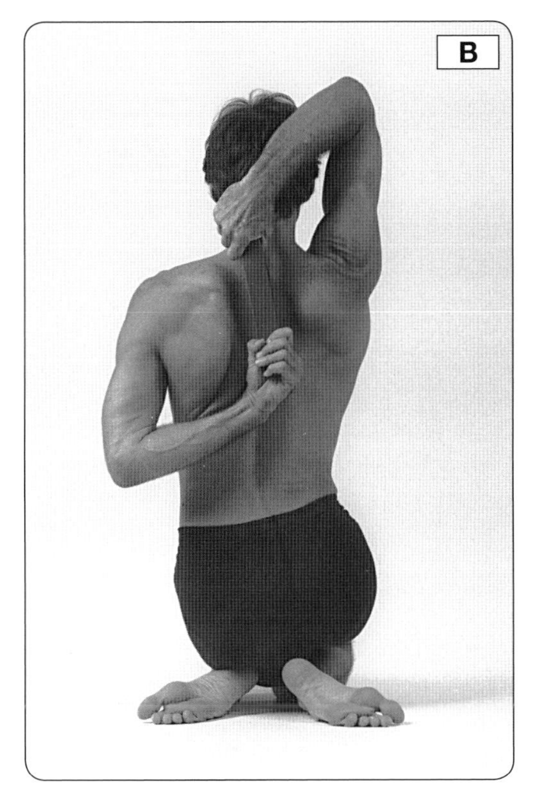

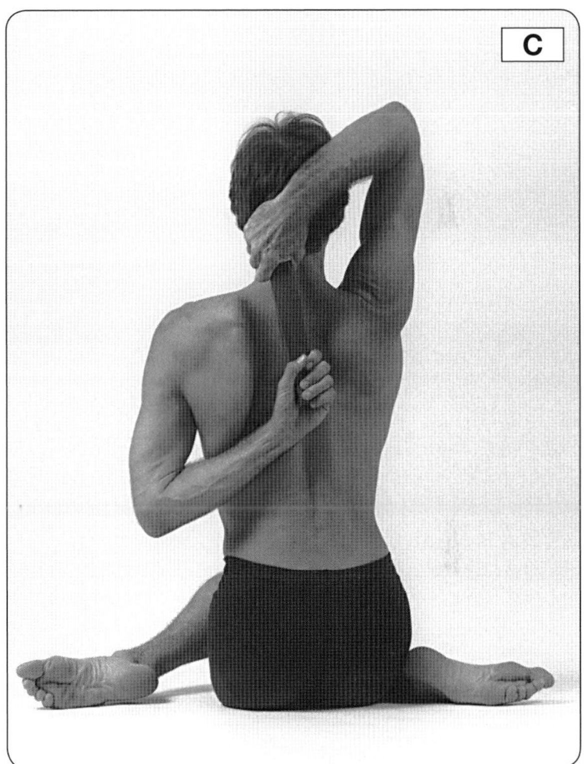

"Practice is the best of all instructions."

Aristotle

Supta Urdhva Pada Vajrasana

Supta = Sleeping Urdhva = Raised Pada = Foot Vajra = Thunderbolt

"Sleeping Raised Foot Thunderbolt Posture"

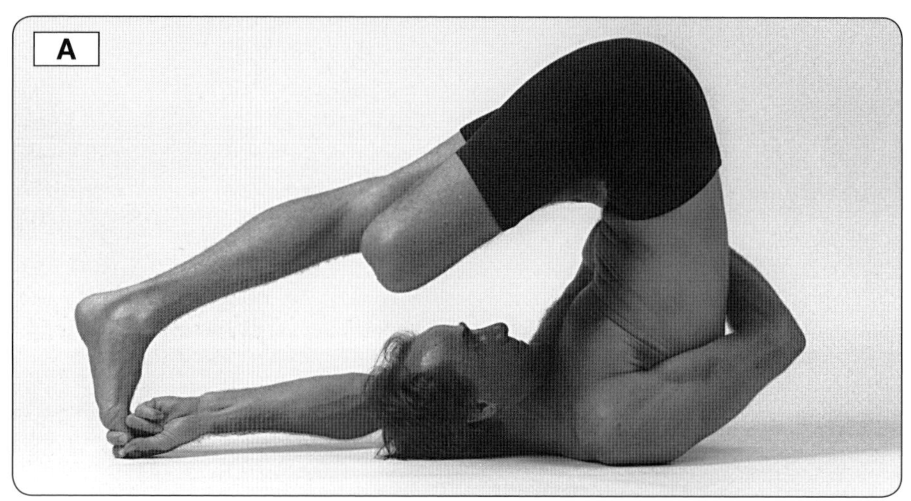

Do not remain in this position. It is only a transition.

1) **Exhale** lie down on your back. Roll up onto your shoulders with the feet on the floor over your head. Place the right foot in half-lotus. Reach the right arm behind the back and grab the right foot. Clasp the big toe of the left foot with two fingers of the left hand while keeping the leg straight **(A)**.
2) **Inhale** roll up. Bend the left leg back as you land in a seated position with the left foot outside the left hip and the right foot still in half-lotus. Release the left foot and place the left fingers under the right knee so that the palm is on the floor with the fingers pointing back under the knee and the heel of the hand pressing down into the floor. Bring the knees toward each other and twist **(B)**. If you cannot clasp the foot that is in half-lotus, use a strap **(C)**. If you cannot take the fingers under the knee, hold it instead **(D)**.

Remain Here for 5 Deep Breaths

~VINYASA~

Repeat On the Left Side

~VINYASA~

Enter the next asana from downward dog

Drishti ~ **Nose**

Comments - To enter this asana the Vinyasa requires you to roll over the arm that is behind the back. If this is too intense you may clasp only the extended foot and wait to clasp the half-lotus foot until after the roll. When practicing the bound approach, roll across the "meaty" portion of the upper forearm just below the elbow. The grip on the extended leg changes in mid transit from a hold on the big toe to a clasp over the top of the other toes. This enables the hand to assist in the movement of the foot to the outside of the hip for the landing. For the seated phase of this asana use the hands to create a spiraling motion in the torso.

Supta Urdhva Pada Vajrasana

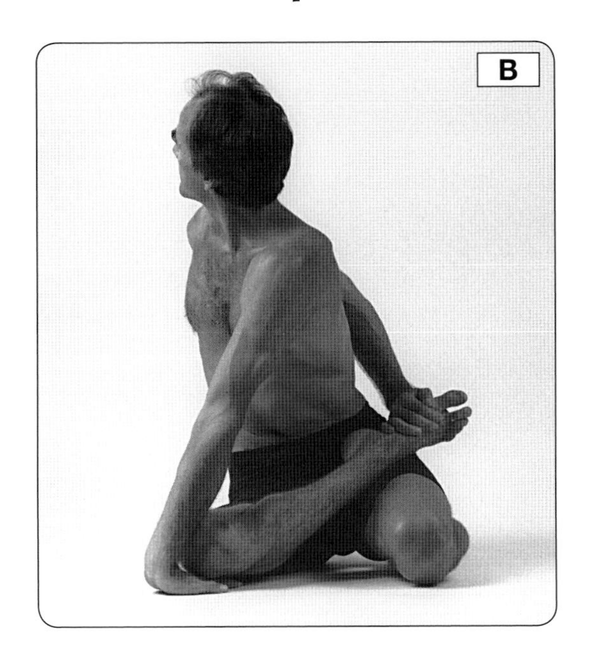

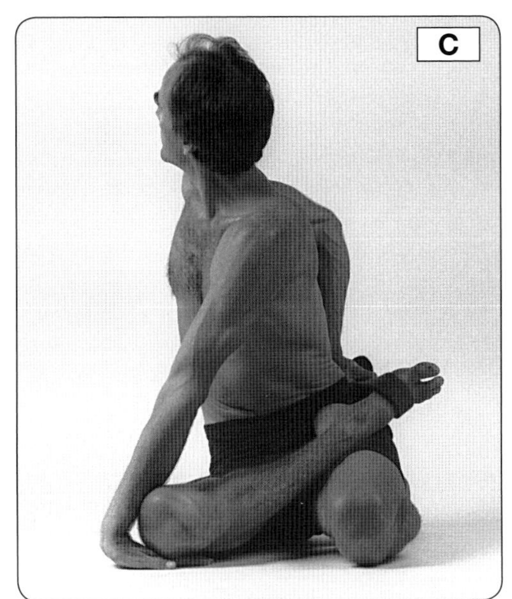

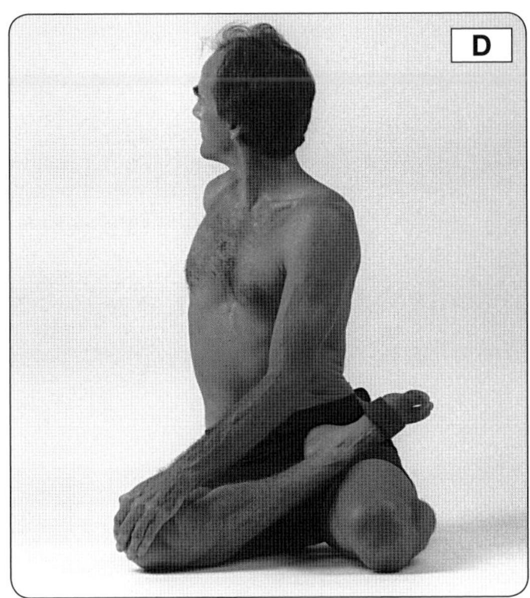

Entering the Seven Headstands

"Finding the Fulcrum"

Following **Supta Urdhva Pada Vajrasana** you will enter the final seven asanas of the Intermediate Series. They are comprised of a variety of headstand variations arranged into two groups. The first group, **Baddha Hasta Sirsasana A, B, C** and **D**, consists of four variations of headstand which utilize the arms for varying degrees of support. The second group, **Mukta Hasta Sirsasana A, B** and **C**, is comprised of three additional headstand varieties which require minimal support from the arms. I am going to illustrate all seven of the headstands in the following pages.

Baddha Hasta Sirsasana A, is the most supported of all. It is present in the finishing sequence of every Series from Primary through Advanced A and B. In the finishing sequence it is referred to simply as "**Sirsasana**". Stability must first be achieved here before moving on to the more advanced varieties. Rather than offer alternatives to the additional six headstands of the Intermediate Series, I feel it is better to repeat **Baddha Hasta Sirsasana A** whenever you find a variation which is too difficult.

As support is removed from the arms it becomes increasingly important to maintain proper alignment. The vertebrae in the neck must be evenly stacked upon one another to avoid undue strain on the cushions which separate them. This requires a high level of postural awareness. The chin should be neither tucked in toward the neck, nor should the head be tilted back. Rather, the neck is positioned as though you are standing on your feet and looking straight ahead while balancing a book on top of your head. While in headstand, the ribs need to be pulled in. The feet should be aligned directly over the hips. When this alignment is not achieved there is a tendency to collapse in the lower back. This misalignment is depicted by the "banana" appearance of the body when viewed from the side. When this occurs, the pressure is amplified along the back side of the cervical vertebrae and the risk of pinching or placing undue strain on the vertebral cushions is increased. This is why I am spending the time to encourage a heightened level of familiarity with **Baddha Hasta Sirsasana A** before moving into the others.

One should be able to remain comfortably in **Baddha Hasta Sirsasana A**, as it is presented in the finishing sequence, for twenty-five breaths without coming out, before attempting the additional headstands of the Intermediate Series. It is best to learn this sequence under the direct supervision of a qualified Ashtanga Yoga instructor. There is a full description of **Baddha Hasta Sirsasana A** in the finishing sequence on pages 226-229. Stability in headstands grows from the ground up. Find the imaginary plumb-line which runs through the center of the body. That is the fulcrum. Grow along that line and balance will manifest. When alignment is found the energy flows freely and physical effort is minimized.

Baddha Hasta Sirsasana A

Baddha = Bound Hasta = Hand Sirsa = Head

"Bound Hands Headstand Posture"

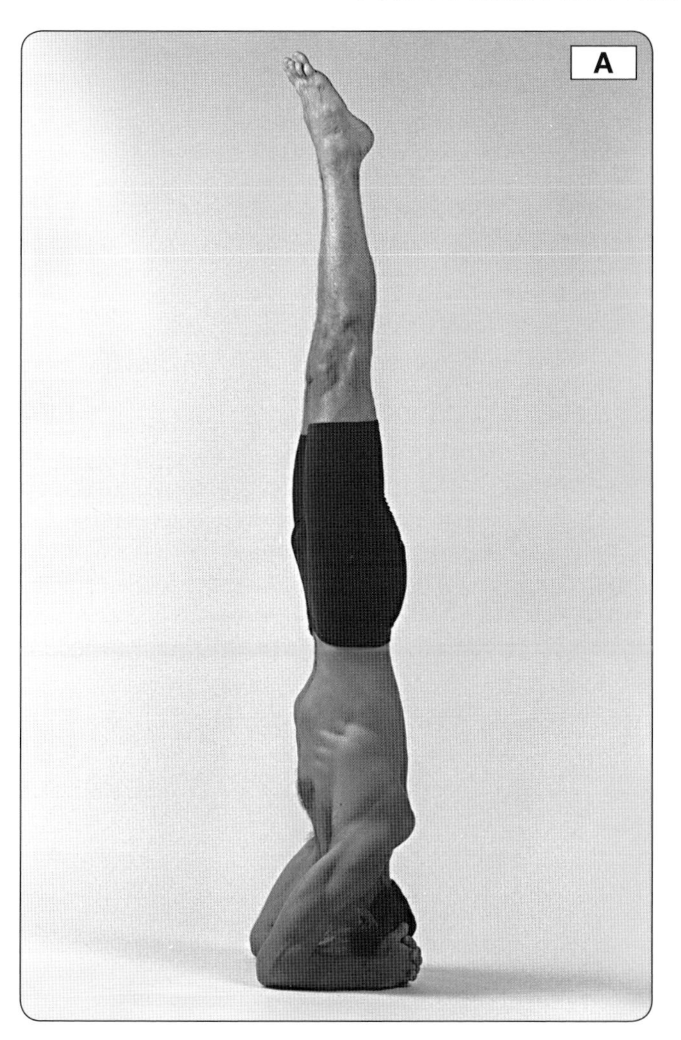

1) **Inhale** and come to a kneeling position from **Downward Dog**.

2) **Exhale** place the outer edges of your forearms on the floor. Lower your head to the floor. Position the elbows so that they are a shoulder's width apart. Interlace the fingers and lower the top of the head to the floor between the hands with the back of the head gently cradled in the hands.

3) **Inhale** straighten the legs and walk the feet toward your face. As you feel the weight transfer from your feet to your head you may bend the knees and lift the feet from the floor. Raise the legs as you straighten them. The body should be perpendicular to the floor. Keep the feet together with the toes pointing toward the sky. (For additional variations of **Baddha Hasta Sirsasana A** refer to pages 226-229.

Remain Here for 5 Deep Breaths

4) Exhale lower your feet to the floor.

~VINYASA~

Enter the Next Asana from Downward Dog

Drishti ~ **Nose**

Comments - This is the most supported of the seven headstands of the Intermediate Series. Take advantage of the position of the arms. Distribute the weight along the outer edges of the hands, the wrists, forearms and elbows. These areas form a perfect trianglular base. Take some of the weight onto the top of your head but avoid the tendency of relying solely on the head for support. You have been practicing this headstand for some time by now since it is an integral part of the finishing sequence. Find your fulcrum. Align your core along that center line. Search for the point of least resistance. Lengthen!

Baddha Hasta Sirsasana B

Baddha = Bound   Hasta = Hand   Sirsa = Head

"Bound Hands Headstand Posture"

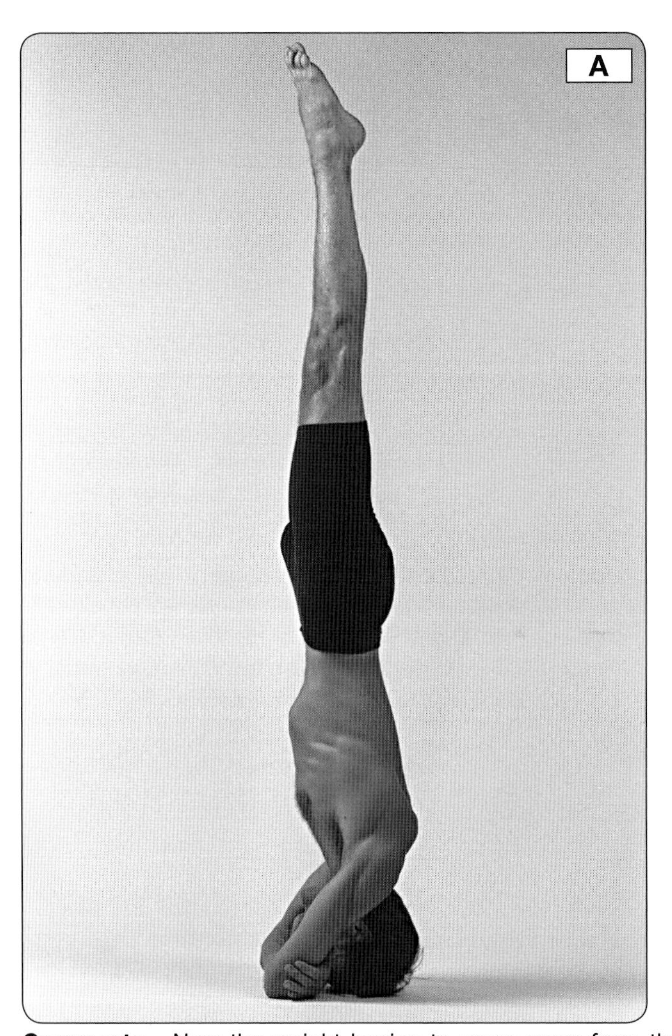

1) **Inhale** and come to a kneeling position from **Downward Dog**.

2) **Exhale** place the forearms on the floor. Reach your fingers around the outside of the elbows. Lower the top of your head to the floor so that the forearms are in front of your face.

3) **Inhale** straighten the legs and walk the feet toward your face. Lift the feet from the floor and raise the legs until the body is perpendicular to the floor. Keep the feet together with the toes pointing toward the sky.

Remain Here for 5 Deep Breaths

If this asana is too difficult you may repeat one of the previous variations or continue on to the finishing sequence.

4) **Exhale** lower your feet to the floor.

~VINYASA~

Enter the Next Asana from Downward Dog

Drishti ~ **Nose**

Comments - Now the weight begins to move away from the arms. Keep a good amount of support distributed across the forearms so that it is not all on the head. It becomes increasingly more important to feel your center line. This is a challenge when the feet are pointed up toward the sky and your line of sight is blocked by the arms. Begin to navigate from your internal awareness. Feel the subtle transferal of weight which occurs from even the most minute movement. Create oppositions of force. As you feel gravity holding you against the earth, use that force as an avenue to lengthen and grow away from as you expand toward the sky.

Baddha Hasta Sirsasana C

Baddha = Bound Hasta = Hand Sirsa = Head

"Bound Hands Headstand Posture"

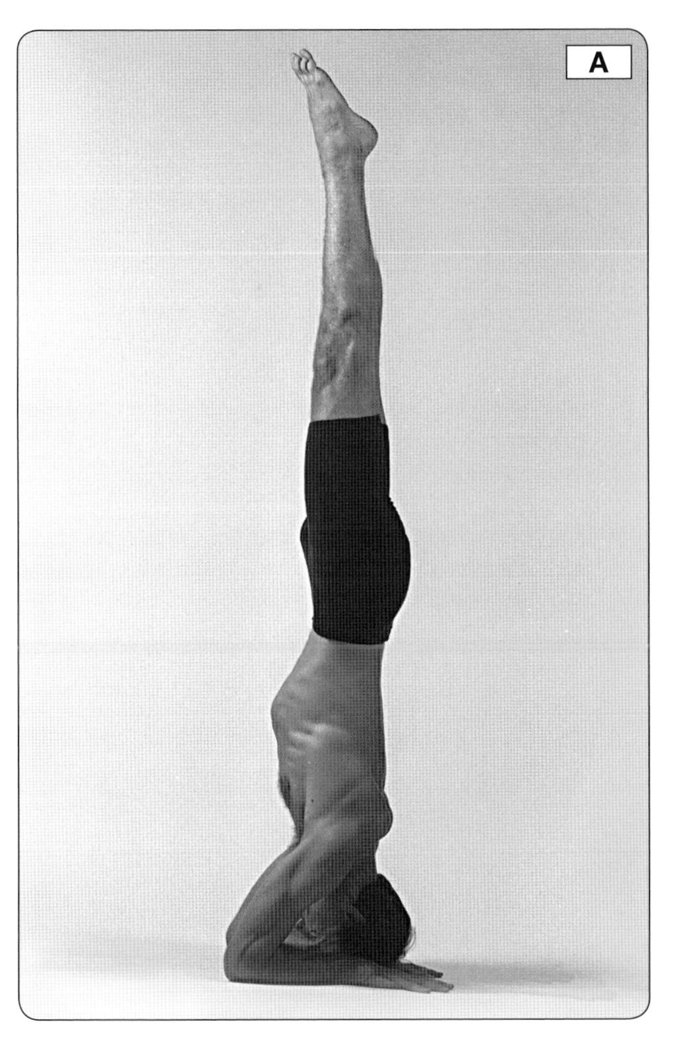

1) **Inhale** and come to a kneeling position from **Downward Dog**.

2) **Exhale** place the forearms on the floor parallel to each other with the palms facing down. Lower the top of your head to the floor between the wrists.

3) **Inhale** straighten the legs and walk the feet toward your face. Lift the feet from the floor and raise the legs until the body is perpendicular to the floor. Keep the feet together with the toes pointing toward the sky.

Remain Here for 5 Deep Breaths

If this asana is too difficult you may repeat one of the previous variations or continue on to the finishing sequence.

4) **Exhale** lower your feet to the floor.

~VINYASA~

Enter the Next Asana from Downward Dog

Drishti ~ Nose

Comments - Here there is a very similar dynamic to **Pincha Mayurasana** which was practiced earlier in the Intermediate Series. The forearms, elbows, palms and fingers may be used as distribution points for weight. Unlike **Pincha Mayurasana**, the head will remain on the floor in this posture. As in all varieties of headstand, the arms are placed in such a way as to provide additional support for the head and neck. Press the wrists down as well as the forearms. There is a tendency for the wrists to want to rise up. That will weaken your support. ***If you feel too much pressure on the neck, Come Down Immediately.***

Baddha Hasta Sirsasana D

Baddha = Bound Hasta = Hand Sirsa = Head

"Bound Hands Headstand Posture"

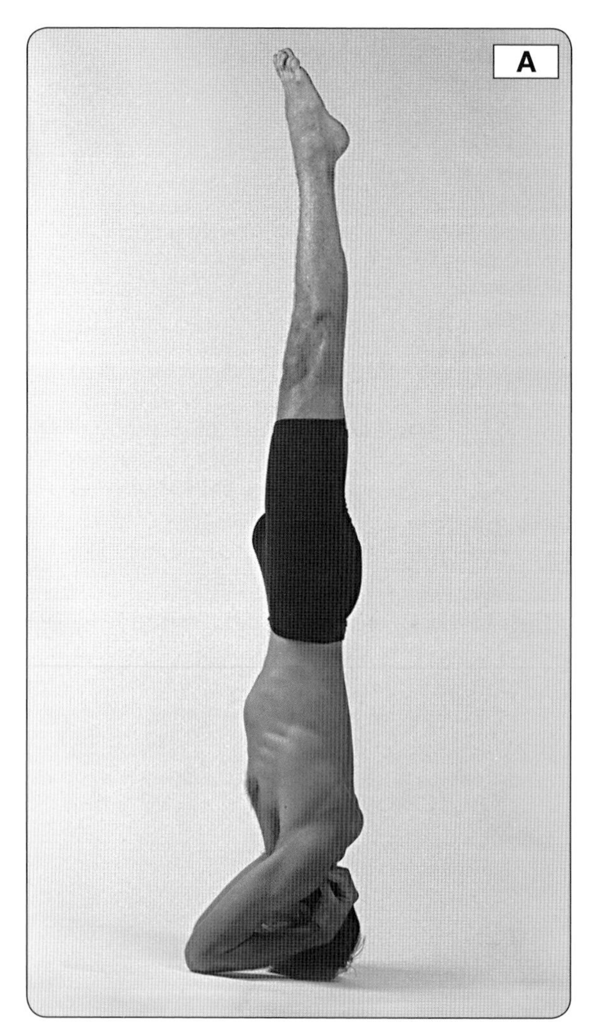

1) **Inhale** to a kneeling position from **Downward Dog**.

2) **Exhale** place your forearms on the floor with the palms facing up. Lower the top of your head to the floor between the wrists. Keep the elbows on the floor as you raise the hands toward the shoulders. Place the fingers so that the tips of each of the fingers are touching in a little cluster. Place that cluster into the small indentation formed on top of the shoulders as seen in **(A)**. If that is too difficult, you may place the fingers behind the shoulders as seen in the illustration below: **Alternate Hand Position**.

3) **Inhale** straighten the legs and lift the feet from the floor. Raise the legs until the body is perpendicular to the floor. Keep the feet together with the toes pointed skyward.

Remain Here for 5 Deep Breaths

If this asana is too difficult you may repeat one of the previous variations or continue on to the finishing sequence.

4) **Exhale** lower your feet to the floor.

~VINYASA~

Enter the next asana from Downward Dog

Drishti ~ **Nose**

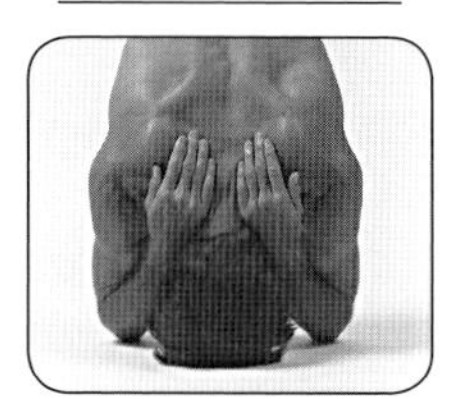

Alternate Hand Position

Comments - This is the last of the **Baddha Hasta Sirsasana** sequence. In this asana the elbows and the top of the head form a tripod. There is a steady progression toward removing support from the arms which creates greater reliance upon the elements of alignment and balance. Whichever hand position you choose you may find it useful to press the wrists in slightly against the head. This will create more stability when learning this asana. Eventually you may keep the wrists free from the head. It is imperative to maintain proper position of the neck. ***Listen To Your Body! If It Doesn't Feel Right, EXIT!***

Mukta Hasta Sirsasana A

Mukta = Free   Hasta = Hand   Sirsa = Head

"Free Hands Headstand Posture"

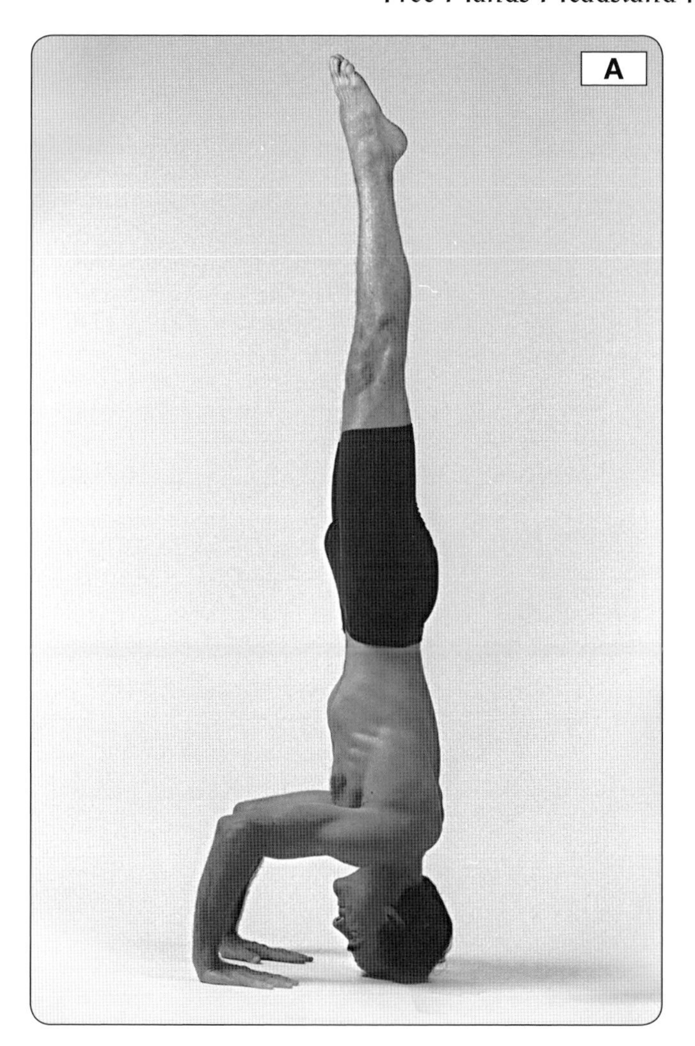

1) **Inhale** jump forward from **Downward Dog** and come to your hands and knees with the hands positioned at a shoulder's width apart.

2) **Exhale** lower the top of your head to the floor out in front of the hands. The palms should remain on the floor with the fingers pointing straight ahead. Keep an equal distance between the head and hands as well as between the hands. These three points will form an equilateral triangle.

3) **Inhale** straighten the legs and walk the feet toward your face. Lift the feet from the floor and raise the legs until the body is perpendicular to the floor. Keep the feet together with the toes pointing toward the sky.

Remain Here for 5 Deep Breaths
If this asana is too difficult you may repeat one of the previous variations or continue on to the finishing sequence.

4) **Exhale** lower your feet to the floor.

~VINYASA~

Enter the next asana from Downward Dog

Drishti ~ **Nose**

Comments - This is the first of the **Mukta Hasta Sirsasana** sequence. The hands and arms continue to move further from the head. For this version there is still a good amount of stability provided by the tripod-shaped base created by the position of the hands and head. This stability can be deceiving. It is possible to stay up there without having proper alignment in the cervical spine. **Remember, You Must Stack the Vertebrae Evenly**. Feel the placement of weight on top of the head. The hands should be a shoulder's width apart with the elbows directly above the wrists so that the forearms are perpendicular to the floor.

Mukta Hasta Sirsasana B

Mukta = Free Hasta = Hand Sirsa = Head

"Hands Free Headstand Posture"

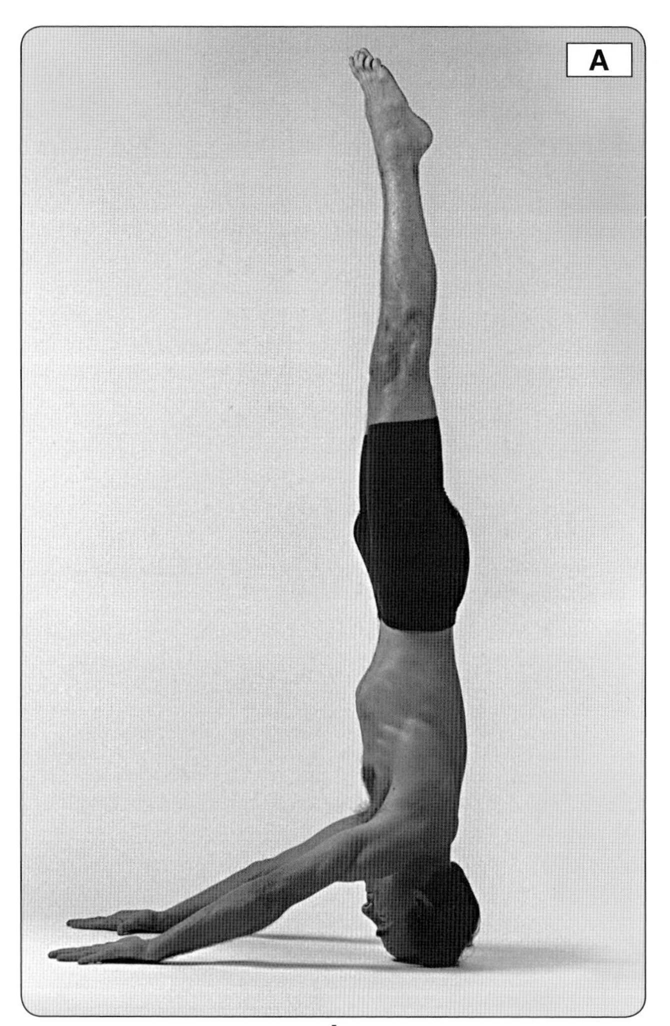

A

1) **Inhale** jump forward from **Downward Dog** and come to your hands and knees.

2) **Exhale** place the top of your head on the floor. Straighten the arms out in front of your face with the palms facing up and the hands positioned with a shoulder's width between them and the thumbs pointing at each other.

3) **Inhale** straighten the legs and lift the feet from the floor. Raise the legs until the body is perpendicular to the floor. Keep the feet together with the toes pointing toward the sky.

Remain Here for 5 Deep Breaths

If this asana is too difficult you may repeat one of the previous variations or continue on to the finishing sequence.

4) **Exhale** lower your feet to the floor.

~VINYASA~

Enter the next asana from Downward Dog

Drishti ~ **Nose**

Comments - For this asana there is once again a triangular base formed between the head and hands. The sides of the triangle have lengthened while the base width has stayed the same. This translates into more weight on the head and greater need for awareness of alignment. Balance may be found in the point of least resistance which is the area closest to your central core or plumb line. I have mentioned this before but it has become increasingly crucial as we progress through these headstands. Press the back of the hands against the floor to create more lift and stability. Listen to your breath. ***If It Is Too Intense, EXIT!***

Mukta Hasta Sirsasana C

Mukta = Free   Hasta = Hand   Sirsa = Head

"Free Hands Headstand Posture"

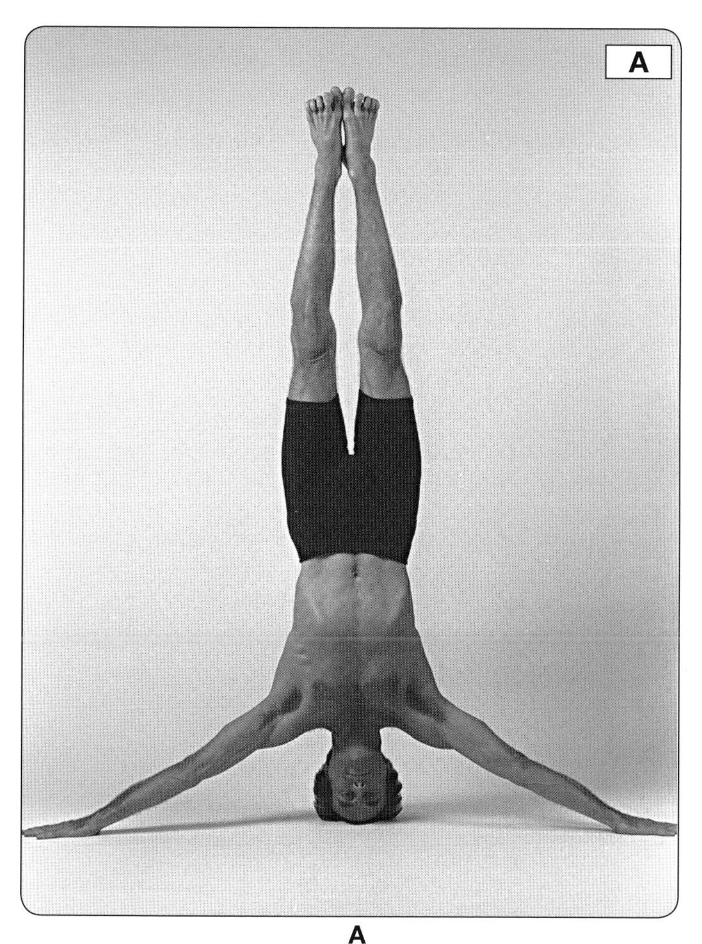

A

1) **Inhale** jump forward from **Downward Dog.** Come to your hands and knees.

2) **Exhale** lower the top of your head to the floor out in front of the hands. Straighten the arms. Place the hands with the palms down and the thumbs pointing behind you. Imagine a line extending out along the floor traveling away from your ears in opposite directions. Your hands should be positioned so that they are slightly in front of that line so that you can just see them in your peripheral vision.

3) **Inhale** straighten the legs. Walk the feet toward your face. Lift the feet. Raise the legs until the body is perpendicular to the floor. Keep the feet together with the toes pointing skyward.

Remain Here for 5 Deep Breaths

If this asana is too difficult you may repeat one of the previous variations or continue on to the finishing sequence.

4) **Exhale** lower your feet to the floor.

~VINYASA~

Take this vinyasa all of the way through to sitting

Drishti ~ **Nose**

Comments - This is the least supported of the seven headstands. The amount of weight on the head has increased. You may find that slightly bending the elbows and/or moving the hands slightly forward will help to gain stability when learning this asana. Once you are able to practice all seven you may work toward moving from one to the next without coming down in between. This requires even more control and should not be attempted without having first become stable while practicing them individually.

Do Not Be In A Hurry! Endurance and Strength Will Come In Time!

Entering the Finishing Sequence

"Keeping the Focus"

The finishing sequence is the second piece of **"bread"** forming the Ashtanga **"sandwich"**. The Sun Salutations and the Standing Sequence are the first slice of bread, and the Primary or Intermediate Series is the **"filling"**. I will now give some general guidelines for the unique dynamics of the Finishing Sequence. The routine is initiated with three backbends which are countered by forward bending.

Backward Bending & Forward Lengthening

When practicing backward bending, it is helpful to think of the forward lengthening which is also occurring. In order to have an effective backbend we must learn to lift and lengthen the front of our body. This lifting and lengthening is made possible by creating a strong foundation with the hands and feet. It is from those four points that our backbends and forward lifts will arise. I will give a variety of backbend choices on pages 208-209. Before picking one, it is crucial to find a solid grounding point for the hands and feet. Many students make the mistake of taking all of the work into the arms and lower back without utilizing the legs. That is asking for lower back pain. The legs and feet must create a harmonious union of effort with the arms and hands.

The triangular base on the bottom of each foot should also be involved. There is a tendency to turn the toes out to the sides like **"Charlie Chaplin"** when entering a backbend. That allows us to feel that we are getting deep into the posture, when in fact, the turning out of the feet creates undue strain in the lumbar area of the spine. It is best to keep the feet parallel to each other. You also want to feel the weight distributed evenly across the entire surface area of each hand. This will help to avoid undue pressure in the wrists.

Back-bending asanas are an incredible tool to keep the spine supple and healthy. The spine houses our nerve core. By keeping it flexible, we allow cleaner pathways for the nerve signals to travel. Choose the option that most suits your needs. Work patiently and move with your breath. It is always wiser to omit a posture, or to work toward it later with supervision, than it is to push too far too fast and become discouraged. Find the joy of backward bending. Feel the exhilaration from prana flowing in the body and the heart opening as the spine arches. Rejoice in the opening of your heart!

Backbending postures are always countered by forward bending, just as upward dog is always followed by downward dog. This helps to bring us back to a neutral point.

Entering the Finishing Sequence

"Keeping the Focus"

Turning Upside Down

Now, it is time to view life from a different vantage point, inversions. The inverted sequence is initiated with the shoulderstand and followed by the headstand. When we turn the body upside down, we create a new and slightly bewildering view of the world. With this perspective there is a natural fear which accompanies it. It is difficult to distinguish right from left and front from back. This confusion of perspective coupled with a feeling that there is a possibility of falling is the seat of our fear. It is a fear of the unknown. Some fear is necessary in life. There are fears that keep us alive and there are fears that keep us from living. The fear that keeps us from taking risks that may harm us is healthy. There are other fears that may keep us from having a wonderful experience. We may create limits far below our potential by remaining strictly within the realms of life which are familiar to us. This type of fear may keep us from living as fully as we might without them. The trick is to identify which is which. We must find a balance.

I have a fear of heights. In Greece I challenged myself to jump from a tall cliff into the ocean. I had fully inspected the area beforehand and knew that the water was deep. I had a friend with me that had made the jump many times. He was able to give helpful hints and encouraging words. It took me hours of contemplating my fears before I finally made the leap. After completing the jump, I was exhilarated. It was a fear overcome, yet I also understood that there is a limit to how high a human may safely jump without harm. We each must determine our boundaries and respect them. We should not persistently seek out that which frightens us. But by confronting an occasional personal challenge, we may discover increased self-confidence by moving past some of our fears. This confidence may filter directly into the very fabric of our daily lives.

If you have no fear of practicing an inversion then this may have no bearing for you. For those who do find this a challenging prospect, then I want to encourage you. I will present safe and effective methods of approach for each inversion with a variety of choices. **Remember: skipping an asana is always a valid option**. Build your confidence over time. It is best to have personal assistance, whenever possible, in learning new asanas. If that is not feasible, then approach them slowly and listen to the body. Keep your breath moving and relax the mind. Inversions are rewarding and full of health benefits. They are however, counter-indicated for certain conditions, such as high blood pressure and retina problems. **If you have any doubts, it is best to consult your physician before practicing inversions**.

The key to inversions is finding our point of balance. We discussed this in the entry into the standing sequence. The same principles apply for inversions. There are opposing forces of rooting and lifting, yet when the world is upside down the application can be confusing. As a general rule keep the ribs drawn in and the legs actively lifting toward the sky. Feel your connection to the earth and grow from there. Use your drishti and the bandhas for additional stability. Avoid sprinting toward the end of your practice in order to reach the "finish line". The beginning is the end. Breathe with awareness and focus. Free the mind. Relish the moment. Capture the magic of life present in each breath. Feel the wonder of consciousness and the pleasure of practicing yoga.

Complete Your Practice One Breath at a Time

Urdhva Dhanurasana

Urdhva = Upward Dhanura = Bow

"Upward Bow Posture"

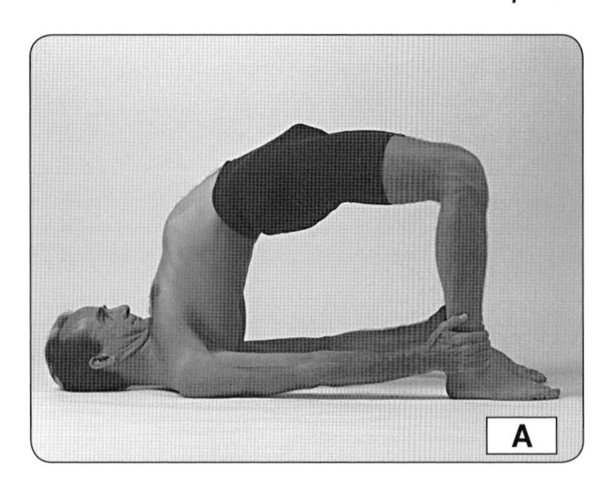

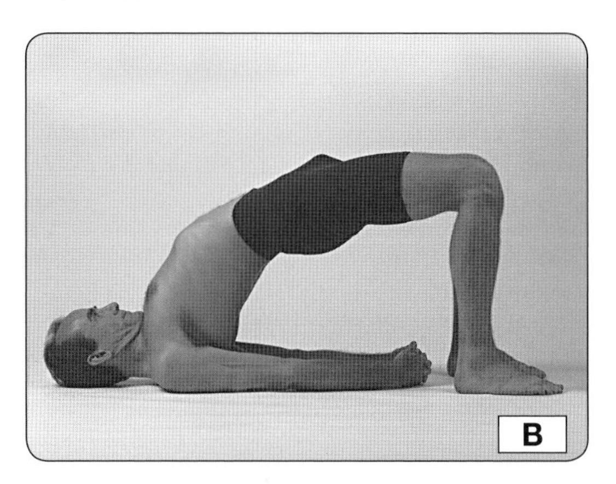

1) **Exhale** lie on your back. Bend the knees and place the feet near the buttocks at a hip's width apart.

2) **Inhale** reach with the hands and grab your ankles. Leave your shoulders on the floor and press the hips up as though you want to touch your navel to the ceiling **(A)**. If you are unable to reach the ankles you may leave the hands on the floor with the fingers interlaced **(B)** or support the hips with the hands **(C)**. If you are familiar with backbends then place the hands under the shoulders **(D)** and press the pelvis toward the sky. Drop the head back. Keep the feet flat on the floor **(E)** or come up onto your toes **(F)**.

Remain Here for 5 Deep Breaths

3) **Exhale** lower to the floor. Remain here for one full breath. **Inhale** and **Exhale**.

Repeat Steps 2 & 3 Two More Times

4) **Inhale** reach around the knees and clasp your hands.

5) **Exhale** give yourself a big hug.

6) **Inhale** and roll up to a sitting position.

Enter the Next Asana from Here

Drishti ~ **Nose**

Comments - If you feel compression of the vertebrae in the lower back then release the posture. This sensation is caused by the lower back being used like a hinge instead of distributing the stretch throughout the spine. Keep the chest open wide by rolling the shoulders back. Engage the legs fully and keep the feet parallel. Feel the balls of the feet pressing down. Open your heart by pushing the feet firmly and evenly into the floor. Rather than focusing on the back, feel the lengthening which occurs on the front side of the body. It is in that lifting that the stretch will find equal distribution. Work with the option that feels most comfortable to you. You may use more than one option since this asana is thrice repeated.

Urdhva Dhanurasana

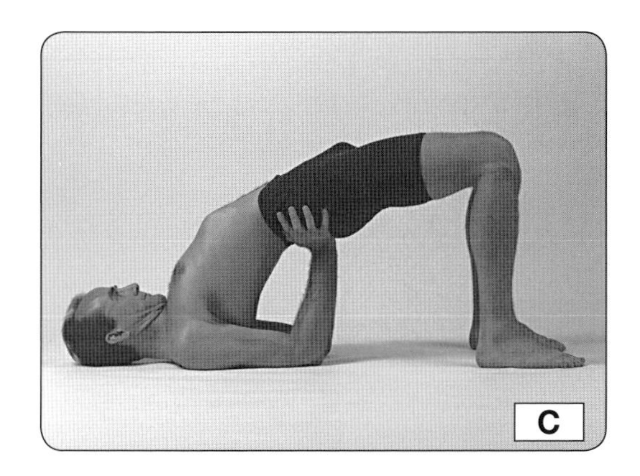

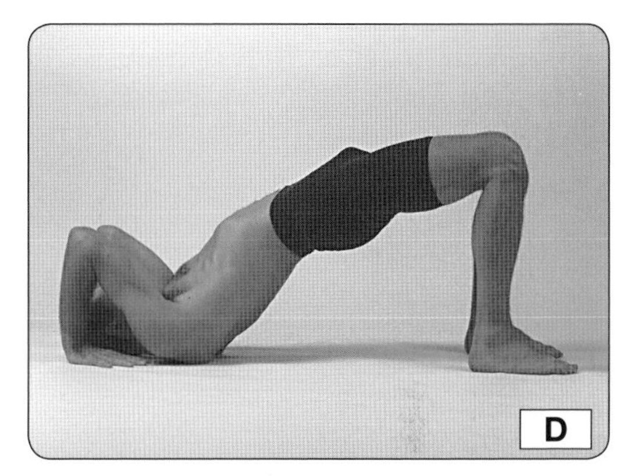

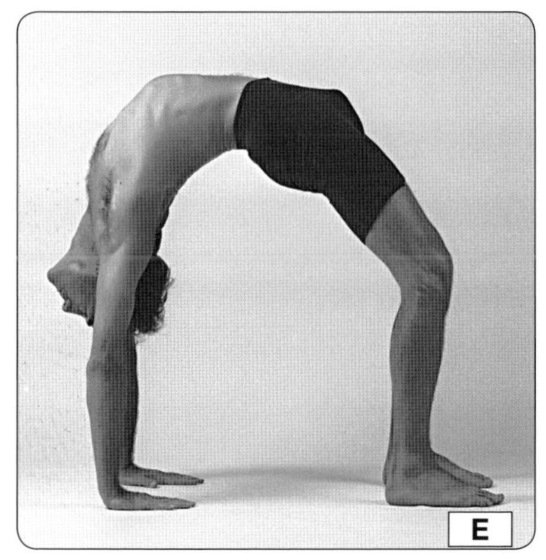

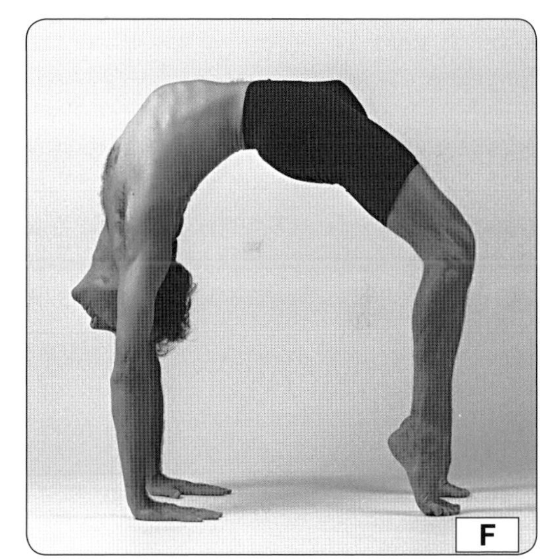

Paschimottanasana A

Paschima = Western   Uttana = Intense Stretch

"Western Intense Stretch Posture"

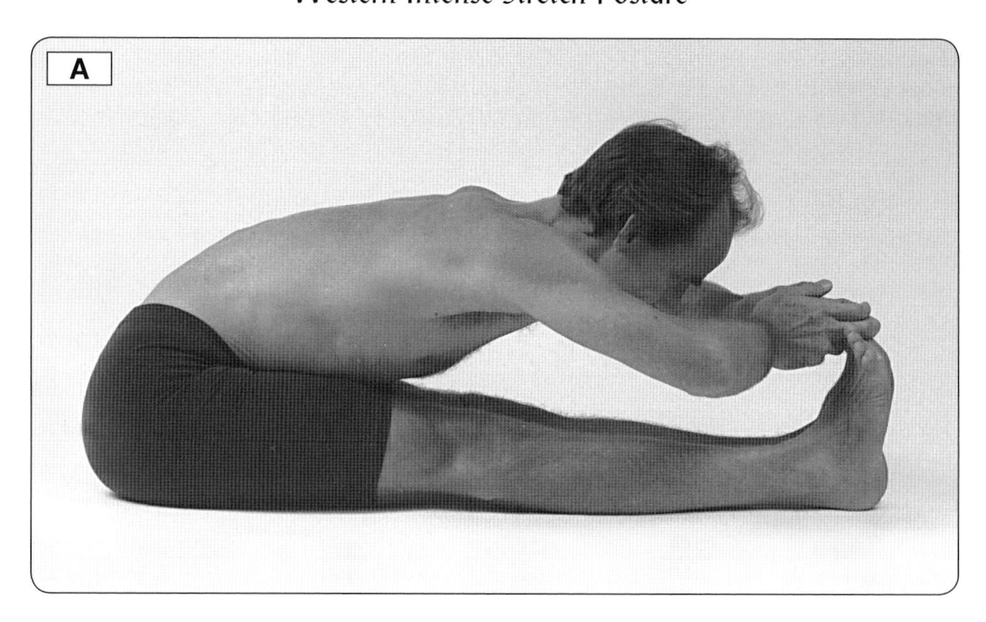

1) **Exhale** fold forward and take the hands to the feet or ankles.

2) **Inhale** lengthen the spine. Gaze to the horizon. Open the chest.

3) **Exhale** fold forward and clasp the big toes with two fingers of each hand **(A)**. If that is too much of a stretch then hold the ankles or shins with the legs straight and the spine long **(B)** or you may bend the knees and either hold the toes or ankles **(C)**.

Remain Here for 5 Deep Breaths

4) **Inhale** lengthen the spine and gaze to the horizon.

5) **Exhale** release the asana.

~VINYASA~

Drishti ~ **Toes**

Comments - This is the same asana as practiced earlier in the Primary Series. Here it is being utilized as a counter-stretch to the three backbends. Fold forward into whichever option is most appropriate and allow the breathing to guide you deeper. Even though the previous asanas are the first ones designated as backbends there are actually many backward bending moments in the practice. Every time that we practice an **Upward-Facing Dog**, during vinyasa, we are engaged in a backbend for that inhale and then the **Downward-Facing Dog** brings us back to a neutral point. While practicing **Paschimottanasana** after backbending, feel the relengthening of the backside of the body.

Paschimottanasana A

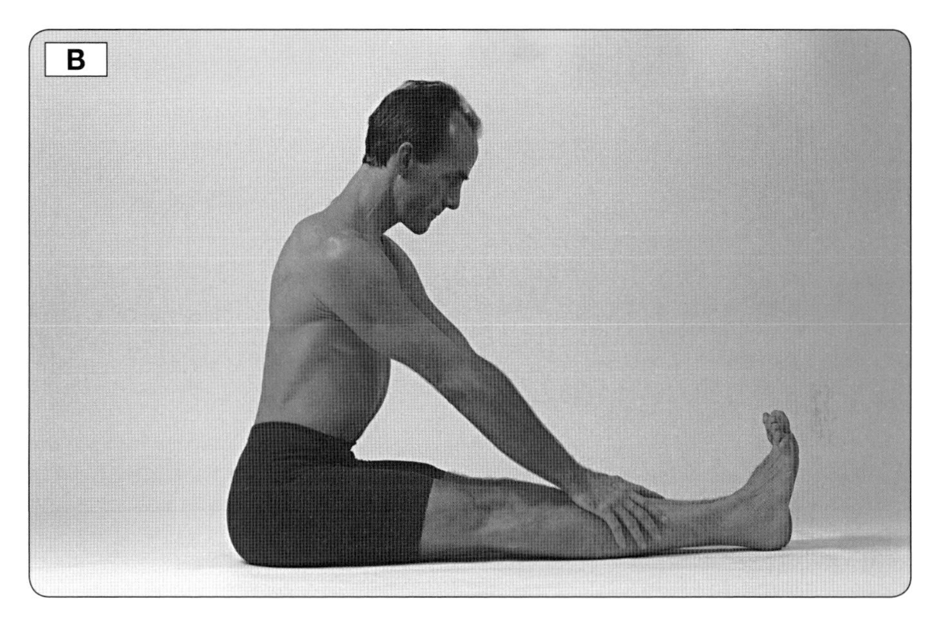

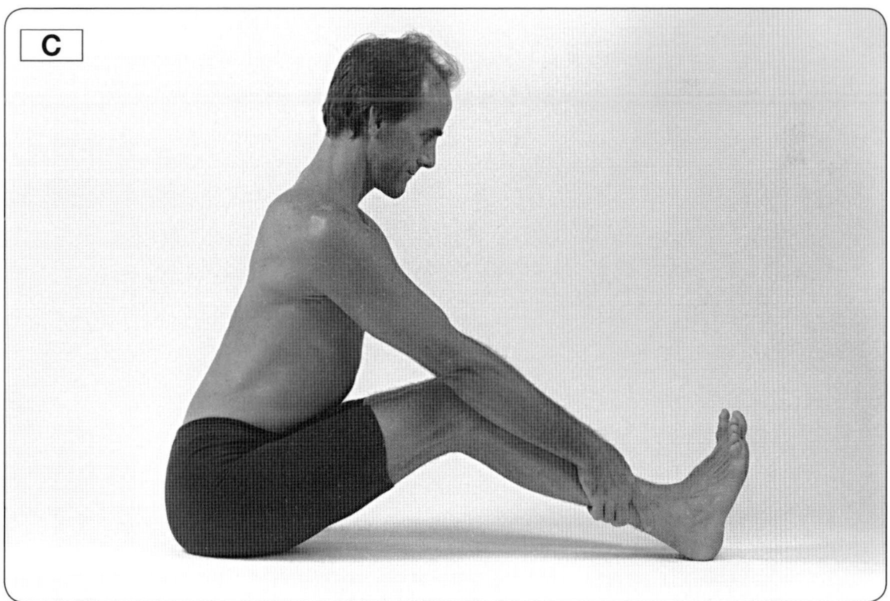

Salamba Sarvangasana

Salamba = Supported   Sarva = All or Whole   Anga = Limb or Body

"Whole Body Supported Posture"

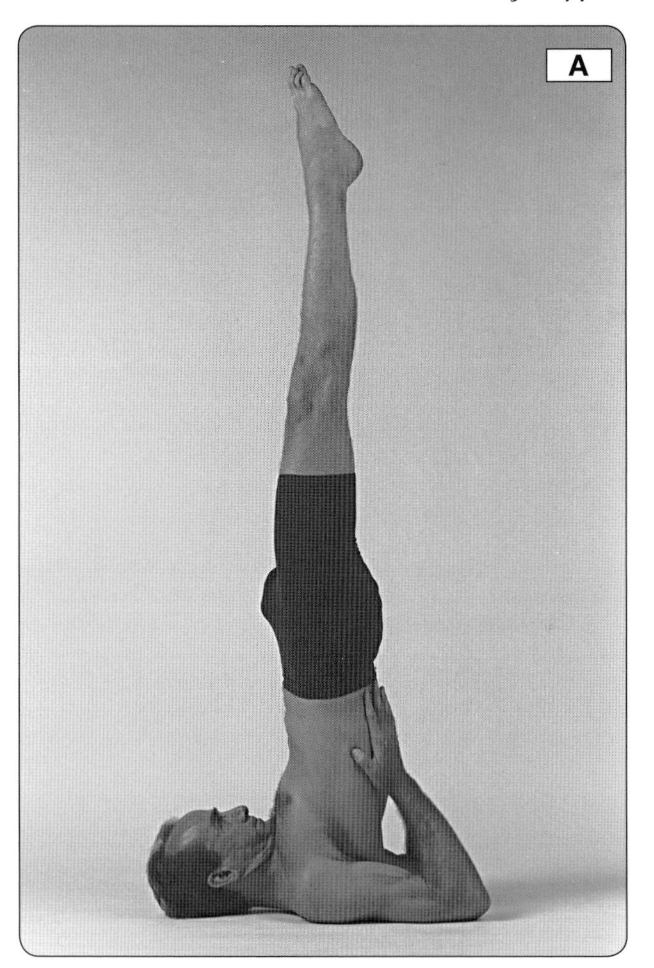

1) **Exhale** roll up onto the shoulders. *(As a preparation for shoulder stand you may take the feet toward the floor over your head. Interlace the fingers behind your back. Straighten the arms onto the floor behind you and then rock from side to side to roll the shoulders together before lifting the feet up. This will assist in keeping the neck free from the floor)*

2) **Inhale** extend the feet toward the sky with the toes pointed. Support the back with both palms close to the spine. Keep the body perpendicular to the floor. Extend from the floor to the sky **(A)**. It may be too extreme to lift the body into such a perpendicular position. If this is so, you may leave the hips in the hands for support rather than higher up the back **(B)**. Another option is to leave the hips on the floor and raise only the legs as you point the toes to the sky **(C)**.

Remain Here for 15 Deep Breaths (or as long as is comfortable)

Enter the Next Asana from Here

Drishti ~ **Nose**

"That which we persist in doing becomes easier
– not that the nature of the task has changed,
but an ability to do it has increased."

Ralph Waldo Emerson

Salamba Sarvangasana

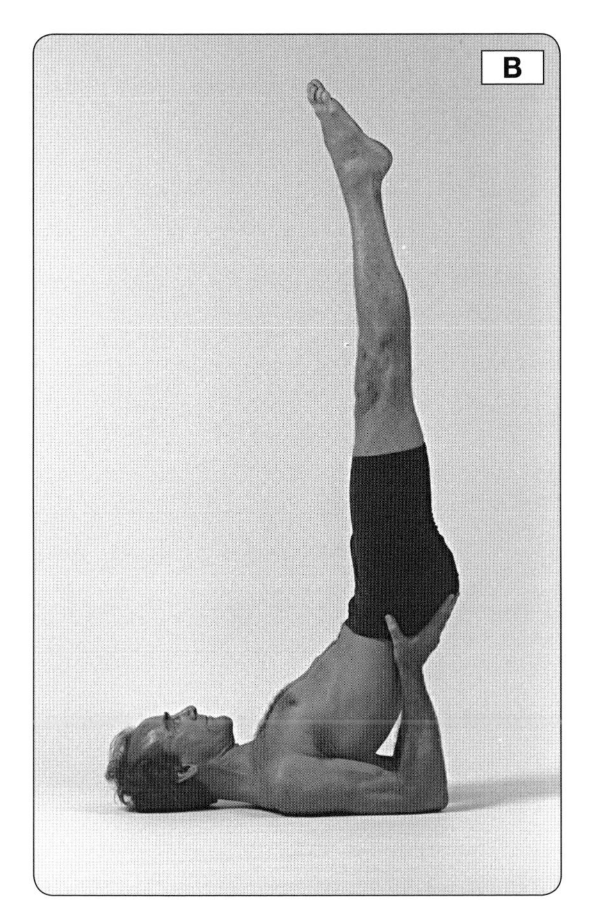

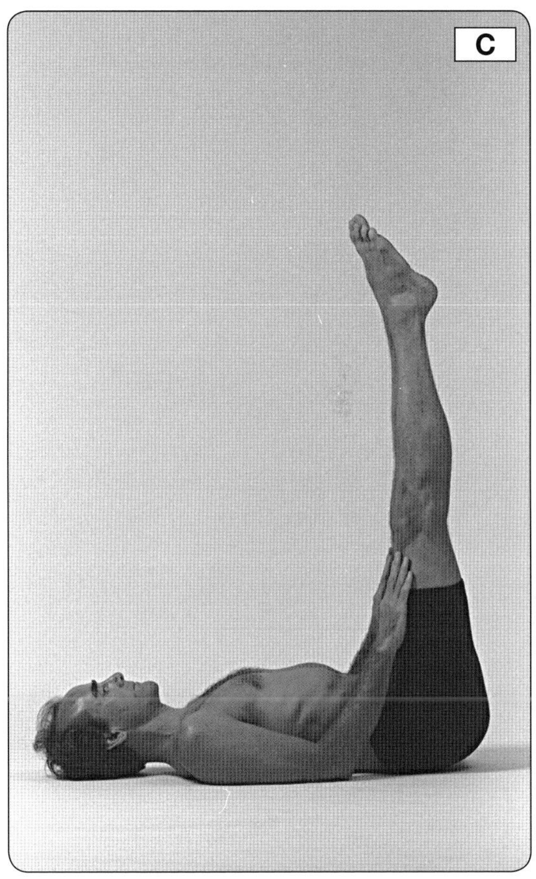

Comments - This asana is generally referred to as the **"Shoulder Stand"**. It is never referred to as the **"Seventh-Cervical Stand"**. The bulk of the weight should be distributed across the shoulders, upper arms and elbows with the vertebrae of the neck free from contact with the floor. That is the reason for the preparatory action of rolling the shoulders under to create lift and space. The natural curvature of the neck should be maintained. ***If you feel discomfort in the neck then back off or come out of the posture***. You may gain full benefits from the inversion without lifting all of the way up. If you are accustomed to using blankets for support the same idea applies to lifting the weight away from the neck. Use the hands against the back to create length in the spine. Distribute the weight across the shoulders, upper arms and elbows.

Halasana

Hala = Plow

"Plow Posture"

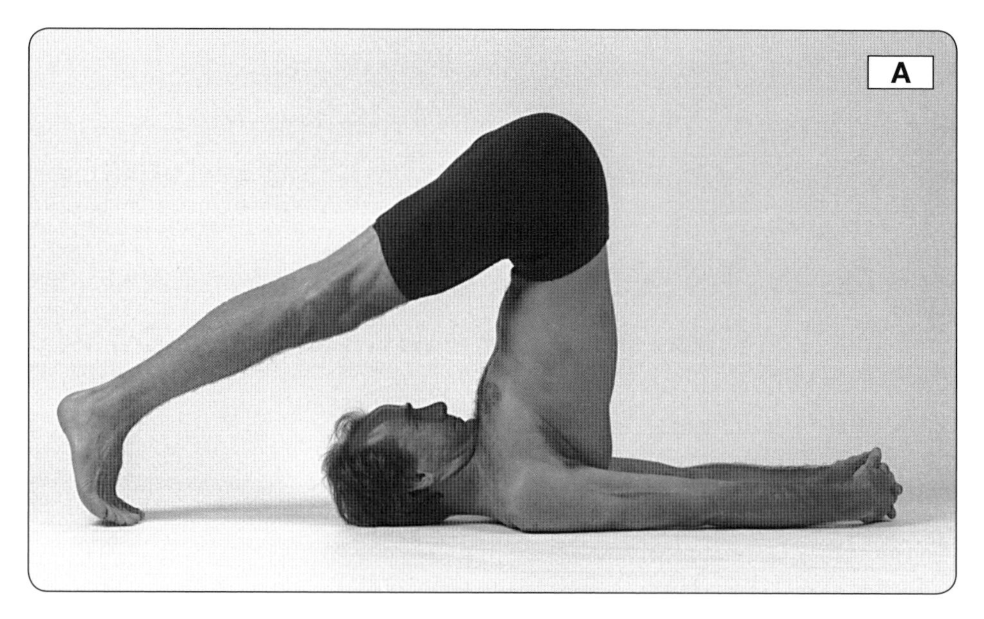

1) **Exhale** lower the feet toward the floor over your head with the feet together. Keep the legs straight and interlace the fingers. Straighten the arms and pull the hands to the floor behind the back **(A)**. If it is too much to take the feet all of the way to the floor you may rest them on a chair behind you as in **(B)** or lower them only halfway to the floor and support the hips with the hands **(C)**.

Remain Here for 5 Deep Breaths

2) **Inhale** release the fingers and place the palms flat on the floor.

Enter the Next Asana from Here

Drishti ~ **Nose**

Comments - ***If you find Halasana and its variations to be too extreme then you may exit after Salamba Sarvangasana and enter Matsyasana on pages 222-223***. If you are continuing into **Halasana** keep the spine lifting as in **Salamba Sarvangasana**. You may maintain a lifting of the neck away from the floor by pulling the shoulders together. If you are practicing option **(A)** push the toes against the floor and lift the sit-bones. These two actions will create a lengthening of the spine. You may also imagine that you are pulling the spine toward the front of the body. The greater spinal length you achieve the more freely the breath will flow. ***If your breath becomes restricted or if you feel discomfort in your neck then come out of the asana***. You may engage all three bandhas throughout the entire **Shoulder Stand** sequence.

Halasana

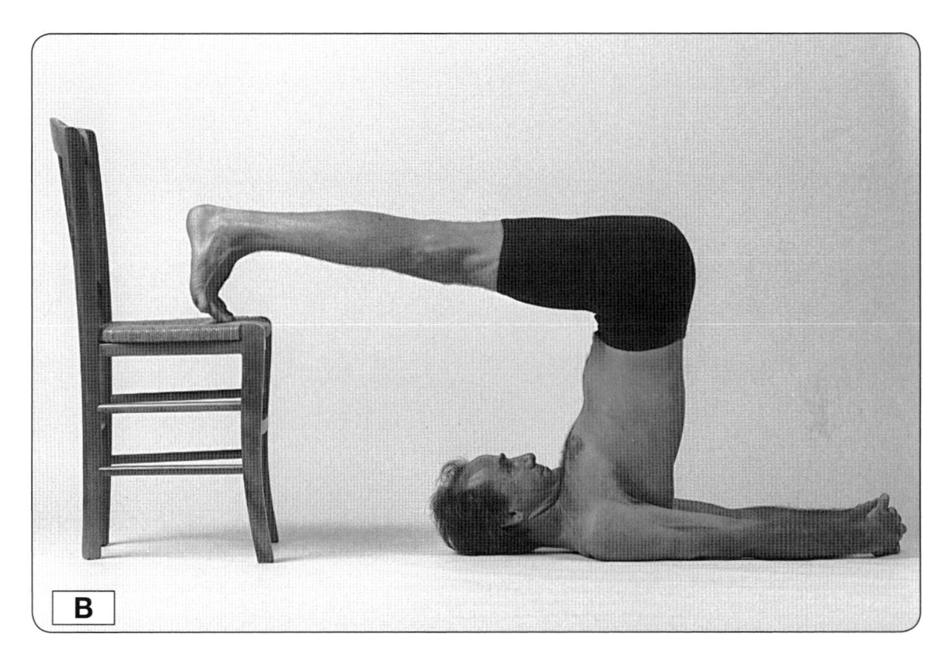

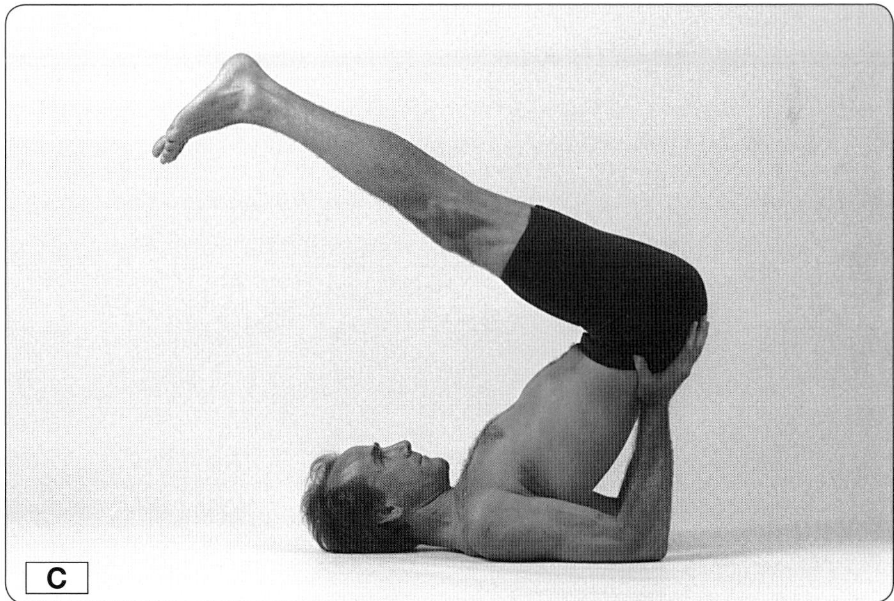

Karnapidasana

Karna = Ear   Pida = Pressure

"Ear Pressure Posture"

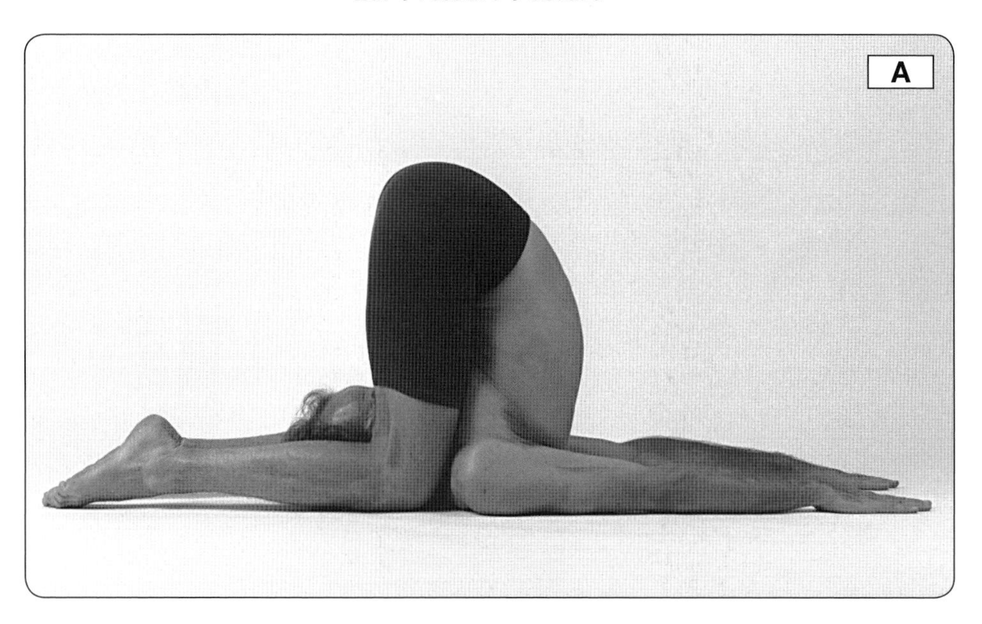

1) **Exhale** as you exit from the previous posture. Lower the knees toward the floor close to the ears. Keep the arms straight. The arms should be outstretched behind you with the palms facing the floor **(A)**. If it is too much to take the knees all of the way down you may take them partially toward the floor and support the back with the hands as in **(B)** or take the hips into the hands for support and bend the knees and draw them in toward the chest **(C)**. If you do not find any options above to be appropriate at this time then repeat one of the previous postures or come out and move into **Matsyasana** on pages 222-223.

Remain Here for 5 Deep Breaths

Enter the Next Asana from Here

Drishti ~ **Nose**

Comments - If you are practicing option **(A)** and your knees are on the floor then you may gently press the knees against the ears. This action is the source of the posture's name, "Ear Pressure". Among its varied health benefits it is thought to relieve ear aches. Whichever option you choose be careful when taking the knees toward the floor. ***Do not force the knees down***. Too much pressure may strain the neck. ***If you feel pain or discomfort in the neck then come out of the posture without delay***. The breath is the guiding factor. Let the inhales and exhales draw you deeper into the asana. If the breath becomes restricted then back off until you can breathe fully without strain. Keep the shoulders rolling in.

Karnapidasana

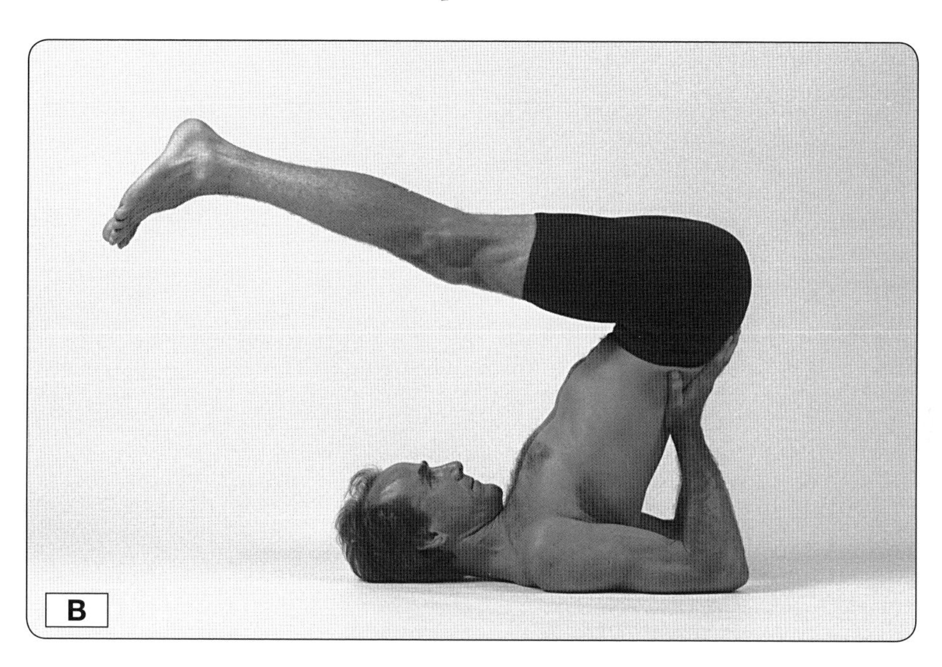

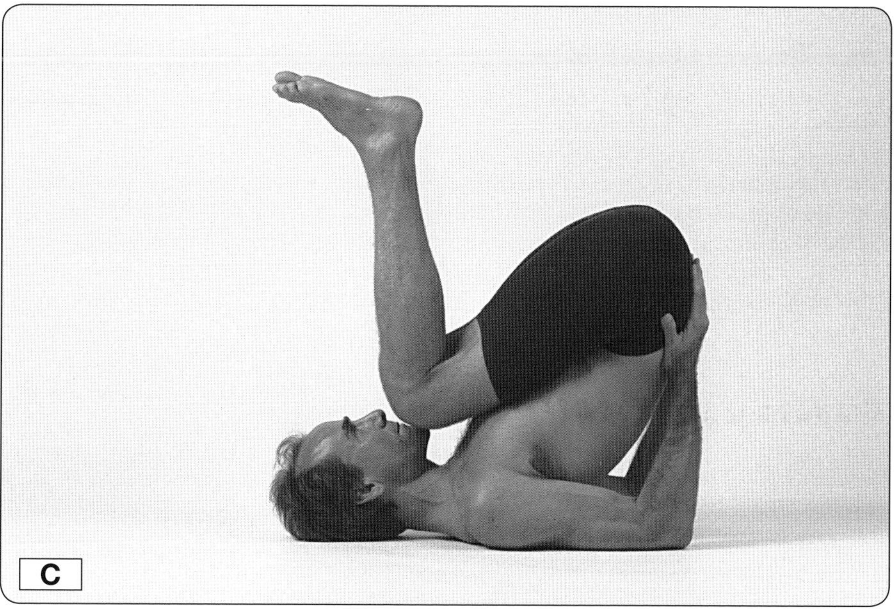

Urdhva Padmasana

Urdhva = Upward Padma = Lotus

"Upward Lotus Posture"

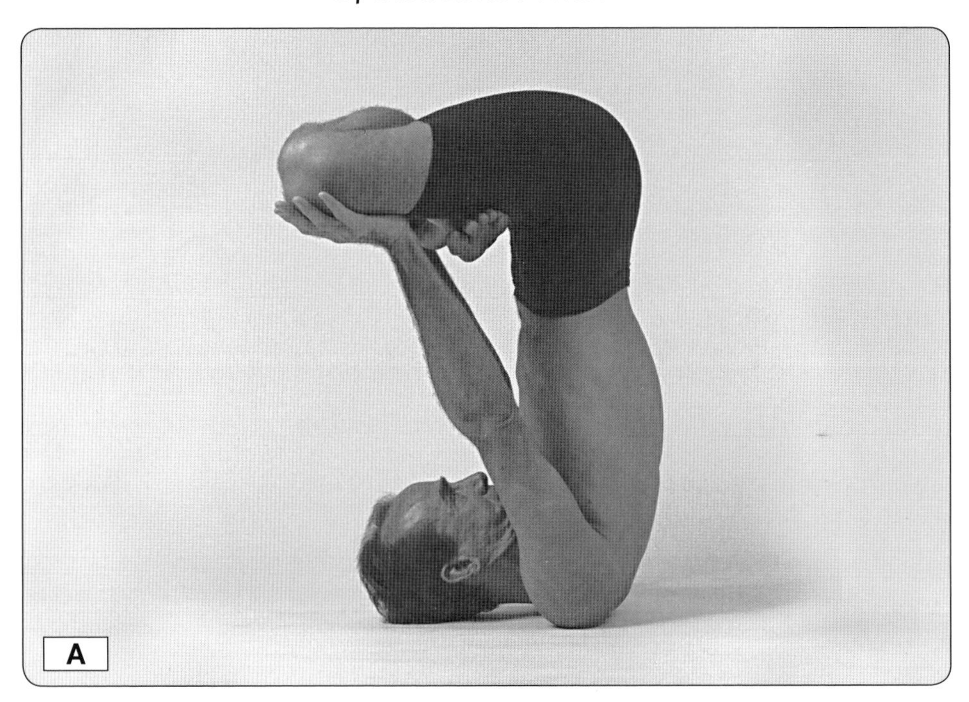

1) **Inhale** lift the feet toward the sky as you return to the **Shoulder Stand** position.

2) **Exhale** take both legs into full-lotus. Place the hands on the knees. Straighten the arms **(A)** or cross the legs without lotus as in **(B)**. If you find that placing the hands on the knees is too difficult, you may support the lower back with the hands while keeping the legs in full-lotus **(C)** or with crossed legs **(D)**. If the above options feel inappropriate, then repeat one of the previous variations of shoulder stand or come out and move into **Matsyasana** on page 222-223.

Remain Here for 5 Deep Breaths

Enter the Next Asana from Here

Drishti ~ **Nose**

Comments - If you are choosing one of the above options you may gain greater lift in the back by extending the arms upward like two stilts and then pressing the knees into the hands. This opposition of force will create a lifting and lengthening of the spine. This lengthening process affords more space for the lungs to expand so that you may maintain deep breathing without hindrance. Keep the shoulders rolling under.

Urdhva Padmasana

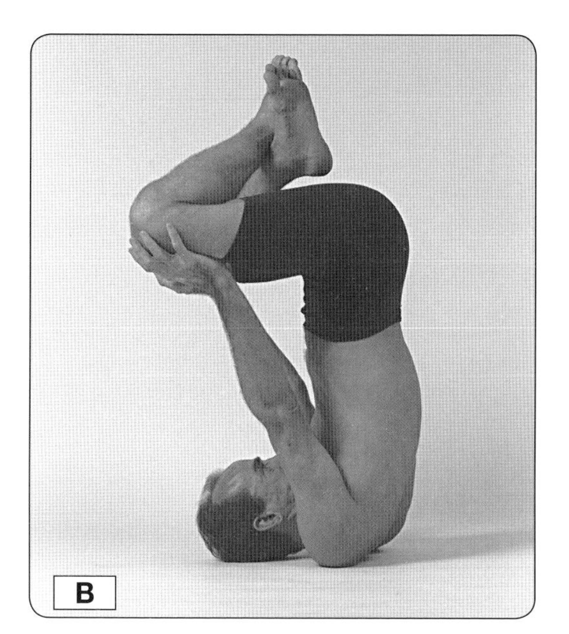
B

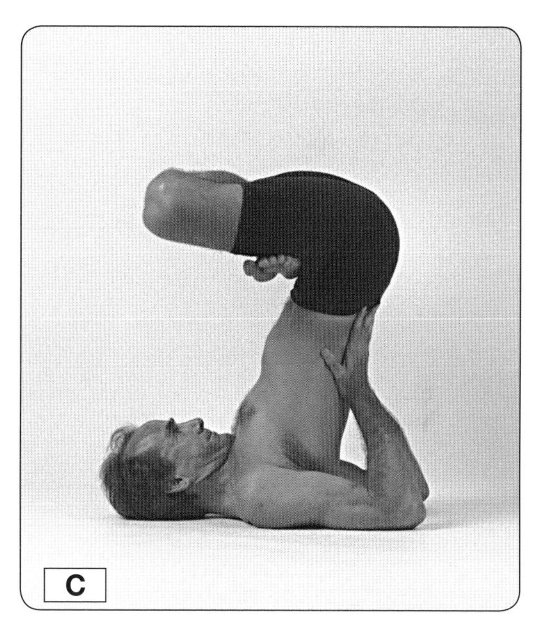
C

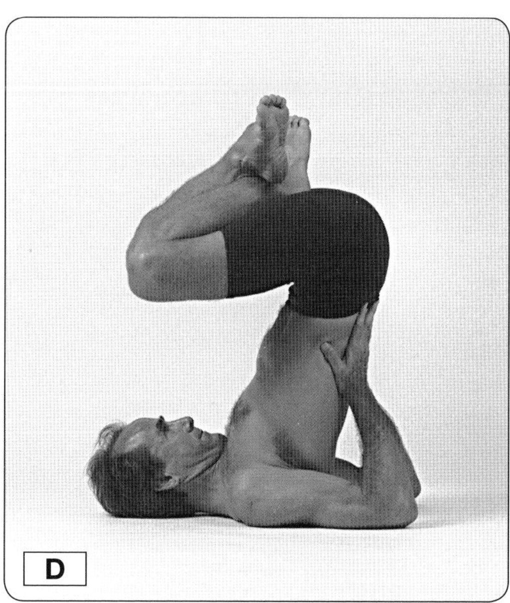
D

Pindasana

Pinda = Embryo

"Embryo Posture"

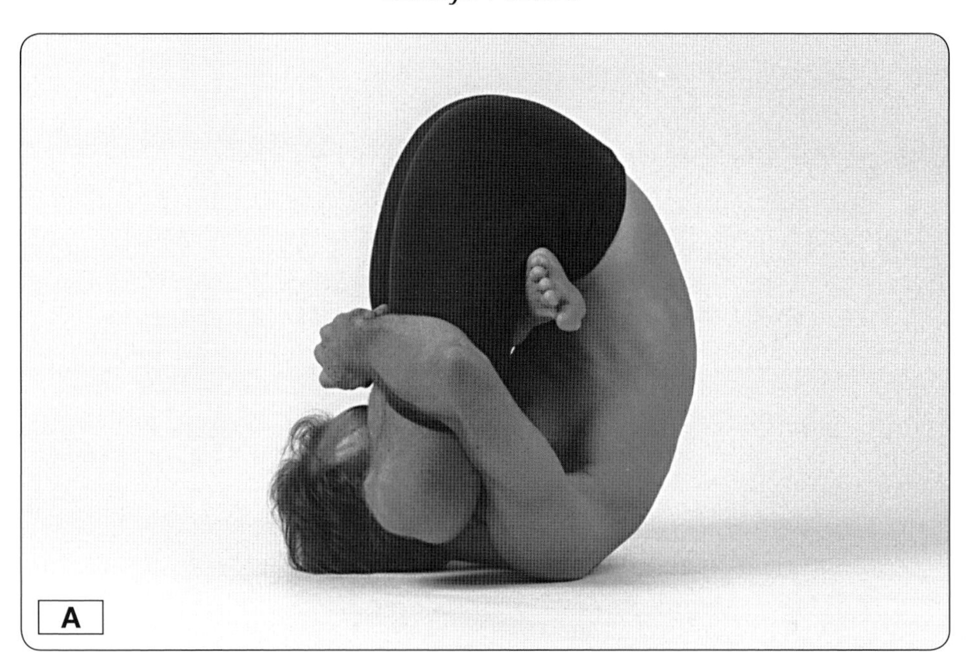

A

1) **Exhale** as you lower the legs toward your chest from whichever option you chose in the previous asana. If you were in lotus then reach around the outer thighs and clasp the hands behind the legs **(A)**. If you are not in full lotus and are unable to clasp the hands you may hold the ankles with crossed legs **(B)** or place the hands on the hips or lower back for support **(C)**. If you choose to omit these options for now, you may come out and move into **Matsyasana** on page 222-223.

Remain Here for 5 Deep Breaths

Enter the Next Asana from Here

Drishti ~ **Nose**

Comments - If you are flexible enough you may rest your legs on your forehead. As usual be careful of your neck. Come out if there is discomfort. Be sure that your breath does not become restricted. For this asana we are to make our body as small as possible just as an embryo is curled within the womb. Be careful that you do not roll back too much onto the head. This may cause strain to the neck. Distribute weight evenly across the shoulders. ***If you feel discomfort in the neck or if your breathing is restricted, Come Out.***

Pindasana

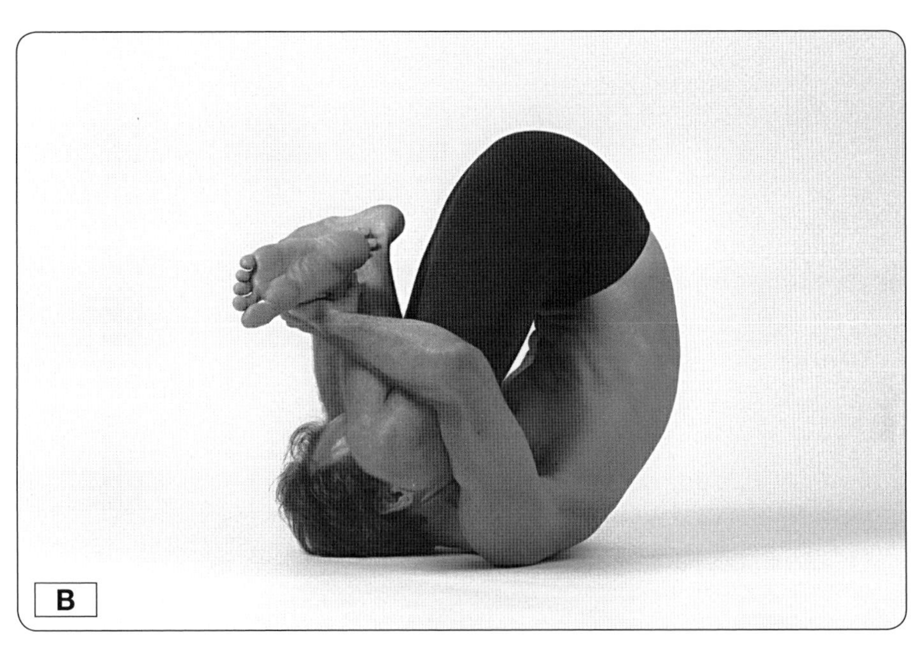
B

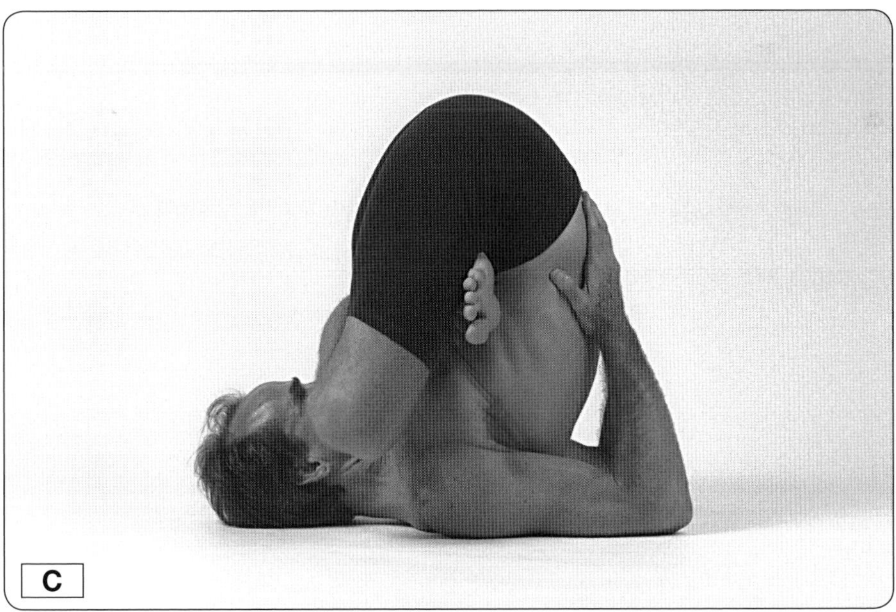
C

Matsyasana

Matsya = Fish

"Fish Posture"

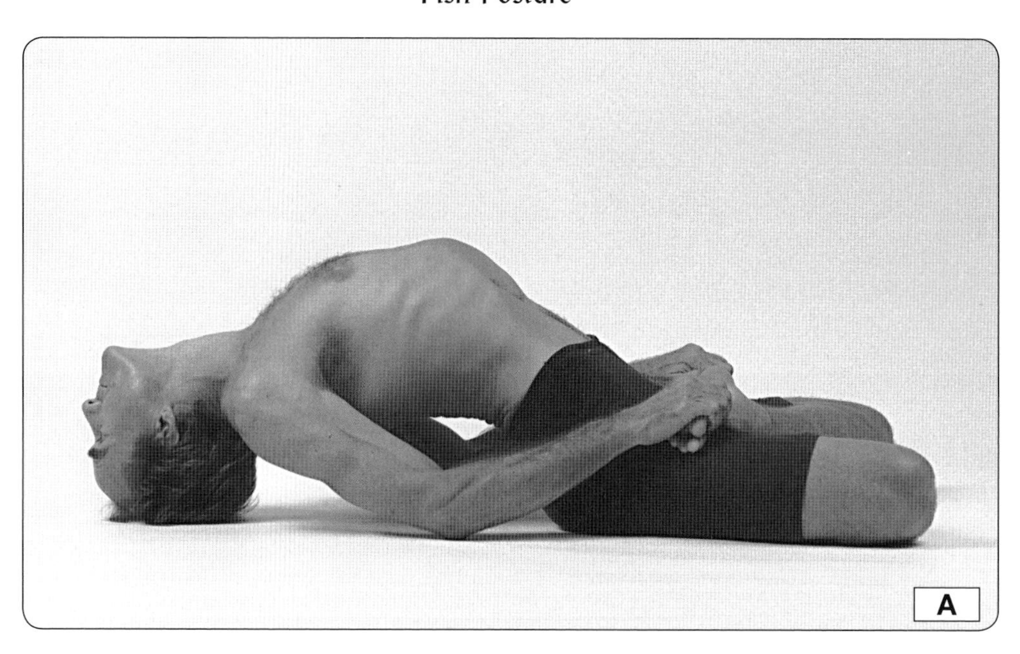

1) **Exhale** as you exit from **Pindasana** by placing the hands on the floor behind the back with arms straight. Roll down slowly using the abdominal muscles to resist until the hips and legs reach the floor. If in full lotus then grab the feet with both hands. Pull the elbows toward the floor without them actually touching down. Lift the chest and drop the head back until the crown touches the floor **(A)**. If you are not in lotus, you may cross the legs and hold the thighs as you press the elbows down to the floor **(B)** or you may keep the legs straight and the hands under the hips as in **(C)**. If placing the head on the floor is too intense, then take it only partially back **(D)**.

Remain Here for 5 Deep Breaths

Enter the Next Asana from Here

Drishti ~ **Nose**

Comments - This asana is the counter-pose for the previous inversions in which the chin has been locked into the chest and **Jalandhara Bandha** has been engaged. By lifting the chin and drawing the head back there is a surge of blood sent to the throat area. This benefits the thyroid. With the chest expanding fully the breath is encouraged. Feel the surge of life force moving through the spine.

Matsyasana

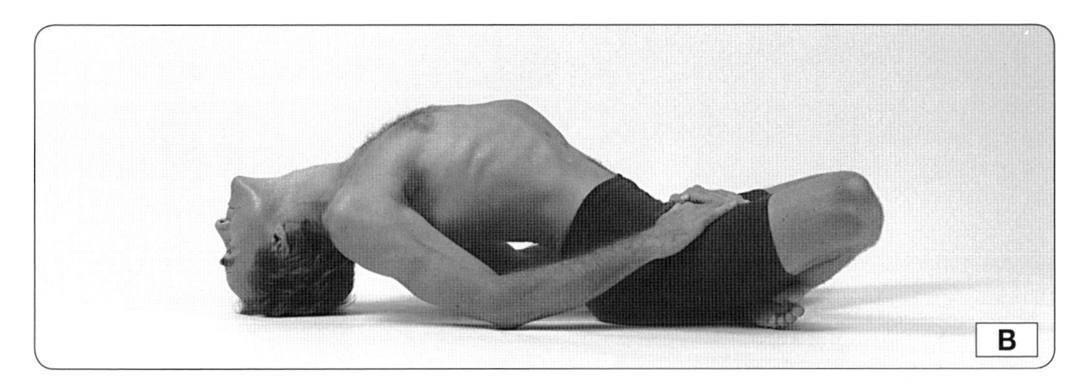

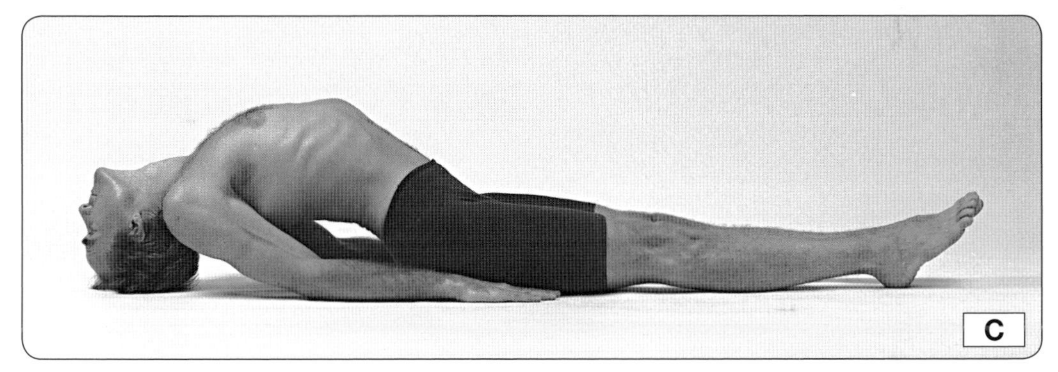

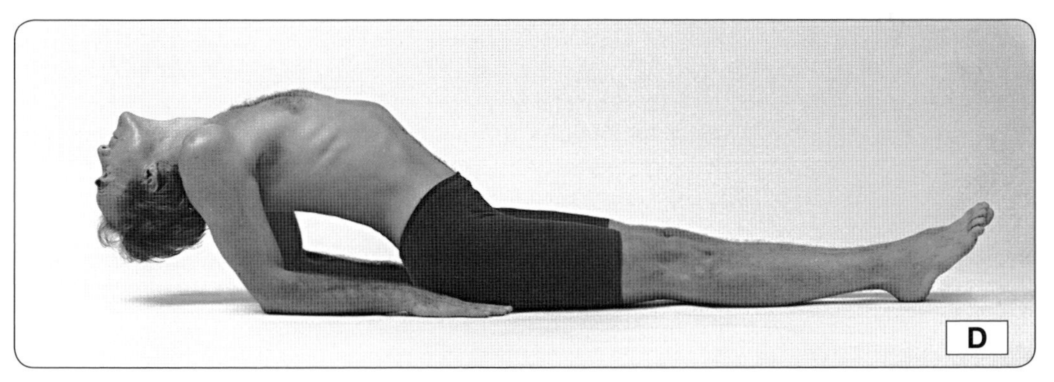

Uttana Padasana

Uttana = Extended   Pada = Leg or Foot

"Extended Leg Posture"

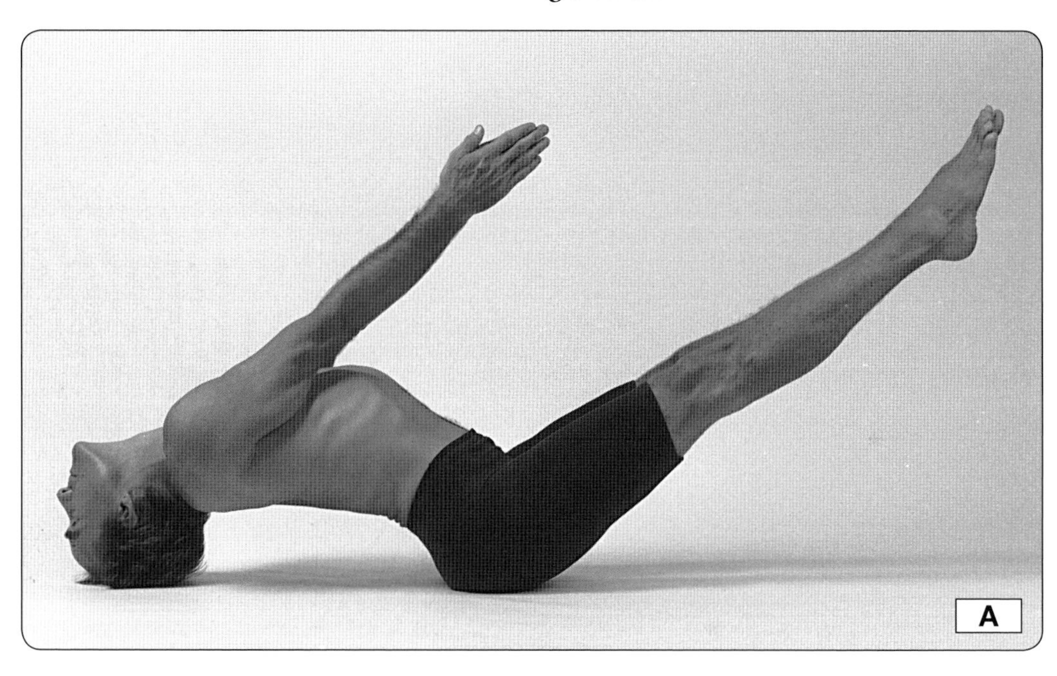

1) **Inhale** straighten the legs as you lift them forty-five degrees from the floor with the toes pointed and the feet together. Raise the arms parallel to the legs with the palms touching **(A)**. If lifting the legs and arms simultaneously is too intense you may place the hands under the buttocks and lift only the legs **(B)** or instead of lifting the feet you may leave the legs on the floor and raise only the arms **(C)**.

Remain Here for 5 Deep Breaths

~CHAKRASANA~

Remember your options for Chakrasana described on pages 120-121

Enter the Next Asana from Downward Dog

Drishti ~ **Nose**

Comments - When lifting the legs it is important that the abdominal bandhas are engaged. This will support the lower back. Keep the legs fully active and extend all of the way through the balls of the feet and toes. When lifting the arms extend fully from the shoulders all of the way through the fingertips. Lift the chest in order to keep excess weight from settling in the neck. Keep the feet glued together and the palms touching.

Uttana Padasana

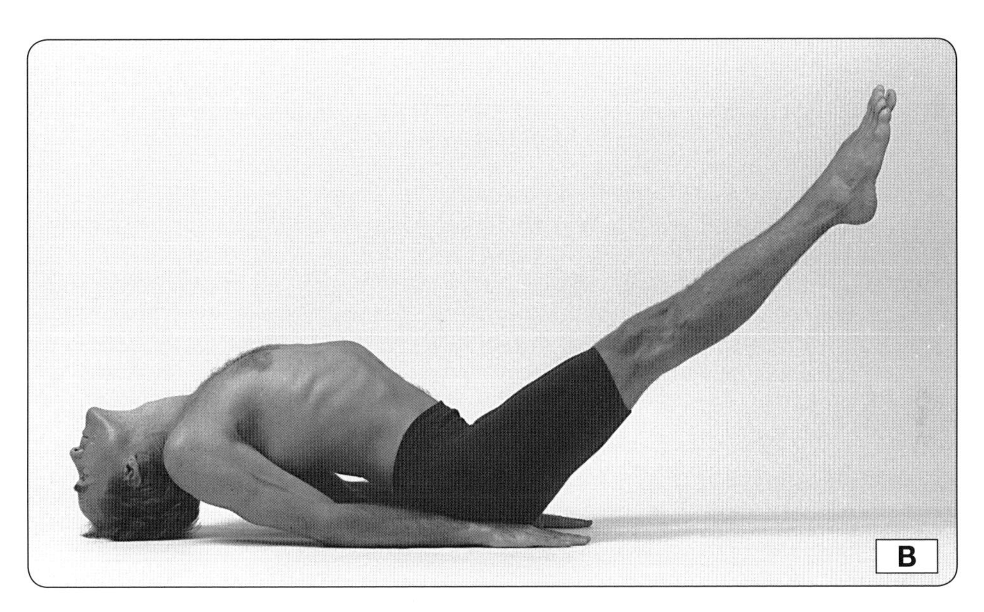

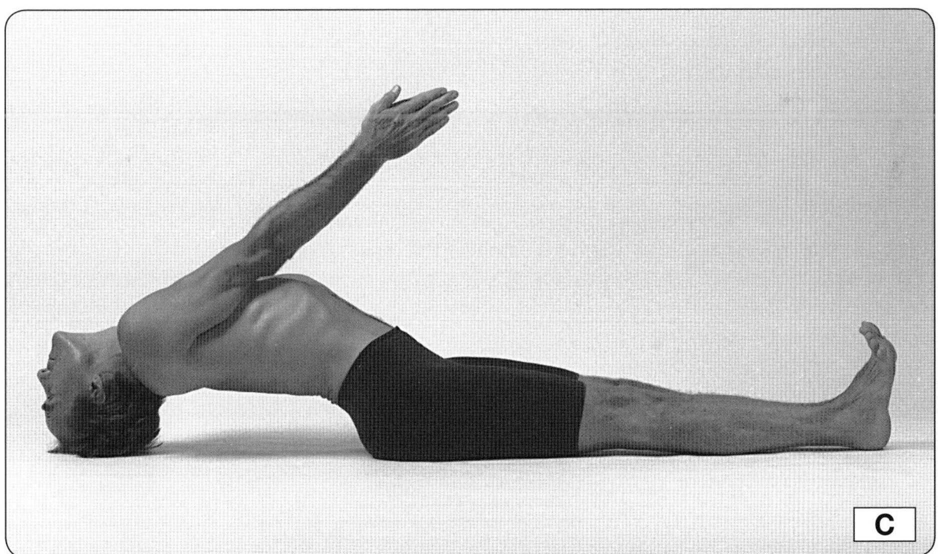

Entering the Headstand

"Support With Confidence"

It is time to enter the headstand. I would like to give some preparatory options and hints as to this asana's unique dynamics. I recommend that you review these steps before entering **Sirsasana**. I mentioned, in the "**Entering the Finishing Sequence**" section, there is a fear factor surrounding inversions. Headstand tends to be a bit scarier than shoulderstand. We must learn the art of supporting ourselves with confidence. The key to practicing headstand with the least amount of energy and the greatest amount of stability is to build a solid foundation. On the next page you will find a variety of suggestions with corresponding photos. **Sirsasana** is one of the most dynamic postures in all of the series! When I find the sweet spot of least resistance there is an exhilaration which accompanies it. This zone of balance is located within our central core. There is an imaginary vertical line around which we may build the headstand. Even though it is called a headstand, **Sirsasana** may truly be considered an arm balance. That is where the vast majority of our weight will be distributed. Below is a step-by-step procedure to build a sturdy base.

Building The Foundation

1) Come to a kneeling position. Place your elbows on the floor, shoulder's width apart.

2) Reach around the upper arms so that the fingers wrap around the outside **(A)**. That is how far apart the elbows should remain. There is a tendency for the elbows to run away from each other. Make a concerted effort to keep them in place.

3) Lace the fingers together. Place the little-finger-side of the hands against the floor **(B)**.

4) Place the center of the top of the head on the floor and allow the back of the head to be gently cradled in the palms **(C)**.

The Feet Begin Their Journey Toward The Sky

5) Straighten your legs. Walk the feet toward you. Lift the hips. Lengthen the spine **(D)**. ***If you have never done a headstand you may remain at this phase and still receive benefits from being inverted.***

6) In order to lift the feet from the floor it will be necessary to transfer your weight behind you. This will actually create a momentary unbalancing. This unbalancing is what will draw the feet upward. The trick is to bring the hips back to the center line as the feet rise. Otherwise, the weight which was lifting the feet will become the same source for the entire body to fall over backwards. It is a matter of getting used to being upside-down and feeling the transferral of weight. As you begin to move your hips back, feel the weight moving from the feet into the arms and bend your knees to allow the feet to rise **(E)**.

7) As you gain control you may begin to straighten the legs. Maintain awareness of the weight distribution in your arms. Spread it evenly from the elbows, across the wrists and to the outer edges of your hands. Keep some weight on the top of your head but ***not*** a disproportionate amount. If you feel the elbows lifting, you will need to lower the legs a bit to regain your balance.

Entering the Headstand

"Support With Confidence"

Be aware of the space around you before going up. It is best not to use a wall when learning headstand. It would be better to remain in one of the options offered with the feet grounded. From there you may gain strength and balance to support yourself in time. When using a wall you may be misaligned. The weight may not be supported sufficiently on your arms yet you will remain upright because of the wall. In the long run it will be safer and you will gain more confidence by building slowly from the ground up. **It is best to have the guidance and hands-on assistance of a qualified instructor when learning yoga**. If this is not possible, then we must do the best we can and move slowly and carefully with awareness. If you have never done a headstand then it is best to keep the feet on the floor. ***There are some physical conditions which are counter-indicated for inverted postures. If you have any doubts, consult your physician first!***

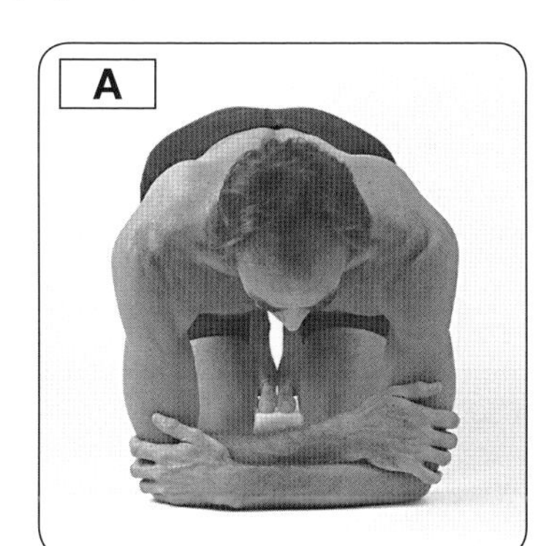

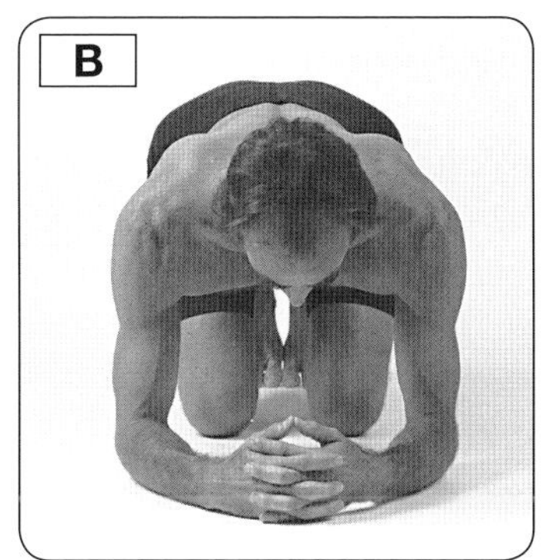

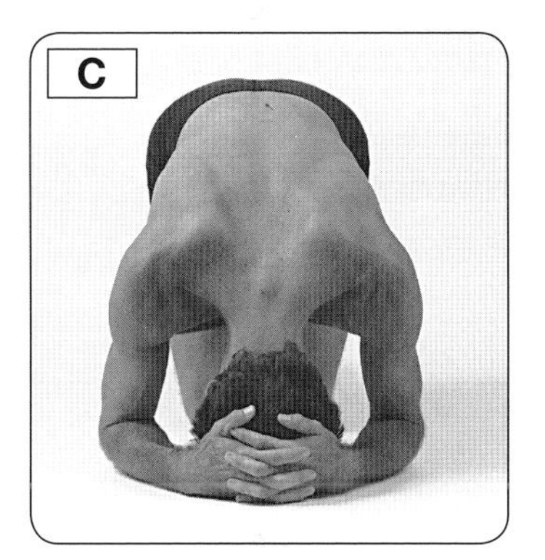

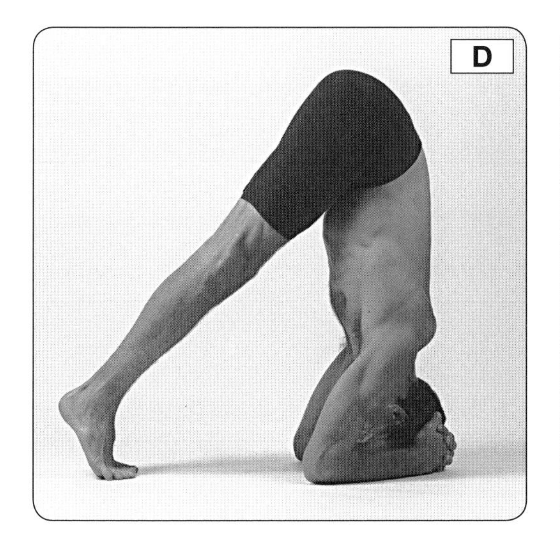

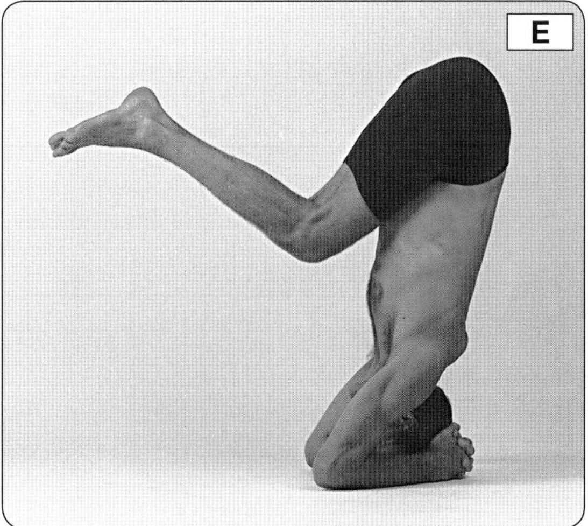

Sirsasana A

Sirsa = Head

"Head Standing Posture"

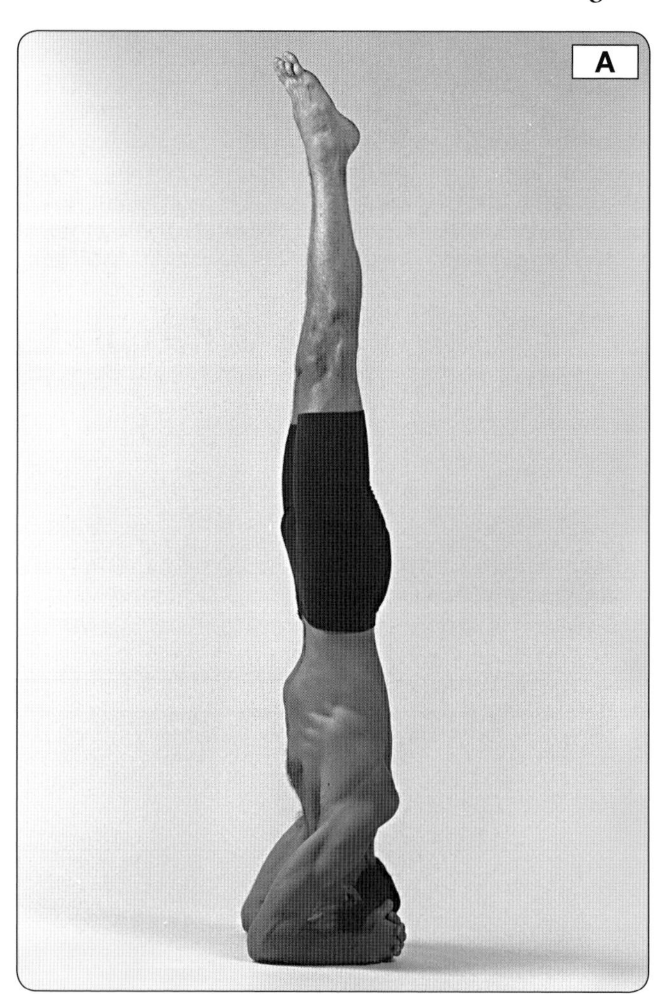

1) **Inhale** from **Downward Dog** and come into a kneeling position.

2) **Exhale** place your elbows on the floor about a shoulder's width apart. Lace the fingers together and put the little-finger-side of the hands on the floor so that the arms form a triangular base. Place the top of the head on the floor between the hands with the back of the head touching the palms.

3) **Inhale** straighten the legs and walk the feet toward your face. Lift the feet away from the floor and take the toes toward the sky with the body fully supported on the elbows, forearms, wrists and head **(A)**. If lifting the feet away from the floor is frightening or too difficult, you may leave the feet on the floor **(B)** or place them on a chair **(C)**. If you would prefer not to bear weight on your head at all, you may keep the feet on the floor and press the forearms down yet keep the head hovering a couple of inches off of the floor **(D)**.

Remain Here for 25 Deep Breaths (or as long as is comfortable)

Enter the Next Asana from Here

Drishti ~ **Nose**

Sirsasana A

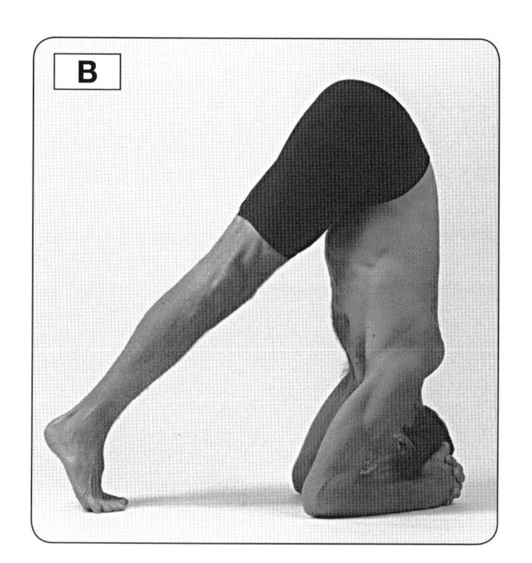

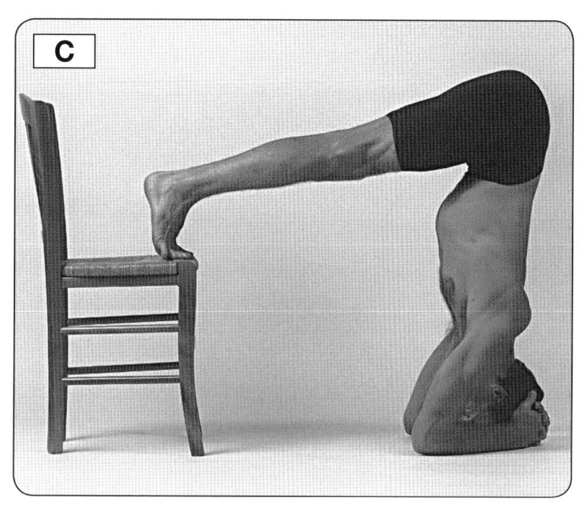

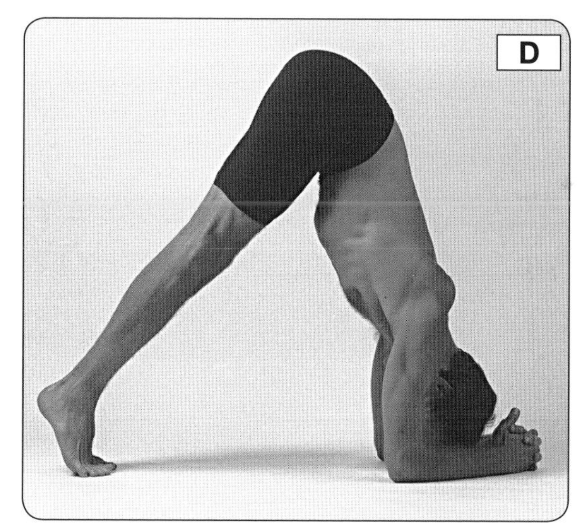

Comments - There is a tendency to push the ribs forward and collapse in the lower back while practicing headstand. Before entering the headstand, stand up and create your best posture with the ribs drawn in and the sit-bones dropped slightly with the legs working. Make a mental note of that feeling of alignment in your body. You may then hold on to that image and reconstruct it when you are in the headstand. Be aware of the contact point on the top of your head. Keep it centered on your crown. Keep the neck straight so that the vertebrae are stacked evenly on top of one another. Remember the majority of weight should be taken by the arms and not the head. Eventually you may take the head fully away from the floor.

Sirsasana B

Sirsa = Head

"Head Standing Posture"

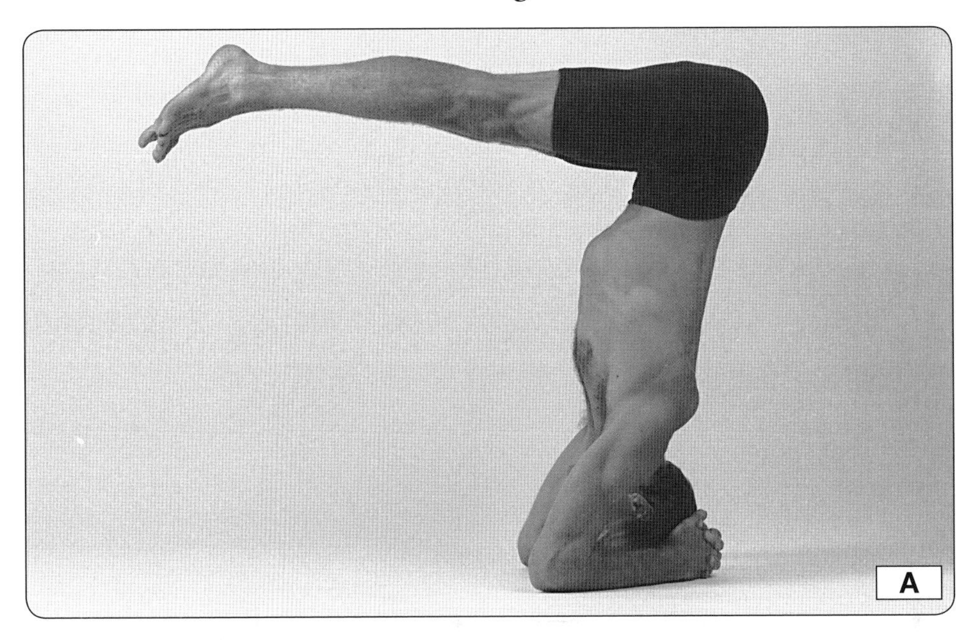

1) **Exhale** lower the legs halfway until they are parallel to the floor. Pause in that position **(A)**. If you find it too difficult to keep the legs straight when lowering them you may bend the knees and lower them part-way toward the chest as in **(B)** otherwise place the feet on a chair **(C)**. If you feel that this asana is too intense then you may exit after **Sirsasana A** and continue on to the final three seated postures.

Remain Here for 5 Deep Breaths

2) **Inhale** go back up to headstand.

3) **Exhale** and lower the feet to the floor.

~VINYASA~

Drishti ~ **Nose**

Comments - As you enter this asana it will be necessary to push the hips back in order to compensate for the legs coming forward. Use the weight distribution as described earlier to find your point of balance. Using weight and counter-weight requires less physical strength. The bandhas must be fully engaged to keep the spine from rounding. Keep the elbows and forearms grounded so that too much weight does not transfer to your head and neck. You should feel the vertebrae stacked evenly upon one another. If the chin is pulled in toward the chest or conversely if the head is tilted back then the vertebral cushions will support the weight more on one side of their circumference instead of evenly distributing it. It is most important to create a strong foundation with the forearms, wrists and outer edges of the hands. If **Sirsasana B** is too intense you may omit it for now and approach it gradually over time.

Sirsasana B

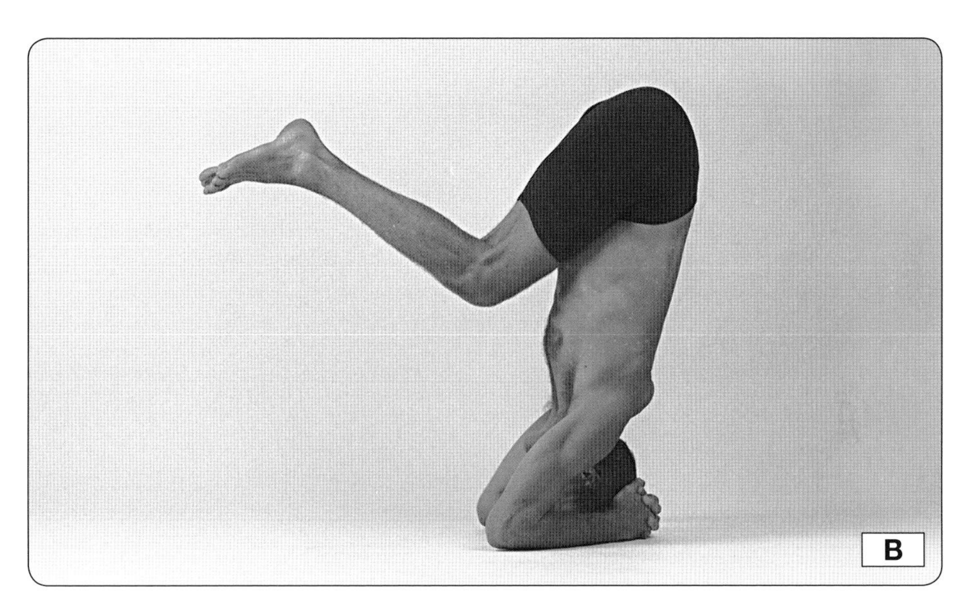

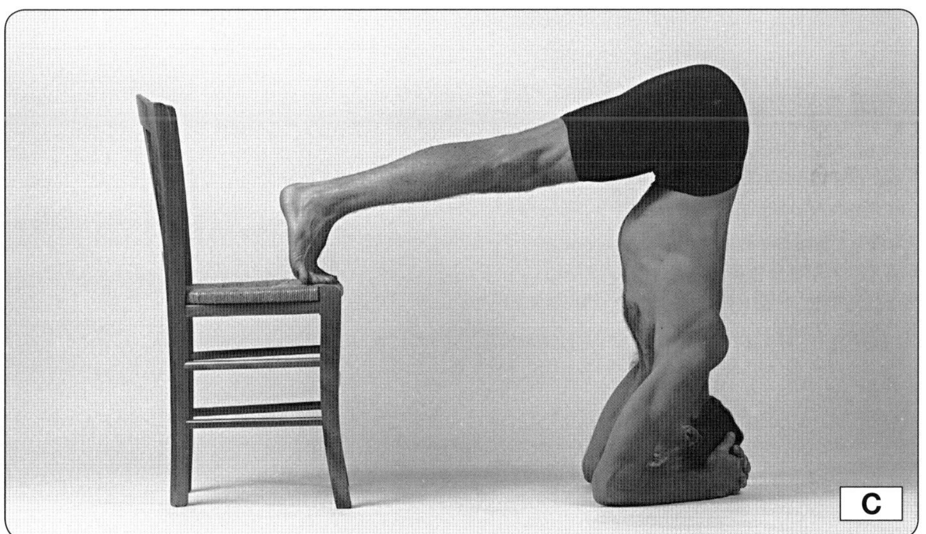

Stillness

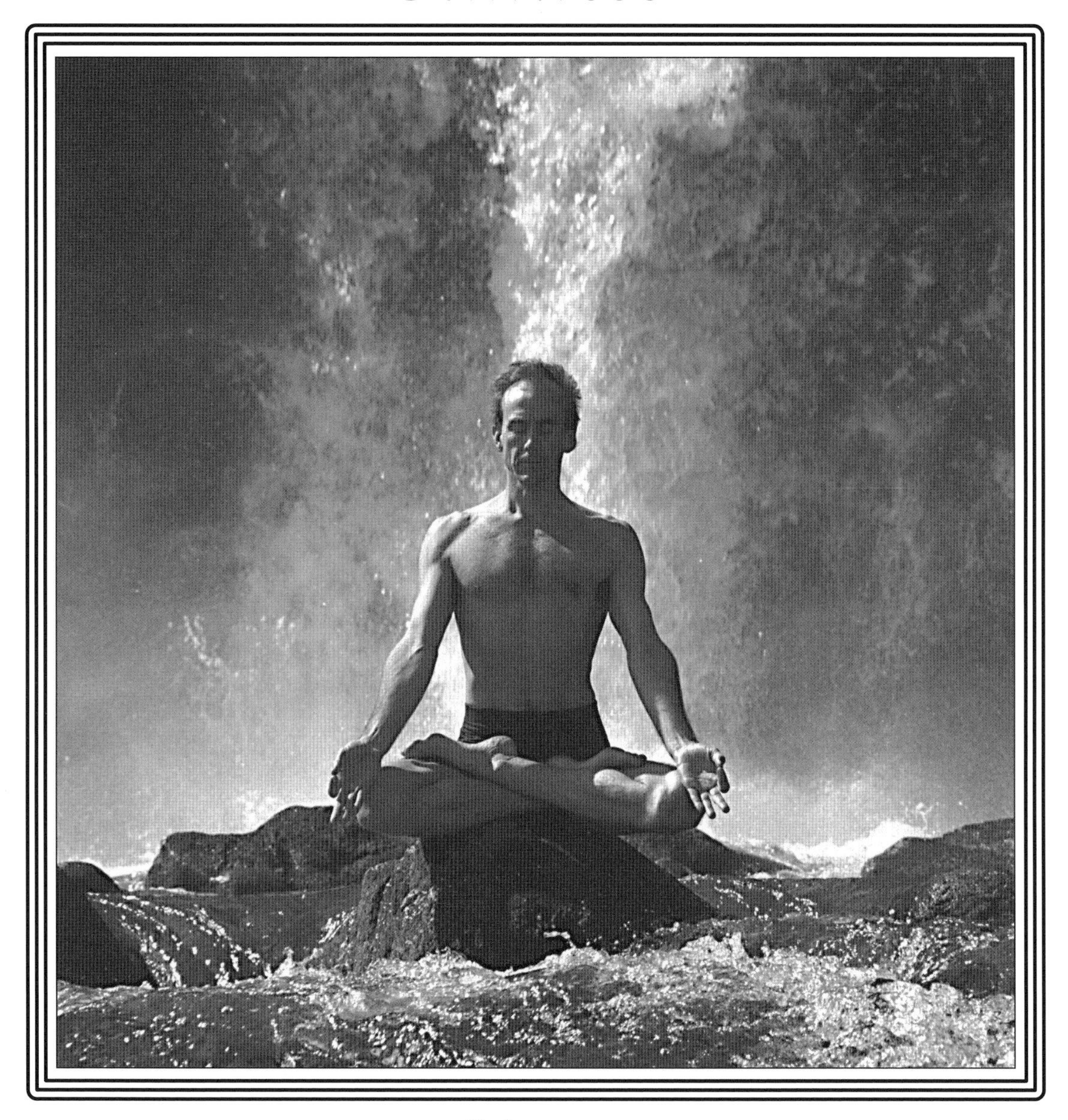

Padmasana
Finishing Sequence
David Swenson ~ Iceland

Three Lotus Flowers

"Completing the Garland"

K. Pattabhi Jois sometimes refers to the vinyasa system as a garland of postures. The asanas are strung together like flowers, one upon the next. These final three asanas, followed by **Savasana**, complete the circle. All of them are practiced in either lotus, half-lotus or "no-lotus", depending upon your capabilities. These asanas bring us back to the root of our practice, the breath and bandhas.

The first lotus flower is **Baddha Padmasana**. Here the arms are clasped behind the back and the torso is drawn forward until the body resembles the bud of a flower waiting to bloom.

In **Padmasana**, the flower opens into a full blown lotus blossom. The breath slows down. Long thin threads of air are drawn into the nostrils to saturate our lungs and spread life giving energy throughout the body. All of the bandhas are engaged and the spine is lifted to invite an open pathway for prana to flow.

Next, **Tolasana** lifts upward like a lotus flower floating free from the surface of a pond. **Tolasana** is meant to be held for **one-hundred breaths**. The breath is more powerful than in **Baddha Padmasana** and **Padmasana**.

Sometimes people question why this dynamic asana is placed here. It seems that the practice has moved into a mellow rhythm with **Baddha Padmasana** and **Padmasana**. Then, **Tolasana** bursts forth with great vigor. I have grown to appreciate **Tolasana**. I sometimes view the entire preceeding practice as nothing more than preparation for this last dynamic asana. The unseen depths of Ashtanga Yoga are present within **Tolasana**. The **breath** and **bandhas** exist at our core, hidden beyond the gross manifestations of our practice. These internal energies are addressed when practicing **Tolasana**. In order to lift the body free from the floor we must engage the **bandhas**. Once they are in place we are prepared to apply full and powerful **ujjayi pranayama**. The nervous system has been cleansed, purified and opened from the preceding asana practice. We have created the utmost fertile environment to receive the pranic life-force from the powerful and extended repetition of breath. This is the essence of the final asana, to cleanse and refine our gross body and senses in order to receive subtle awareness of our core identity.

There is no end to the refinement of practice and growth of understanding. Yoga has no limit or finality. If we speak to those that are considered masters of any particular system, I am certain that in each instance the adept will not consider themselves to have reached a final plateau. Rather: the greater the depth of knowledge obtained, the greater the understanding that there is infinitely more to know. As our realizations mature, we may find new and refined ways of applying the magic and beauty of yoga within the context of our daily lives.

Baddha Padmasana

Baddha = Bound Padma = Lotus

"Bound Lotus Posture"

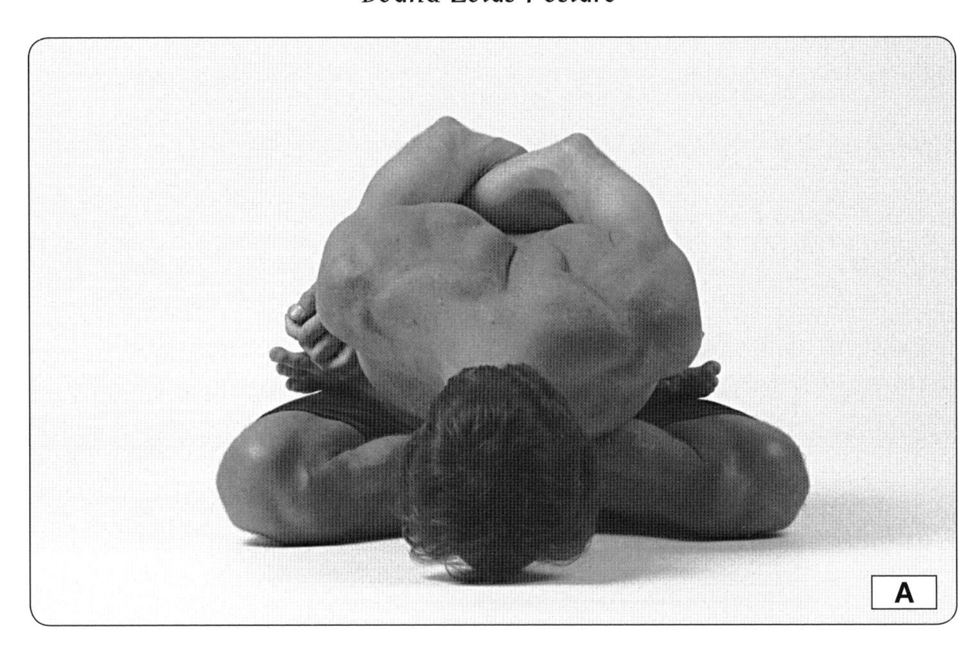
A

1) **Exhale** place the legs in full-lotus position with the right foot up first. Reach behind the back with the left hand and grab the left foot. Then reach behind and clasp the right foot with the right hand **(A)**. If you are able to sit in full lotus yet are unable to clasp the feet, you may use straps to wrap around each foot. You may then hold the straps with the hands behind your back as in **(B)**. If full-lotus is too much then you may practice half-lotus by placing the right foot on top of the left thigh or simply cross your legs. Take the arms behind the back without clasping the feet **(C)**.

2) **Inhale** after arranging your grip. Lengthen the spine.

3) **Exhale** fold forward into **(A)**, **(B)**, or **(C)**.

Remain For 5 Deep Breaths

4) **Inhale** sit up.

Enter The Next Asana From Here

Drishti ~ **Third Eye**

Comments - Be cautious with your knees when approaching the lotus position. Choose the appropriate option. Open from the hips so you do not take undue pressure into the knee joints. If you find that your breath becomes restricted when leaning forward then back off until you are able to breathe fully.

Baddha Padmasana

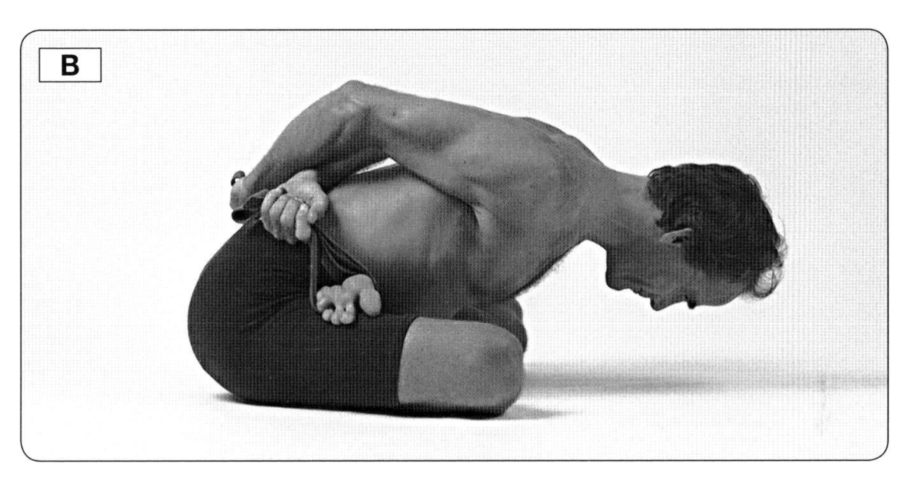

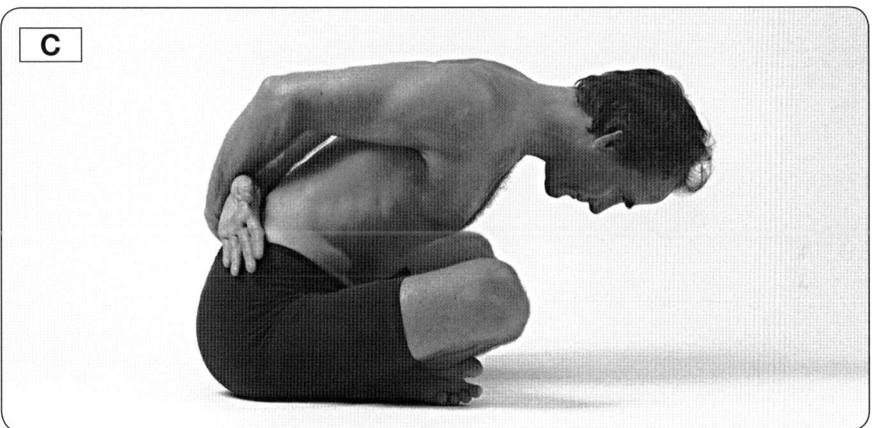

"Your hand opens and closes and opens and closes.
If it were always a fist or always stretched open, you would be paralyzed.
Your deepest presence is in every small contracting and expanding,
the two as beautifully balanced and coordinated as birds wings."

Rumi

Padmasana

Padma = Lotus

"Lotus Posture"

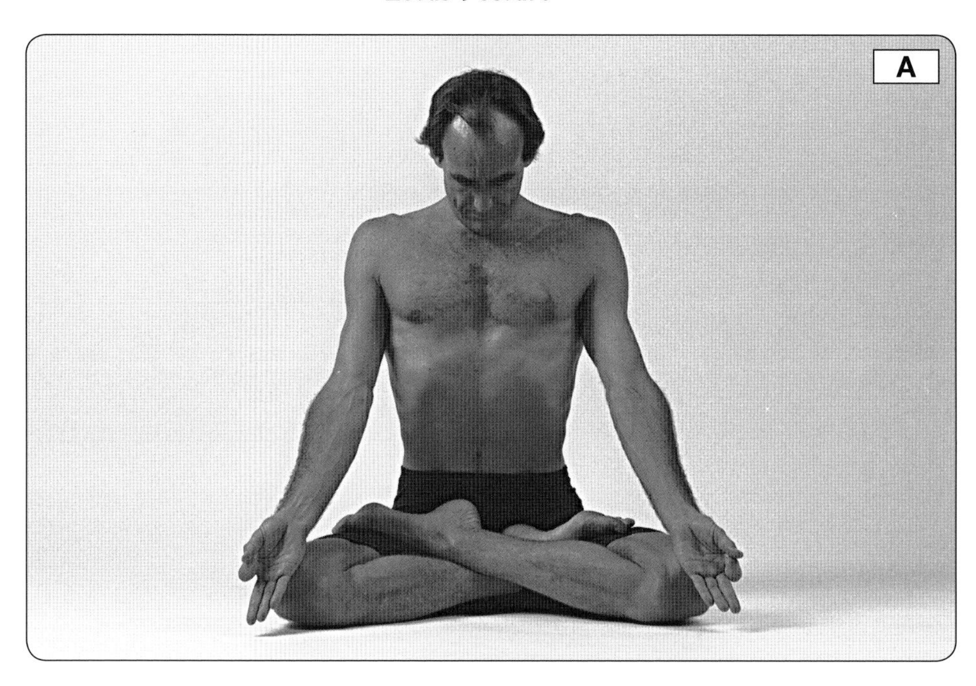

1) **Exhale** place the back of the hands on the knees with the legs in full-lotus position and the thumb and forefinger touching **(A)**. If you are unable to sit in full-lotus you may sit in half-lotus with the right foot on top of the left thigh (you may alternate the foot on top each time that you practice) with the hands on the knees as in **(B)**. If half-lotus is too much then cross the legs with the feet under the opposite ankles **(C)**. If you find it too difficult to sit up straight when the hips are on the floor you may elevate the hips with a block or cushion as in **(D)**.

Remain For 10 Deep Breaths

Enter The Next Asana From Here

Drishti ~ **Nose**

Comments - Choose the option above in which you may sit most comfortably. It is important to keep the spine lifted and the shoulders back so that the lungs have the optimum amount of space for expansion. The spine and shoulders act as a "coat-rack" for the body. The lower back is supported by engagement of the abdominal locks. **Jalandhara bandha**, the chin lock, is also utilized here. Slow the breathing down by creating long thin threads of air to enter through both nostrils. Saturate the entire body with oxygen and life giving prana. Listen to the sound of your breath. Keep it rhythmic and soft. Feel the stillness and the unseen forces moving within. This is the seat of yoga. Free the mind from wandering. Remain present and calm.

Padmasana

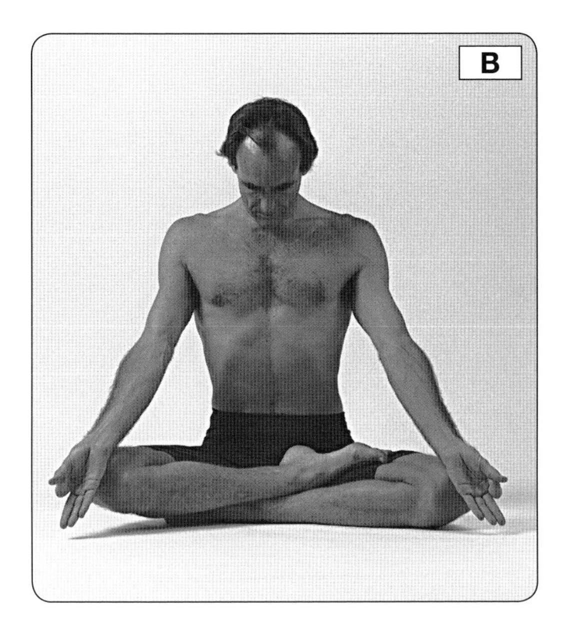

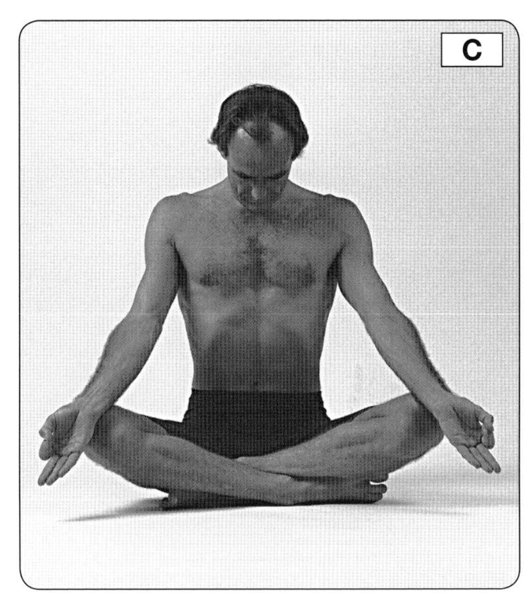

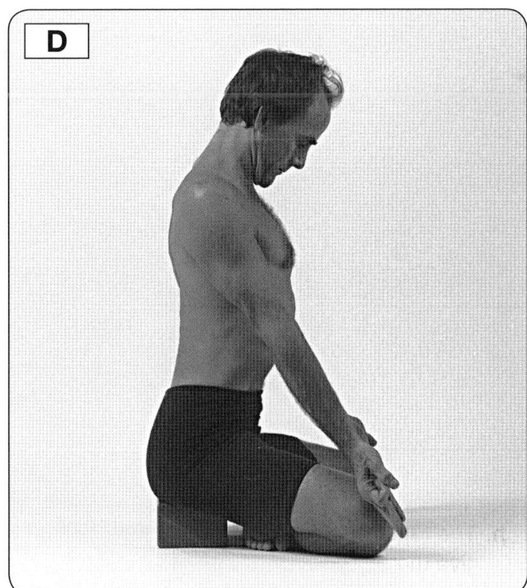

Tolasana

Tola = Scale

"Scale Posture"

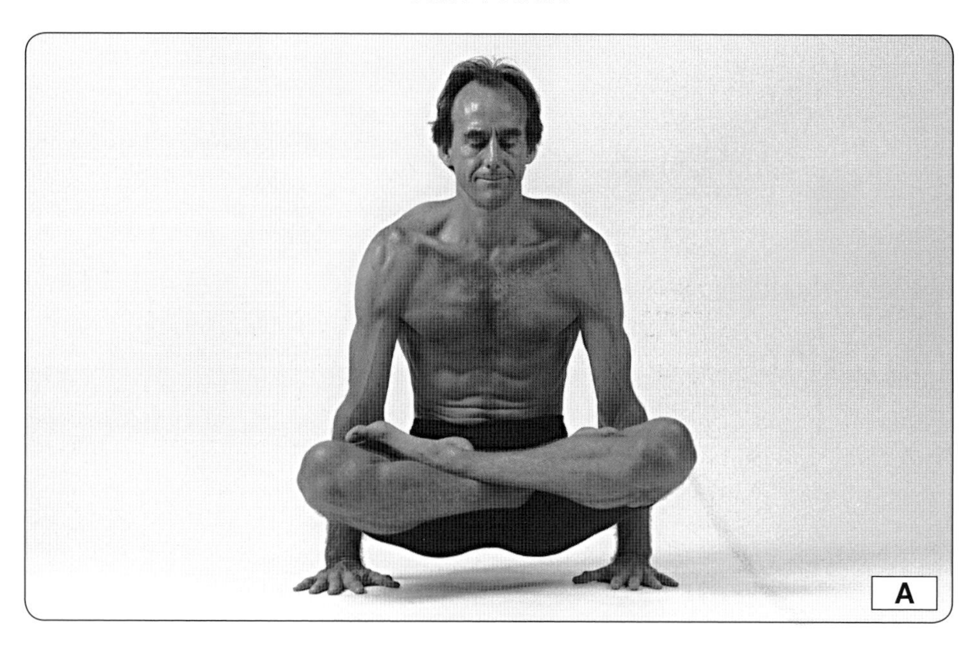

1) **Exhale** place the hands on the floor beside the hips with the legs in full-lotus.

2) **Inhale** lift the body away from the floor and hover in that position **(A)**. If lotus if too much then lift up from a cross-legged position and hold that position with the feet and hips away from the floor **(B)**. If you do not achieve "lift-off" when attempting to lift up you may remain seated and draw the knees toward the chest without lifting up **(C)**.

Remain For 100 Deep Breaths (or as long as you can hold it without straining)

~VINYASA~

Drishti ~ **Nose**

Comments - The breath in this asana is much more powerful than the rest of the practice. Each inhale and exhale should be consciously drawn in and pushed out through the nose with a full and deep ujjayi sound. Keep the sound in the back of the throat. The sound is like a steam engine train. Two opposing forces work powerfully to create the dynamic lifting action present here. The arms must extend as the hands press fully into the earth. The hips lift as the torso shortens by the engagement of **mulabandha** and **uddiyana bandha**. I did not give the option of half-lotus because the foot that is on top will push the other leg toward the floor and this creates instability. The breath count of **one hundred** is not a misprint. It is the prescribed length to remain in this posture. That level of endurance will obviously take many practice sessions to achieve. Hold for as long as you like and increase the duration gradually. Focus on your breath quality.

Tolasana

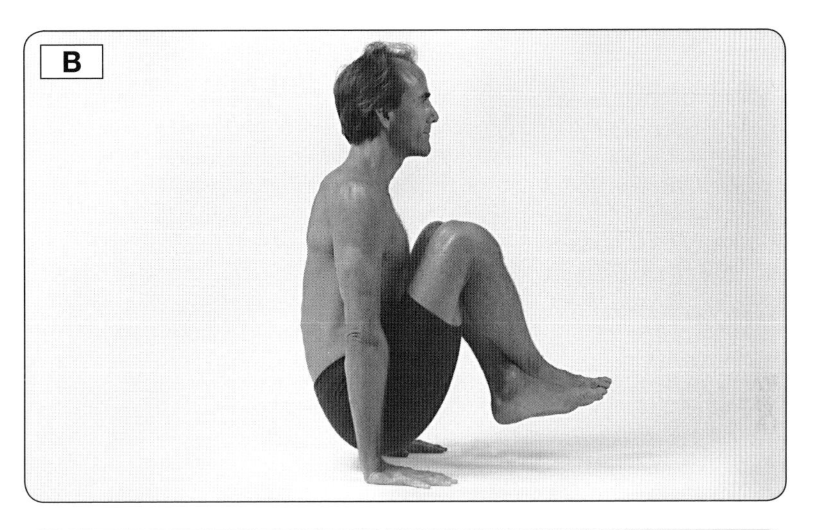

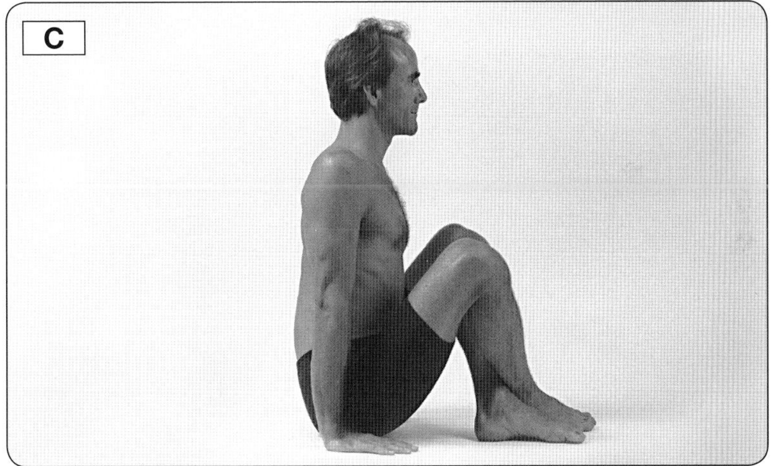

"We shall not cease from exploration.
And the end of all our exploring
Will be to arrive where we started.
And know the place for the first time."

T. S. Eliot

Entering Savasana

"The Death of a Practice"

We give birth to each practice session when we take our first breath in **Surya Namaskara**. There is a beginning, middle and end in the life of each practice series. There are obstacles which are confronted. There are joyful asanas and challenging ones. There are times when we are able to flow along without difficulty and times when the mind runs us ragged and the body feels heavy and unresponsive. When we have completed our routine for the day, it is time to wind down and finally to stop. To return to stillness. It is here that we enter into **Savasana**, the death of our practice. In this "**dying**" we may let go of the session and remain still and unattached. In this stillness we allow the gross and subtle body to absorb and assimilate prana. The final asana in the finishing sequence, **Tolasana**, has prepared us for this moment by engaging the bandhas, contracting the muscles and pumping the breath to saturate every cell with vital life-force.

When we release **Tolasana**, we may easily sink into a deep stillness beyond the physical realm. We may visit that place, deep within, which is a sanctuary of tranquillity. As we enter **Savasana**, we may release all of the locks and let the breath flow freely. It is best to remain in **Savasana** for as long as your schedule permits. The minimum duration should be to stay until the heart rate slows down and the breath finds a natural soothing rhythm. In this place of stillness you may experience the revitalizing and nurturing effects of **Savasana**. Allow yourself the time to absorb the energy. Bathe in the vital forces of life and relish the stillness. Soak it up like a flower drinking in the sun's rays.

When it is time to come out of **Savasana**, it is as though we enter a new birth. A renewal of energy, vitality and spirit has taken place. The body has been cleansed and the mind relaxed. The myriad benefits accrued through practice may then be carried with us for the rest of our day. Really experience the depths of relaxation offered by **Savasana**. Enjoy the sacred journey to inner harmony. Yoga is a divine gift and the opportunity to practice it is a blessing.

Savasana

Sava = Corpse

"Corpse Posture"

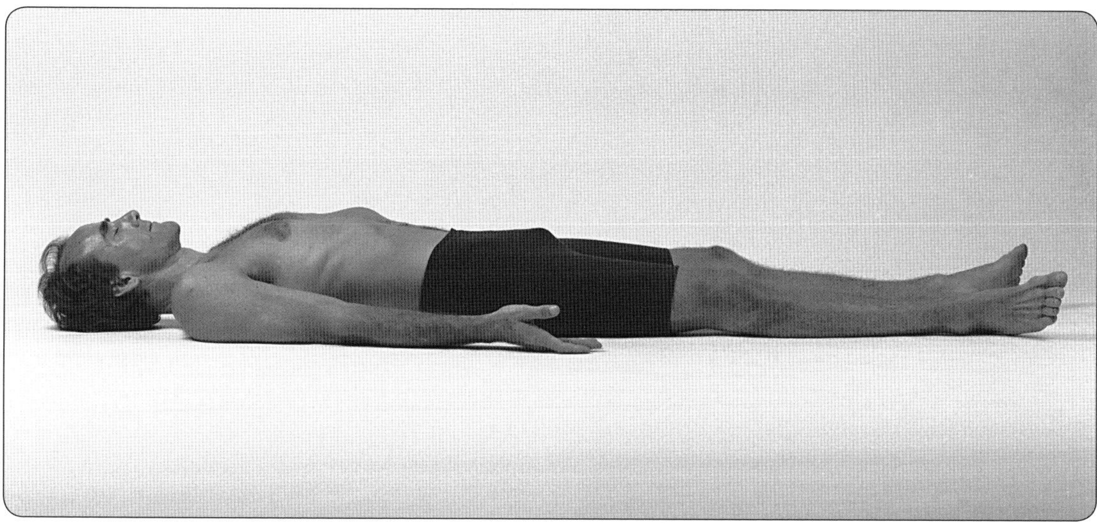

1) **Exhale** lie down on your back. Close your eyes and completely relax.

"At the still point of the turning world. Neither flesh nor fleshless;
Neither from nor towards; at the still point, there the dance is,
But neither arrest nor movement. And do not call it fixity,
Where past and future are gathered. Neither movement from nor towards,
Neither ascent nor decline. Except for the point, the still point,
There would be no dance, and there is only the dance."

T. S. Eliot

Poise

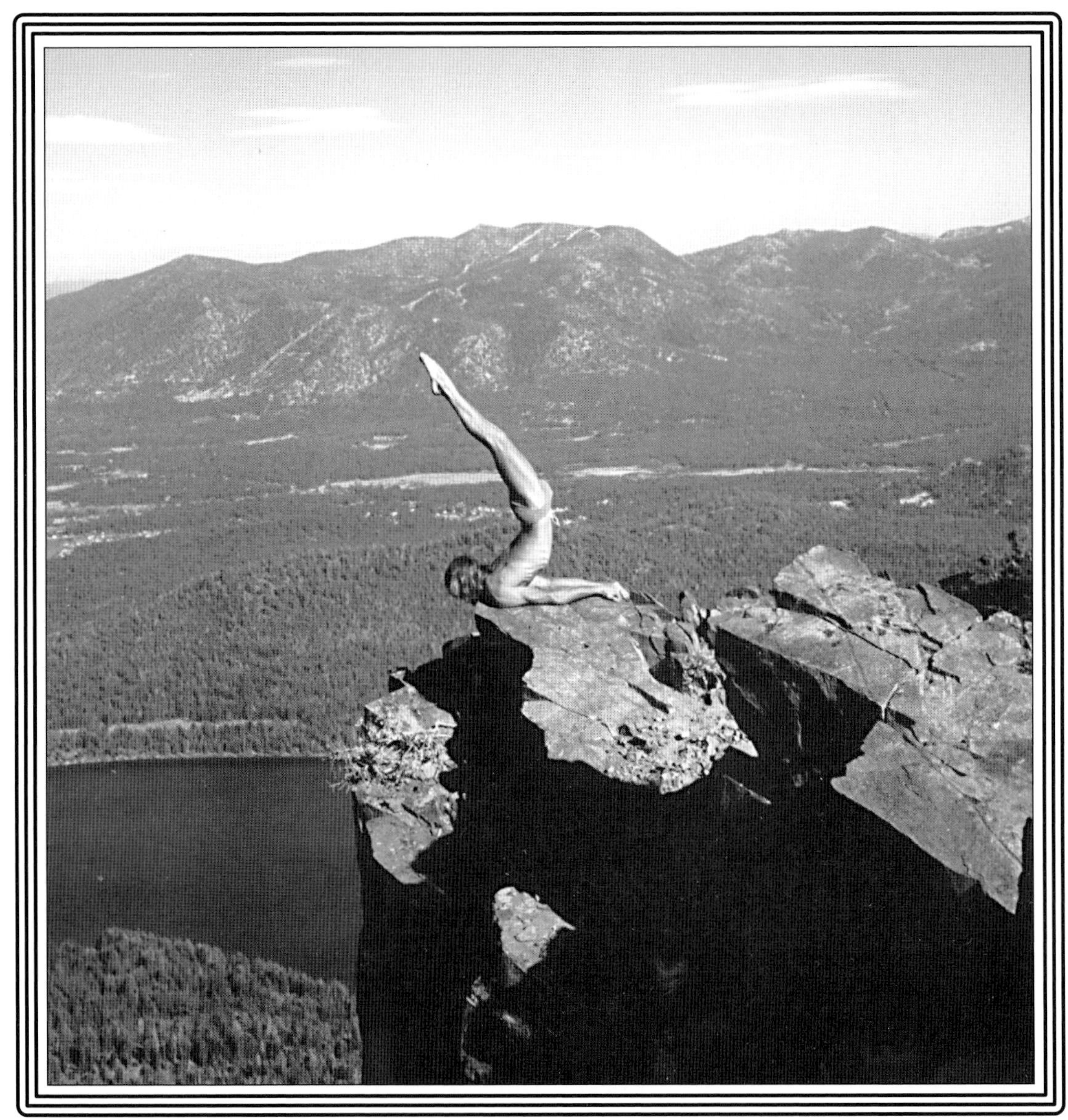

Viparita Shalabhasana
Advanced 'A' Series
Doug Swenson ~ Mt. Talac, Lake Tahoe, CA

The Full Flow

"Viewing the Mandala"

Ashtanga Yoga is a colorful tapestry in motion. It is a mandala of movement. In order to understand it, it must be viewed in its entirety rather than in a segmented form. On the following pages you will find the complete Primary and Intermediate Series including the standing sequence and the finishing postures. It is meant to be a visual reference to enable you to see large blocks of the practice. This section is comprised of photos and the Sanskrit name of each asana. Through regular practice you will become familiar with the sequential pattern inherent within Ashtanga Yoga. Work toward committing the sequence to memory. Your personal practice will grow from that seed. You may then carry it with you and partake of its fruits at any time without the need for visual tools or outside prompting. This system is designed to wean the practitioner from dependence upon any external stimulus. The practice becomes your personal guide and teacher. With regulation the asanas become intimately familiar and a relationship develops which will mature and mellow over time. Yoga is a benevolent friend that is always there to greet us with a smile. Practice is a journey to our inner selves. Ashtanga has been an invaluable tool within my life and I hope that you enjoy this dynamic, magical system and find the fruits of the Ashtanga tree to be sweet and nourishing to your body, mind and soul.

Namaste,

David Swenson

"Nothing would be done at all
if we waited until we could do it so well
that no one could find fault with it."

Cardinal Newman

Surya Namaskara A

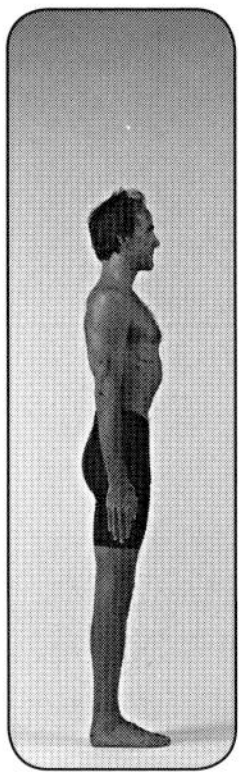

Samasthiti

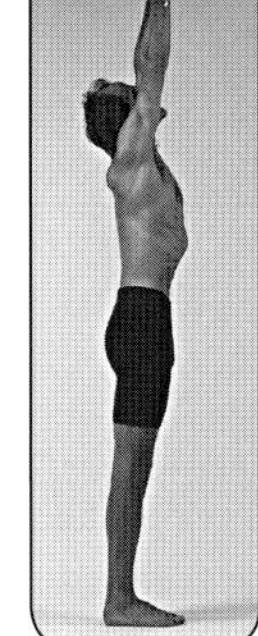
One

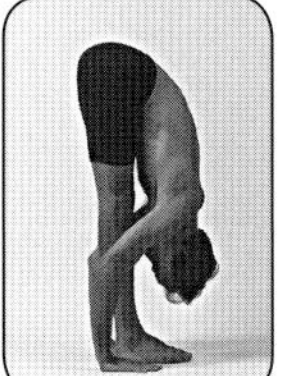
Two

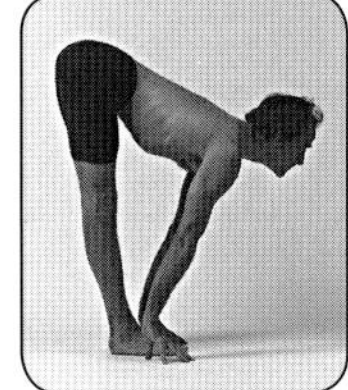
Three

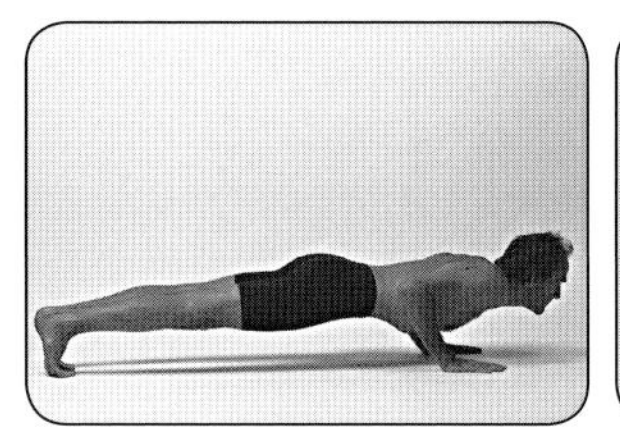
Four

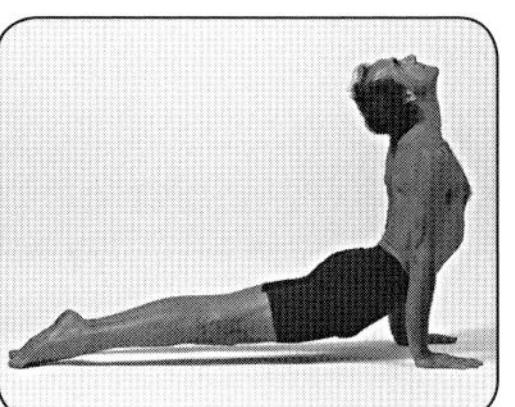
Five

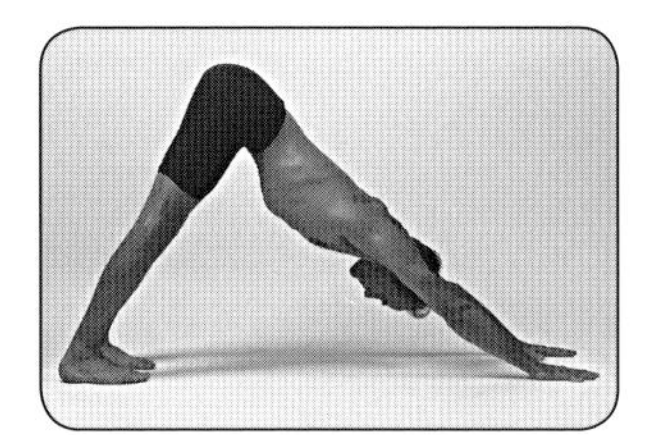
Six
(Hold For 5 Breaths)

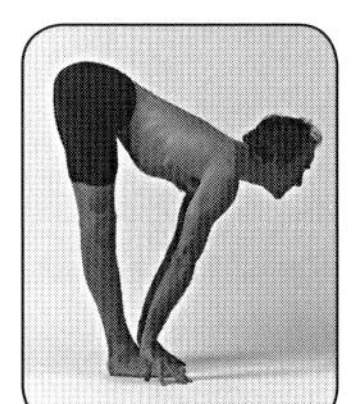
Seven

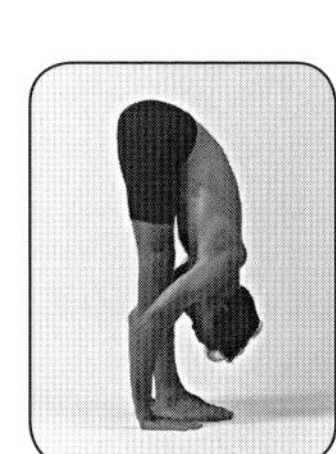
Eight

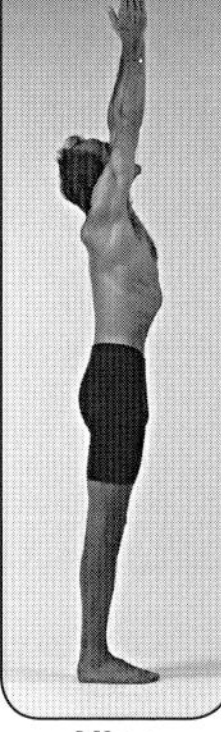
Nine

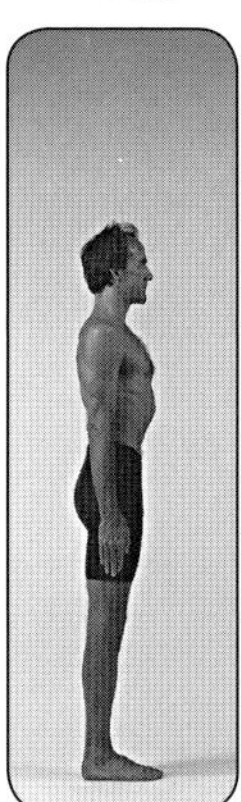
Samasthiti

vina vinyasayogena asanadin na karayet
(Oh Yogi, do not practice asana without vinyasa.)

Vamana Rishi

Surya Namaskara B

Samasthiti

One

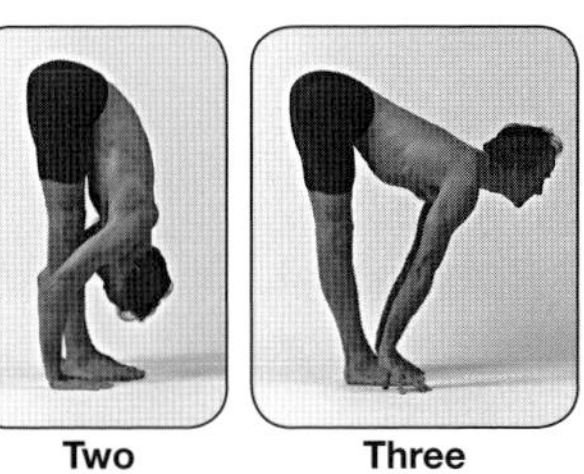

Two

Three

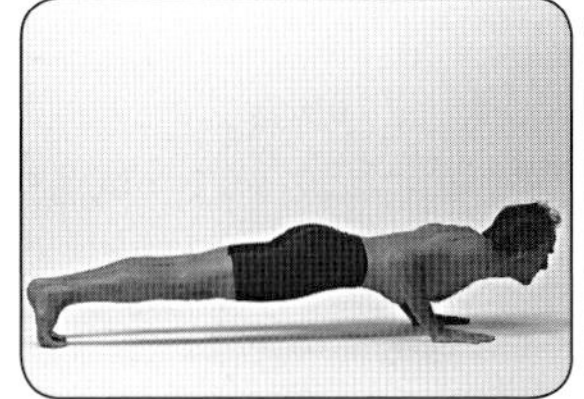

Four

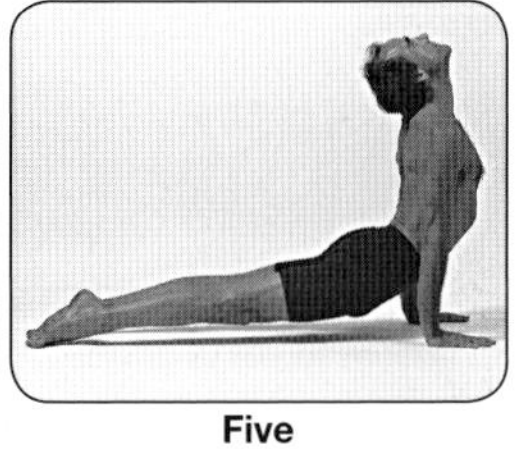

Five

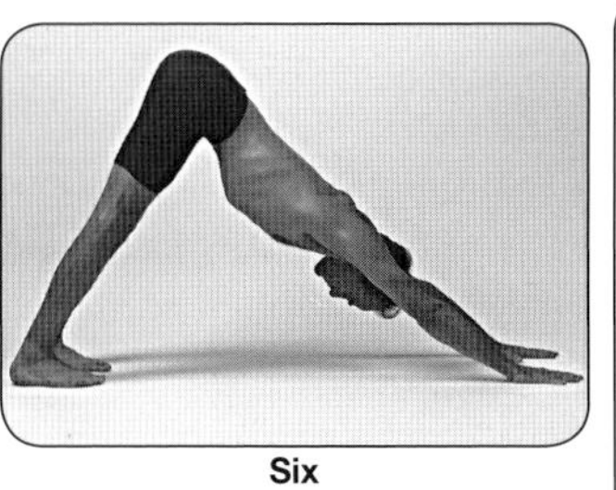

Six

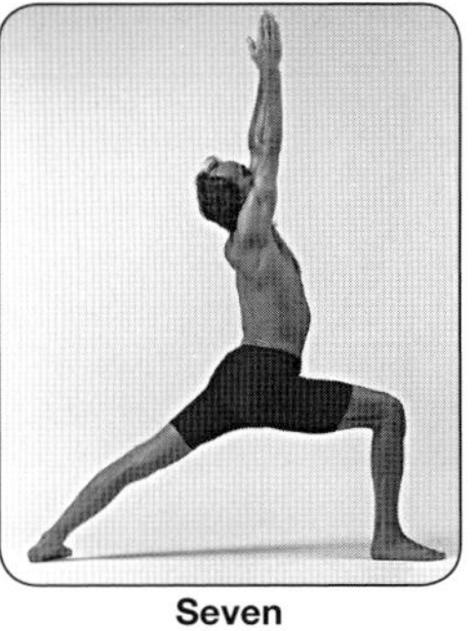

Seven

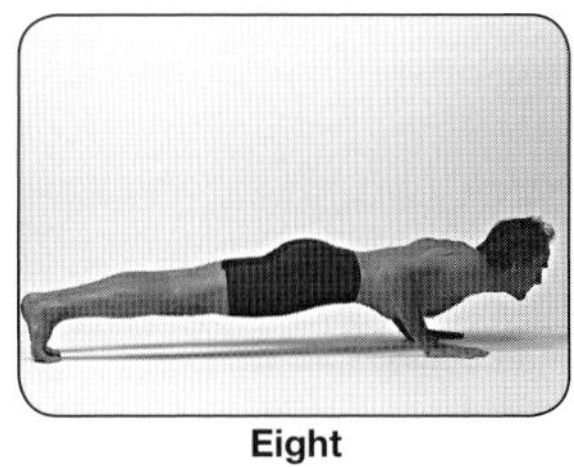

Eight

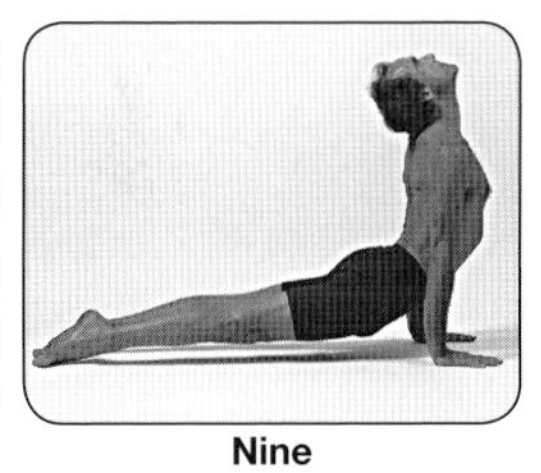

Nine

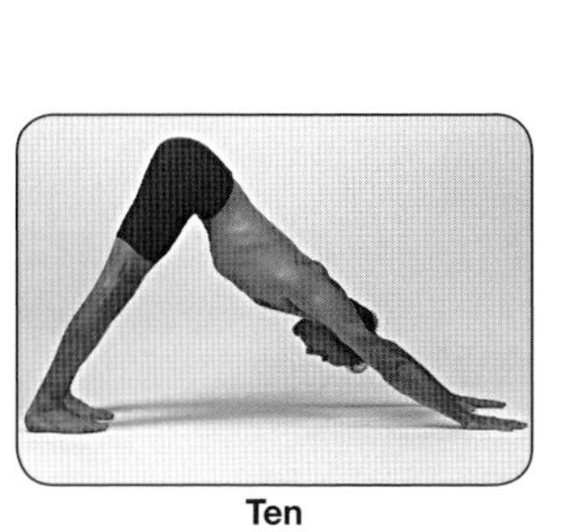

Ten

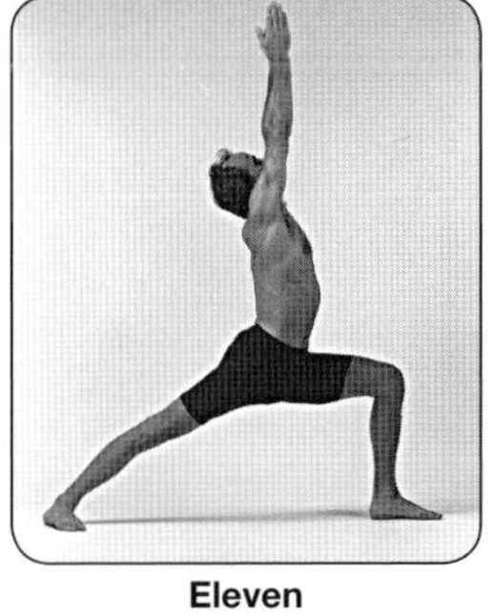

Eleven

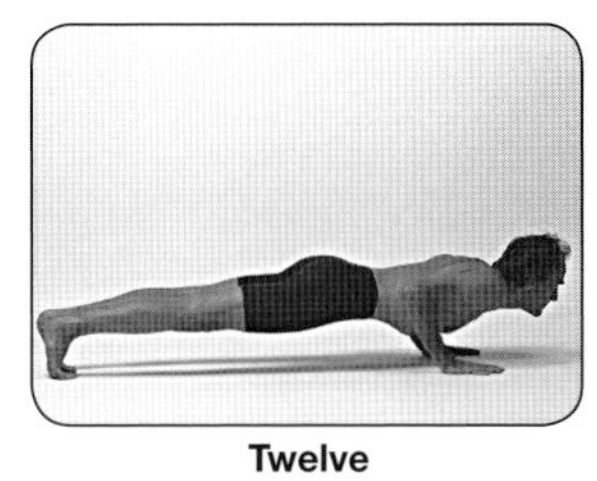

Twelve

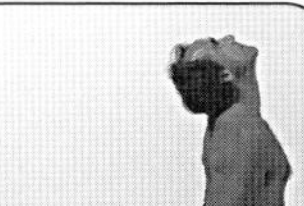

Thirteen

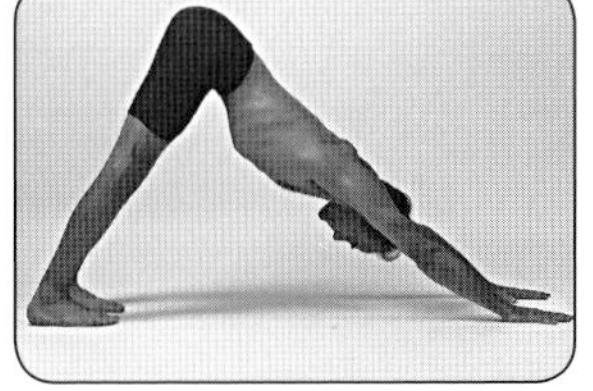

Fourteen
(Hold For 5 Breaths)

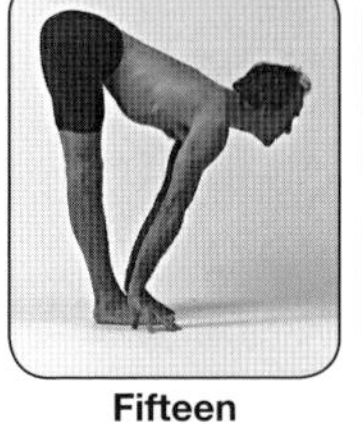

Fifteen

Sixteen

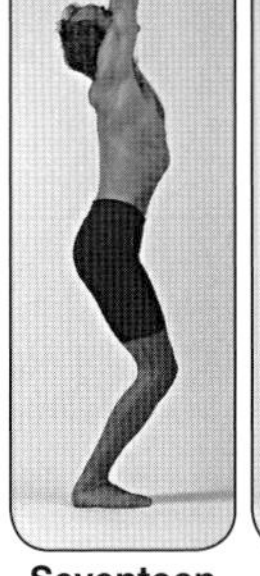

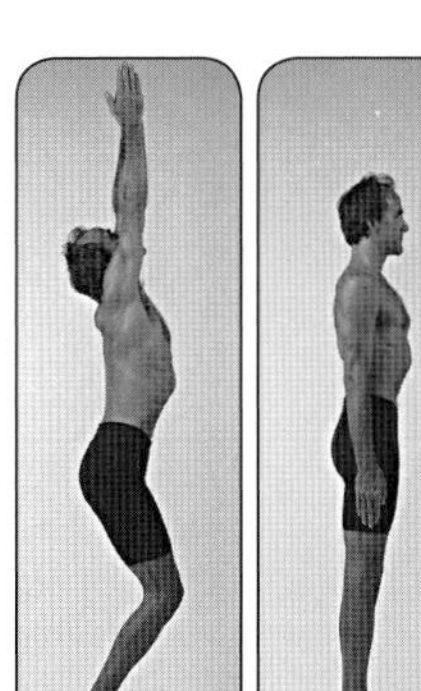

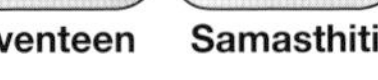

Seventeen

Samasthiti

The Standing Sequence

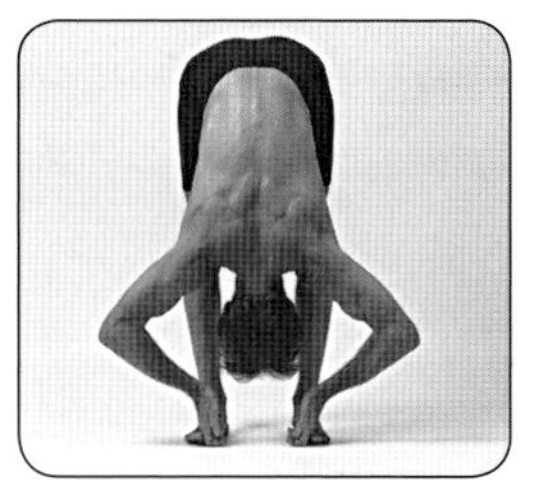
Padangusthasana

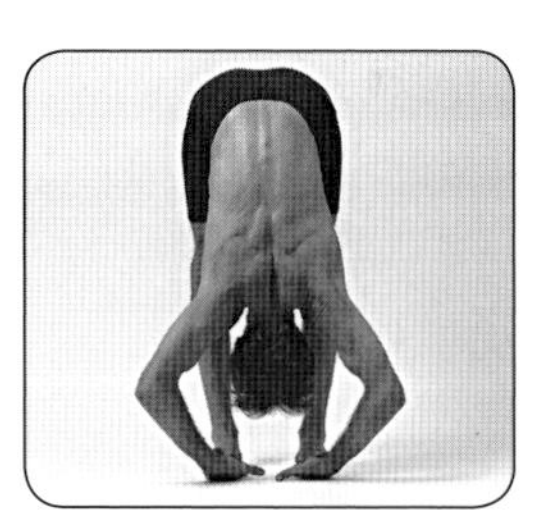
Padahastasana

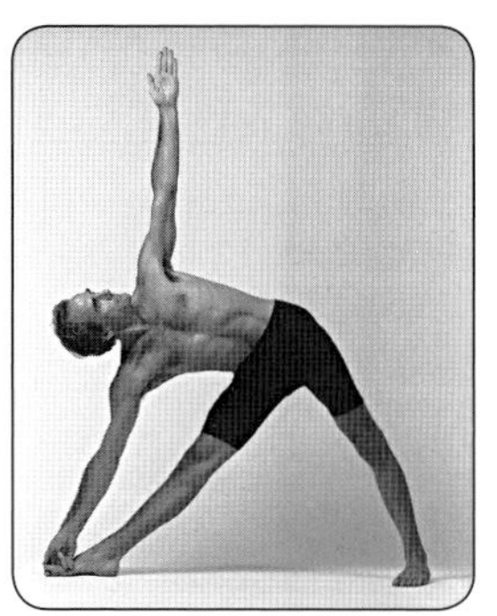
Utthita Trikonasana

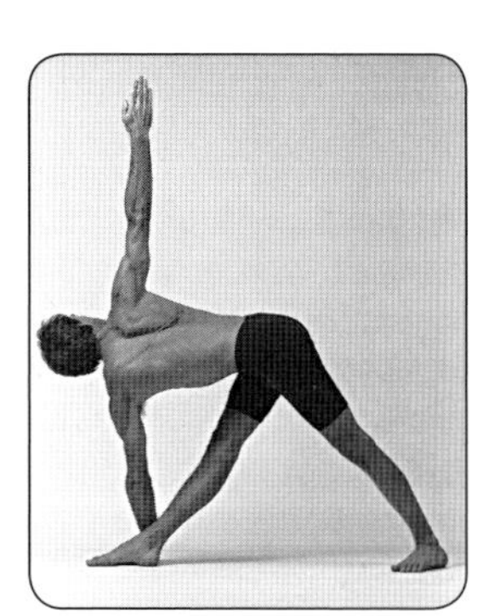
Parivritta Trikonasana

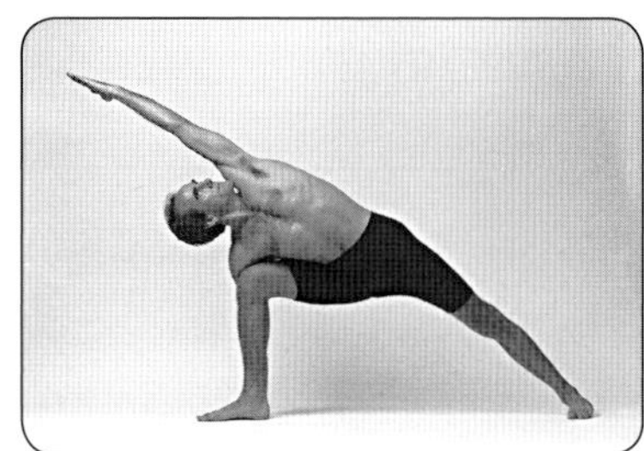
Utthita Parsvakonasana

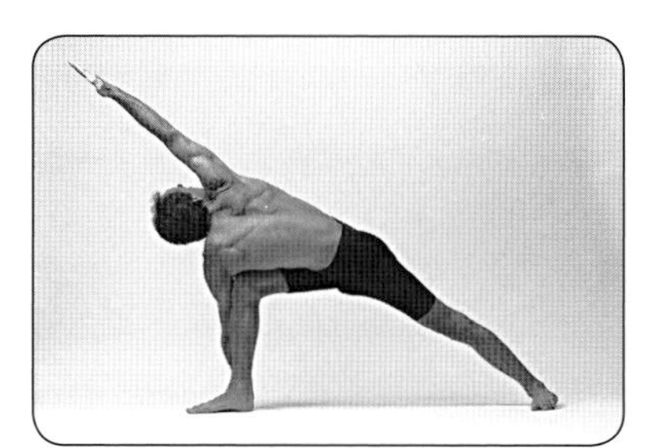
Parivritta Parsvakonasana

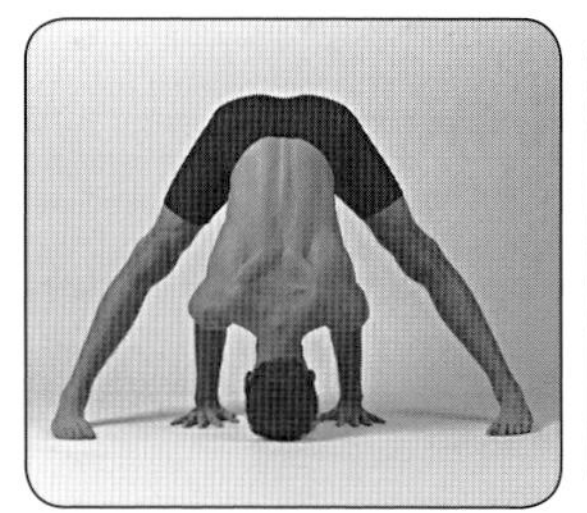
Prasarita Padottanasana
A

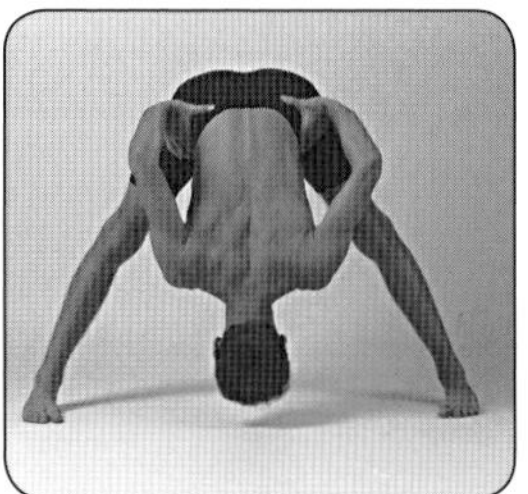
Prasarita Padottanasana
B

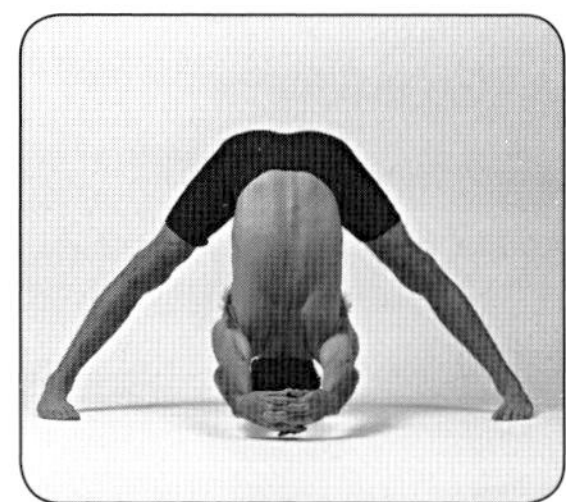
Prasarita Padottanasana
C

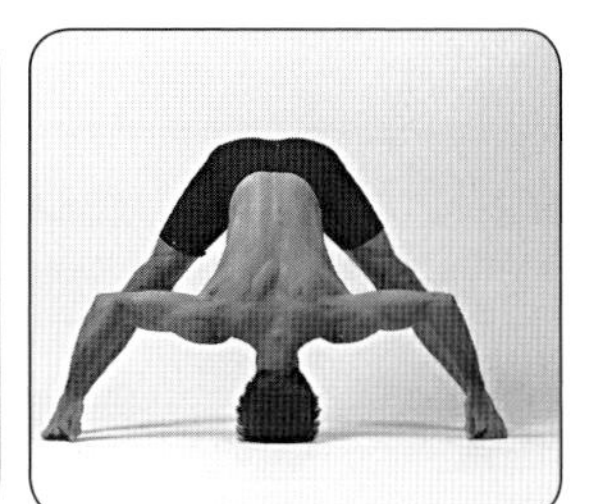
Prasarita Padottanasana
D

Balance = a weight, force, or influence counteracting the effect of another

Webster's Dictionary

The Standing Sequence

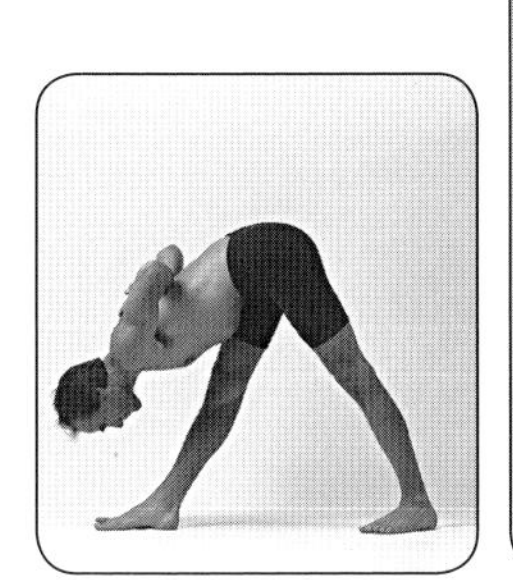
Parsvottanasana

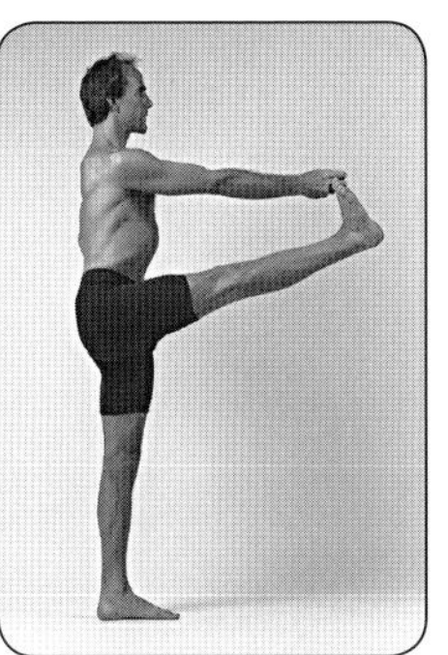
Utthita Hasta Padangusthasana A

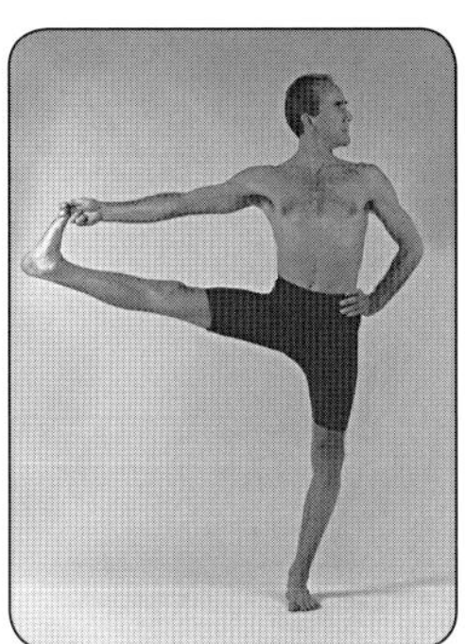
Utthita Hasta Padangusthasana B

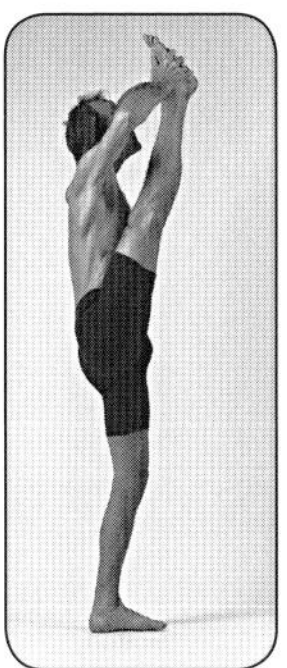
Utthita Hasta Padangusthasana C

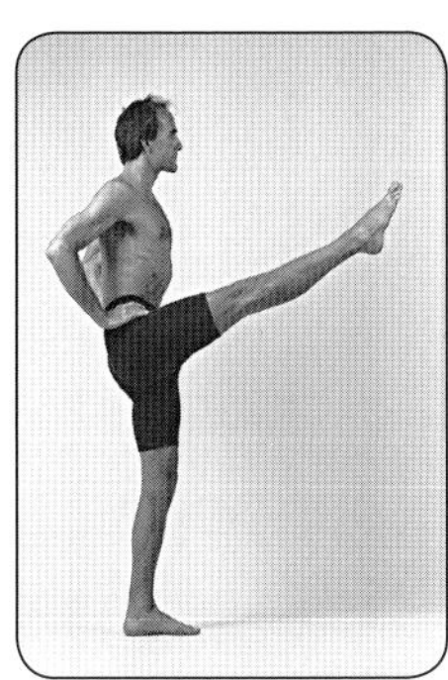
Utthita Hasta Padangusthasana D

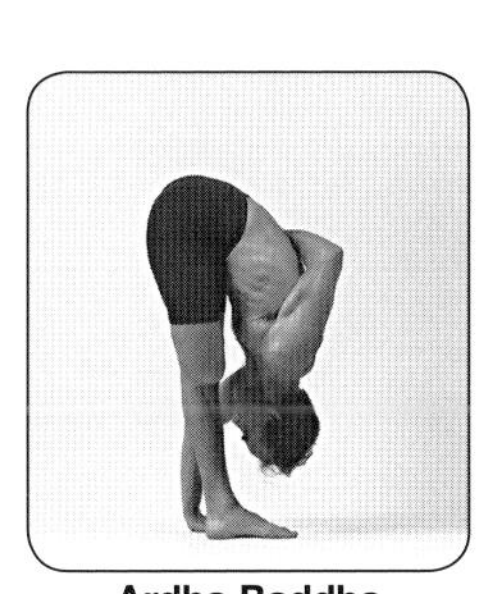
Ardha Baddha Padmottanasana

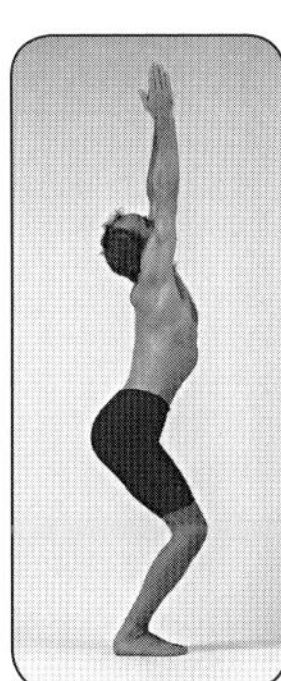
Utkatasana

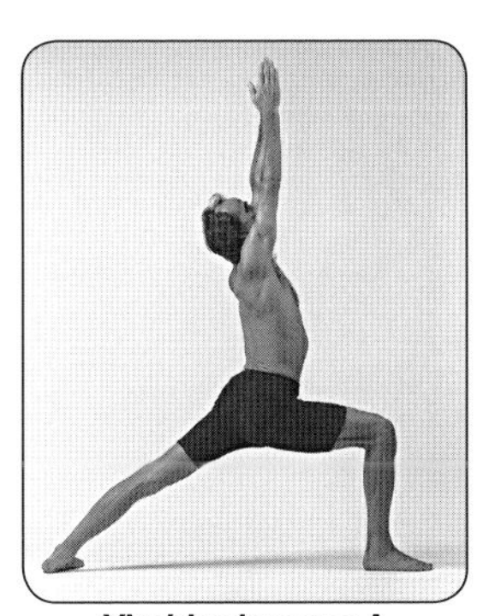
Virabhadrasana A

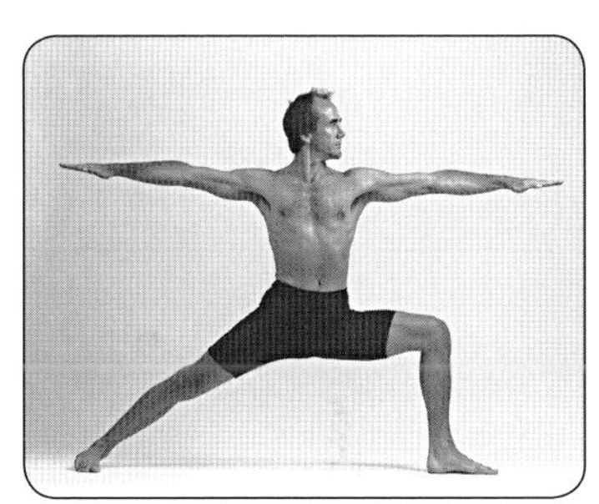
Virabhadrasana B

"The Only Journey Is The Journey Within."

Rainer Maria Rilke

The Primary Series

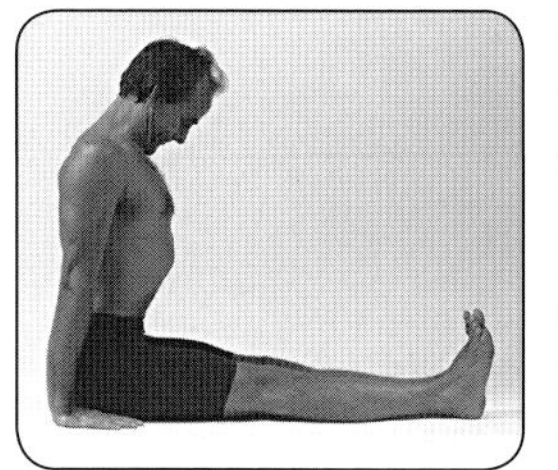
Dandasana

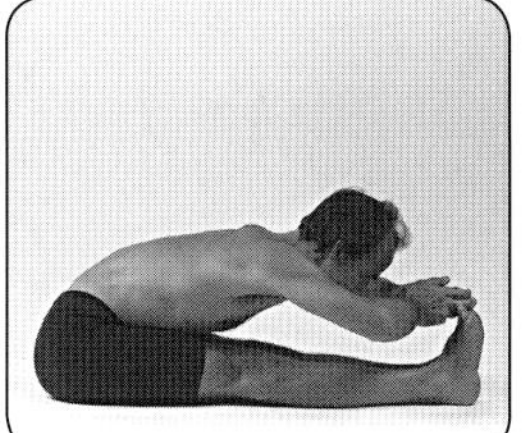
Paschimottanasana A

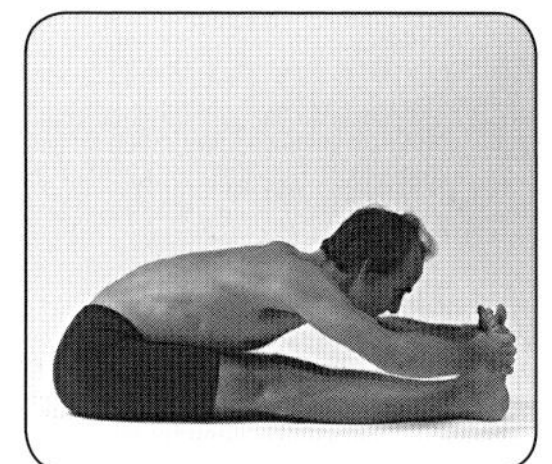
Paschimottanasana B

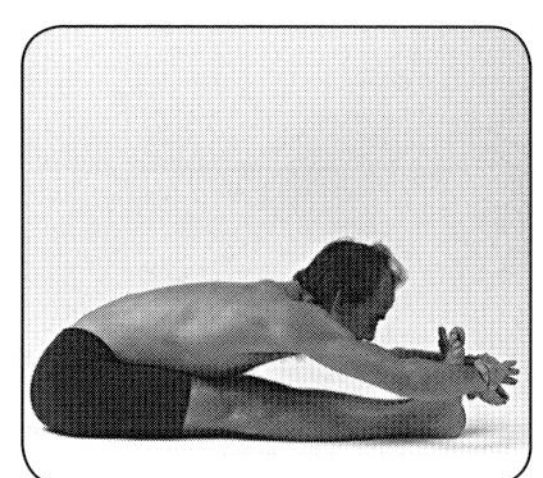
Paschimottanasana C

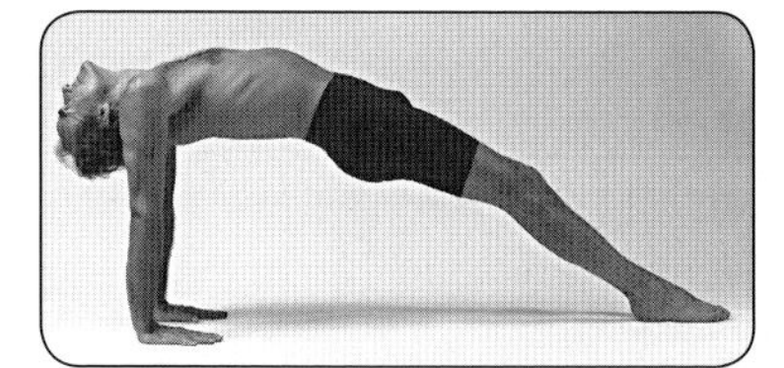
Purvottanasana

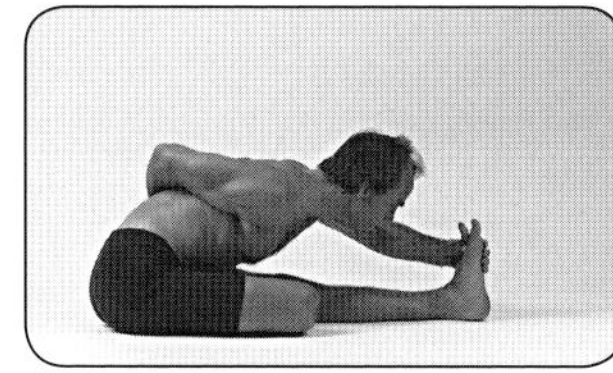
Ardha Baddha Padma
Paschimottanasana

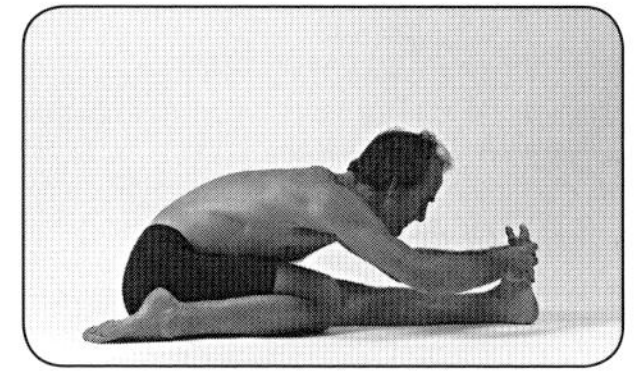
Trianga Mukhaikapada
Paschimottanasana

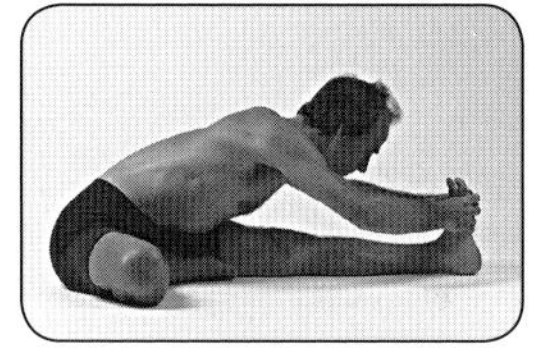
Janu Sirsasana A

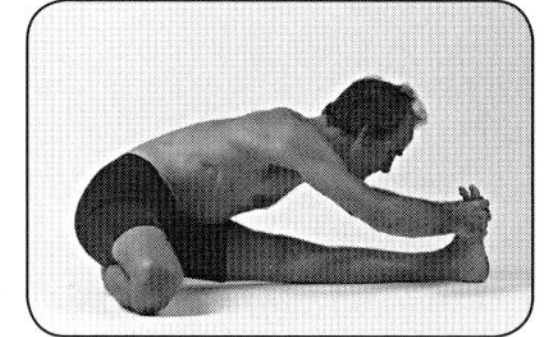
Janu Sirsasana B

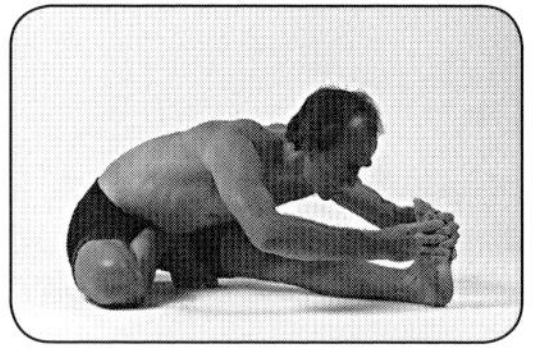
Janu Sirsasana C

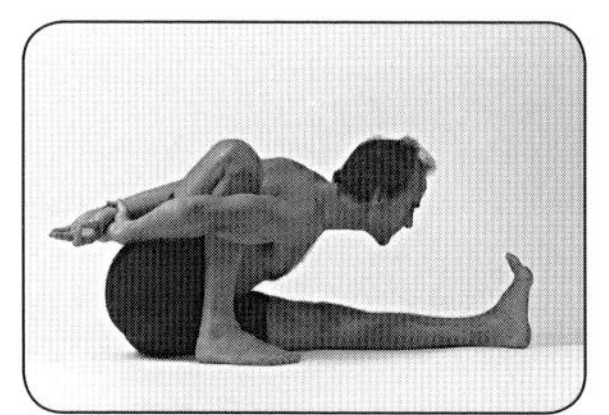
Marichyasana A

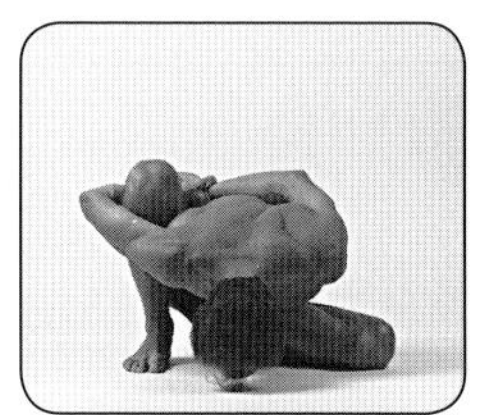
Marichyasana B

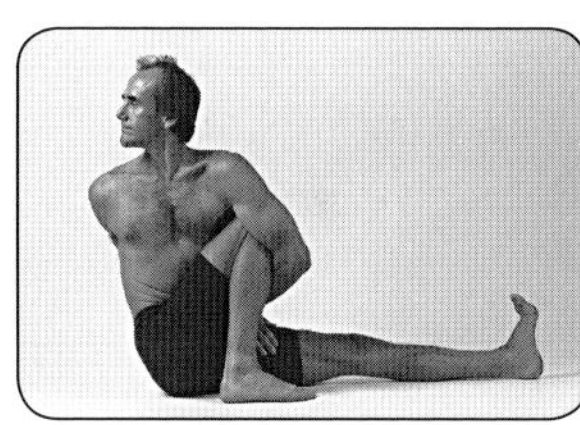
Marichyasana C

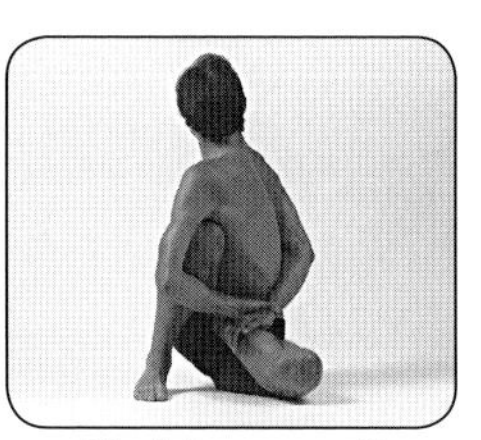
Marichyasana D

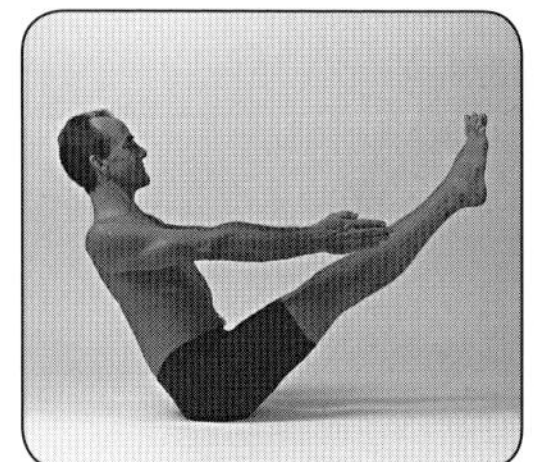
Navasana
5 Times

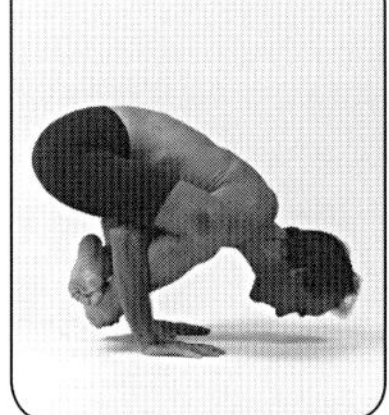
Bhujapidasana

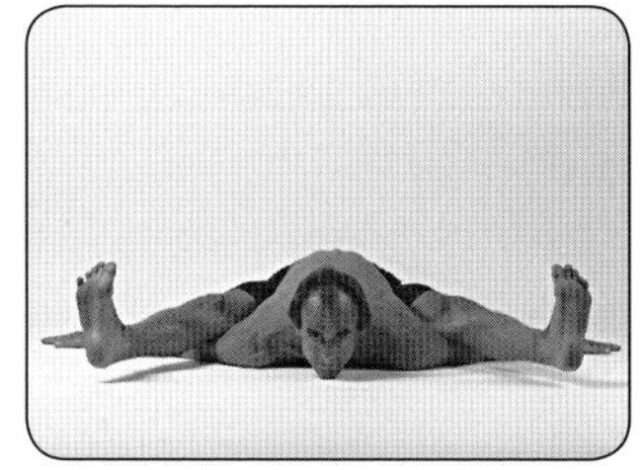
Kurmasana

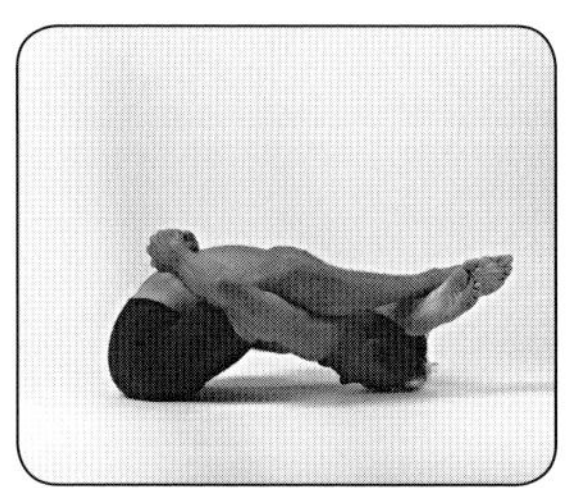
Supta Kurmasana

The Primary Series

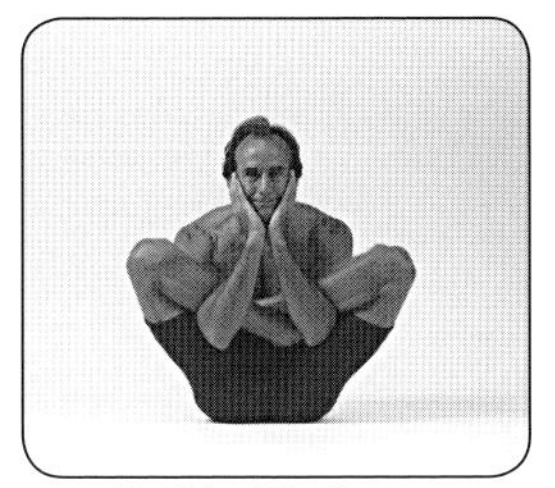
Garbha Pindasana

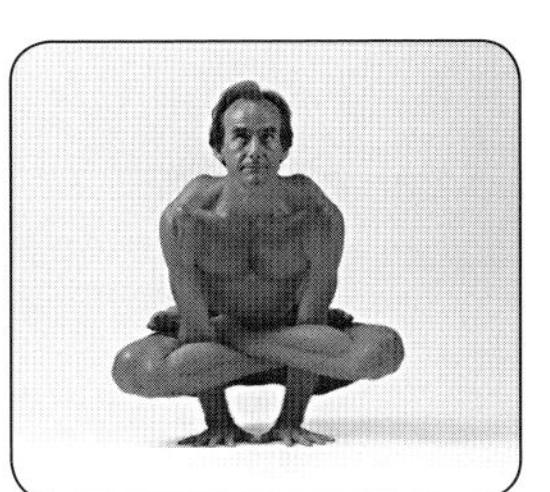
Kukkutasana

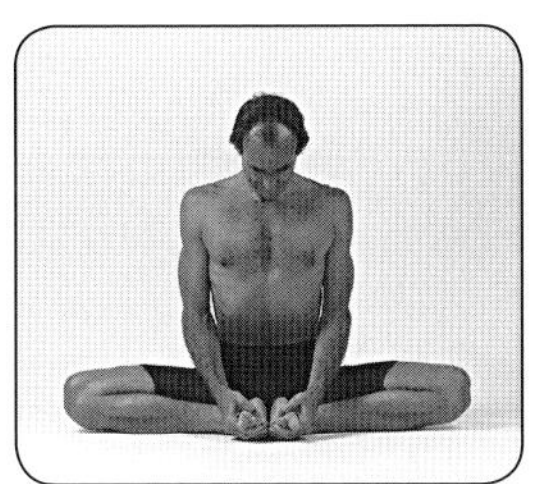
Baddha Konasana A

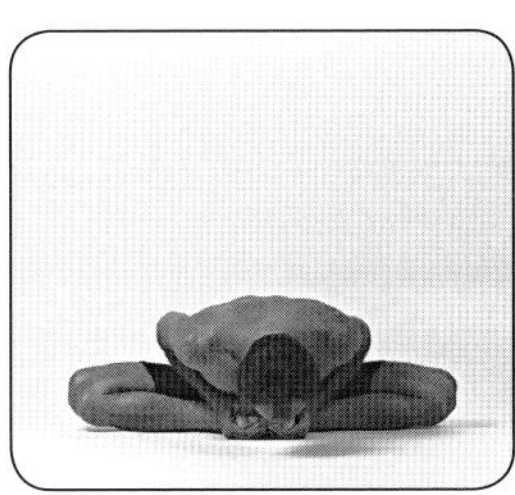
Baddha Konasana B

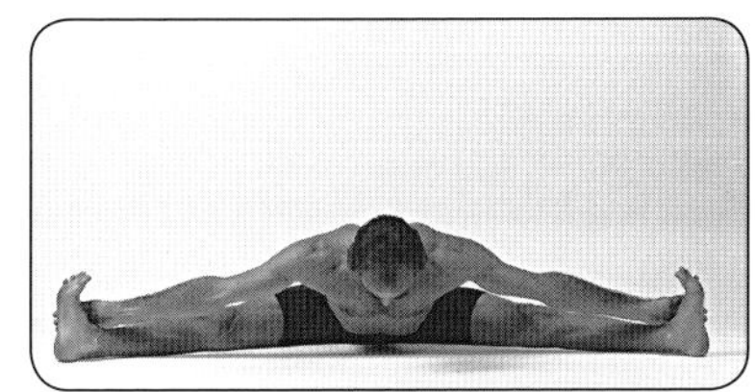
Upavishta Konasana A

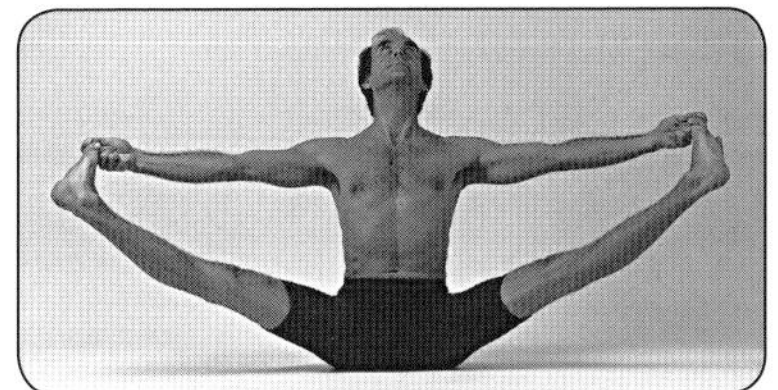
Upavishta Konasana B

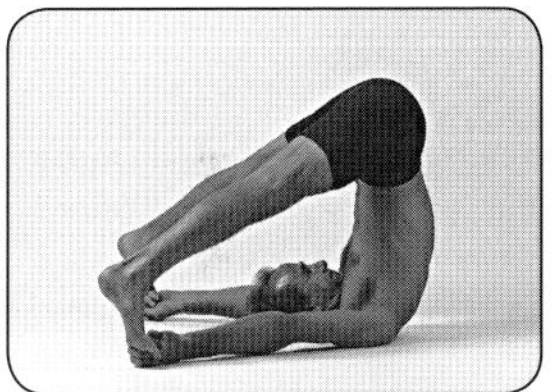
Supta Konasana

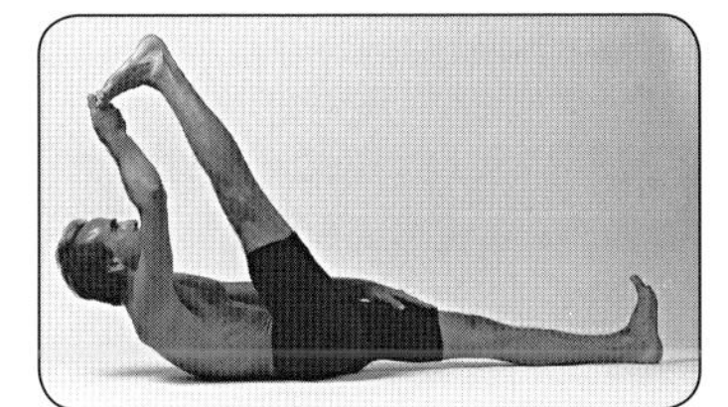
Supta Padangusthasana A

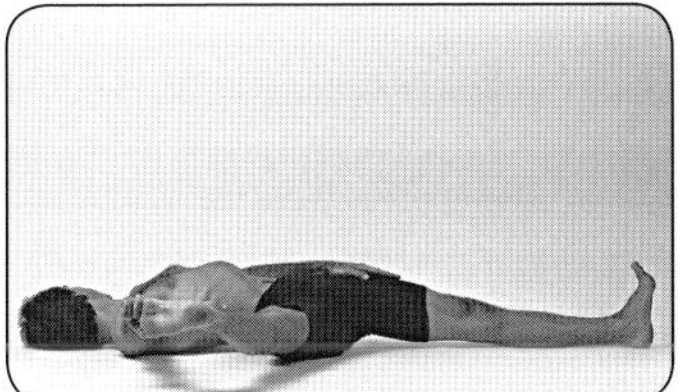
Supta Padangusthasana B

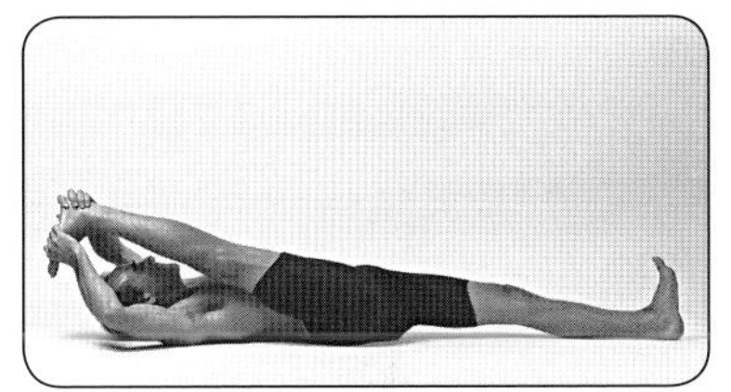
Supta Padangusthasana C

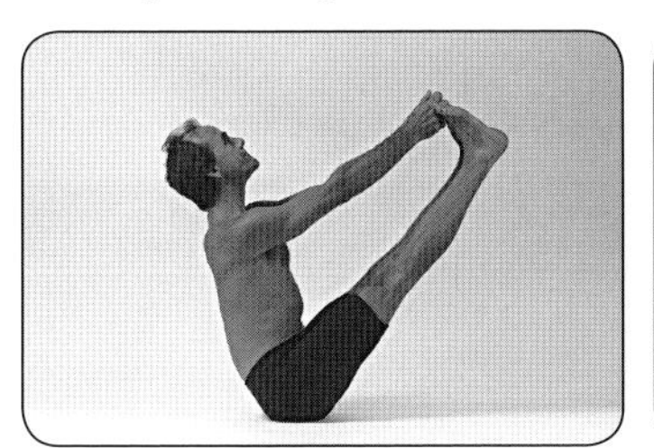
Ubhaya Padangusthasana

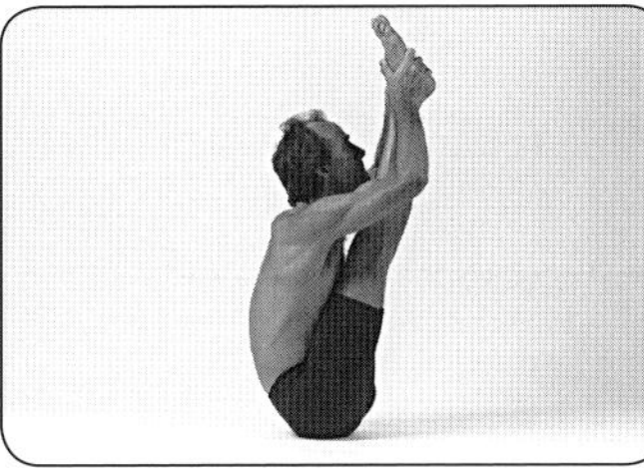
Urdhva Mukha Paschimottanasana

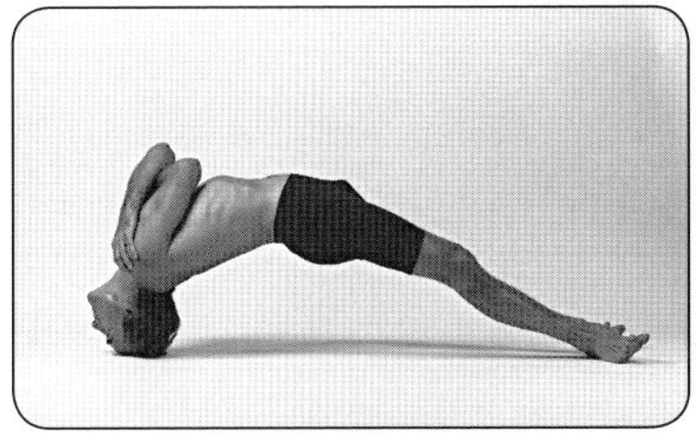
Setu Bandhasana

"99% Practice – 1% Theory"

K. Pattabhi Jois

The Intermediate Series

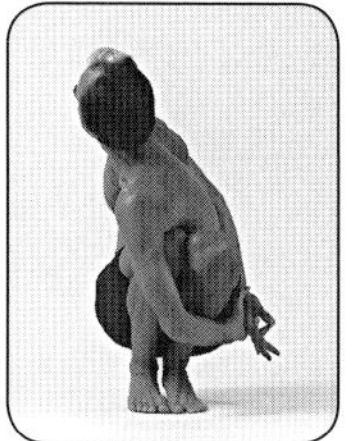
Pashasana

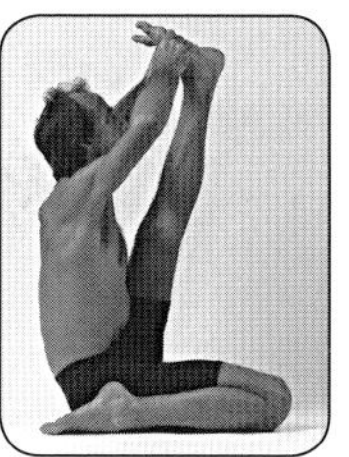
Krounchasana

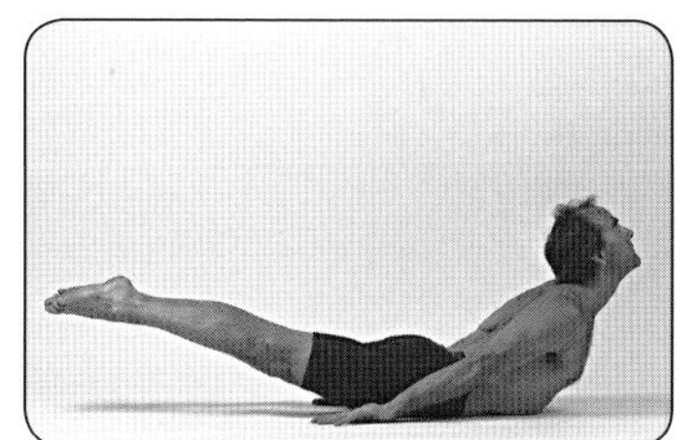
Shalabhasana A

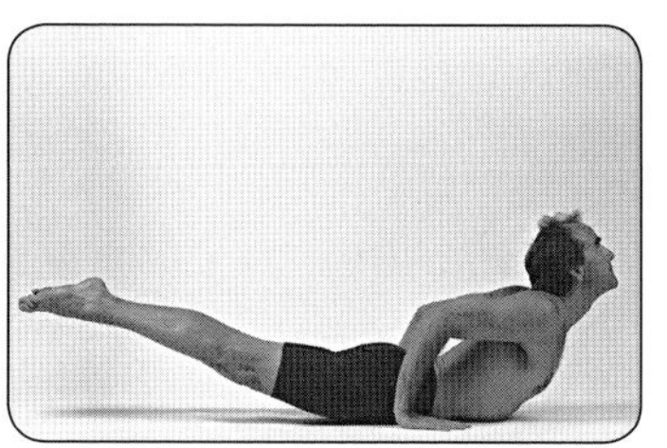
Shalabhasana B

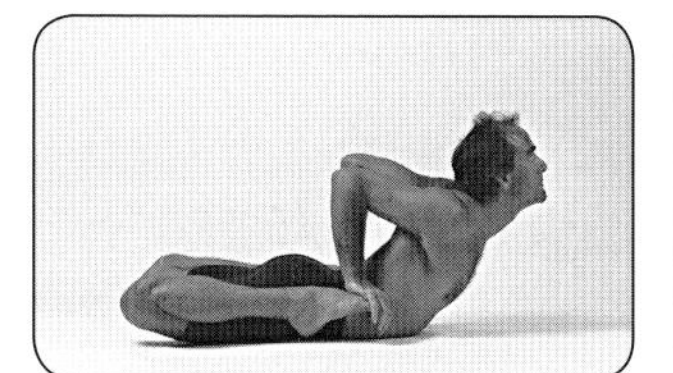
Bhekasana

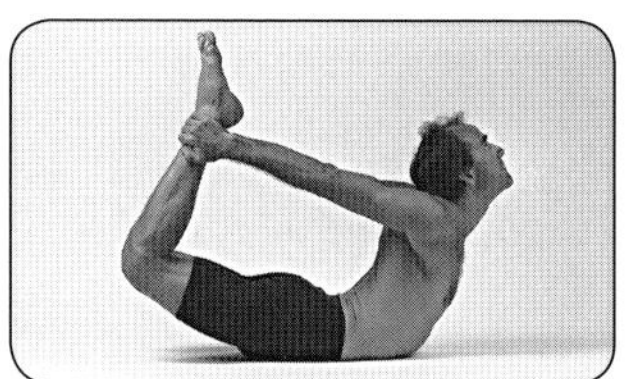
Dhanurasana

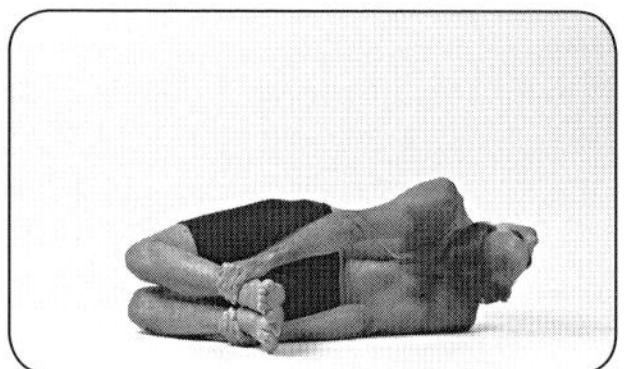
Parsva Dhanurasana

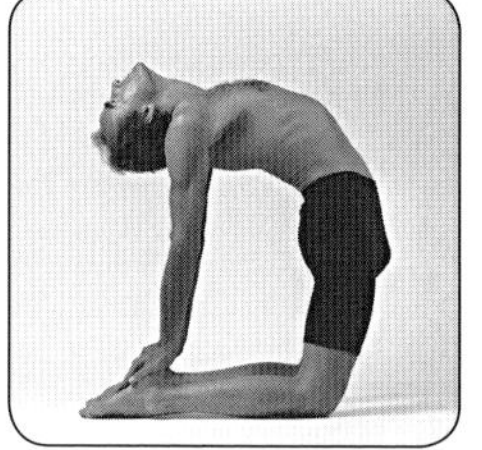
Ushtrasana

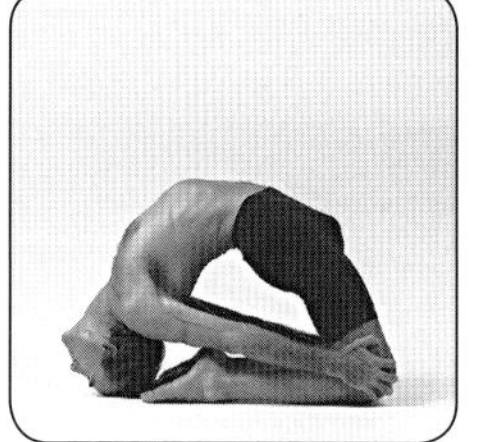
Laghuvajrasana

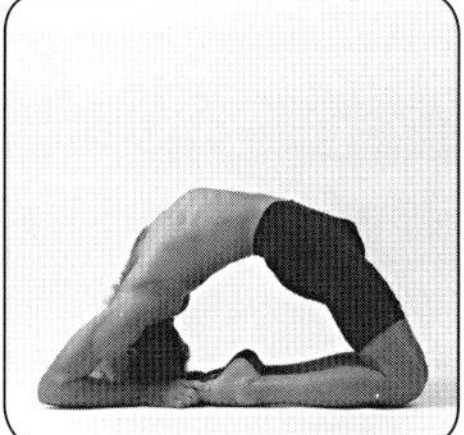
Kapotasana

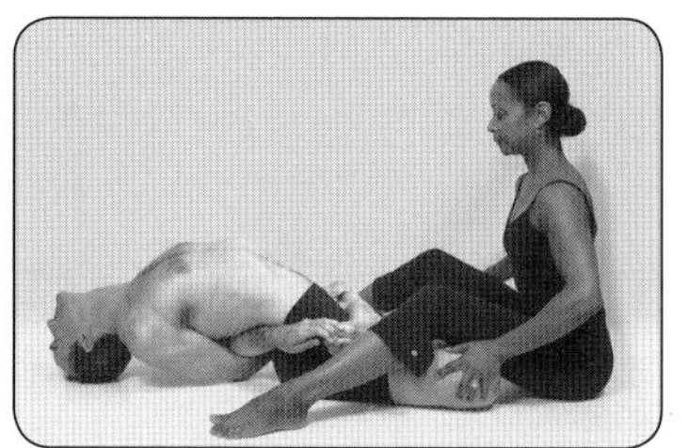
Supta Vajrasana

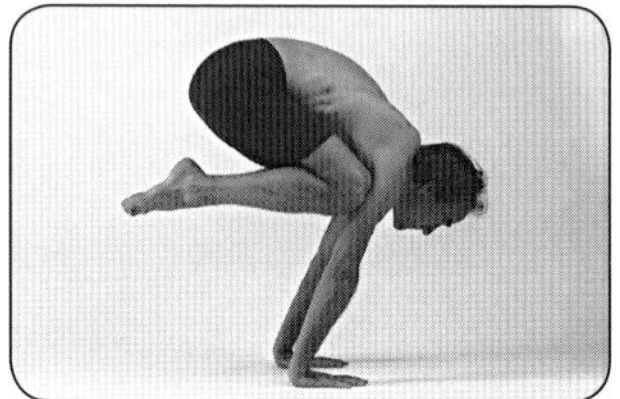
Bakasana (Two Times)

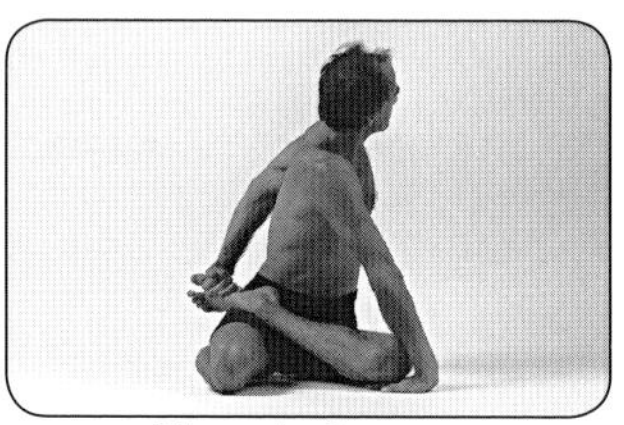
Bharadvajasana

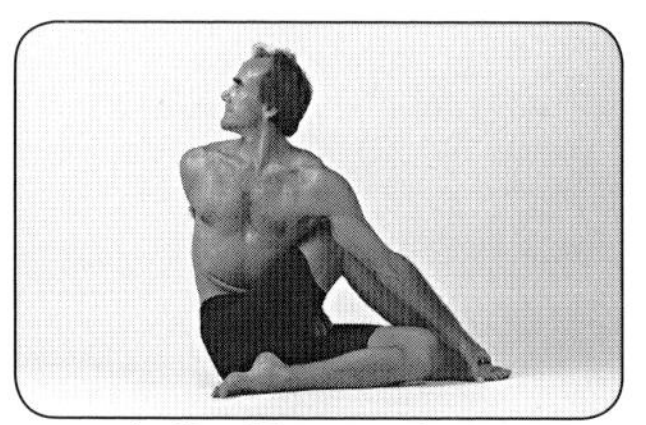
Ardha Matsyendrasana

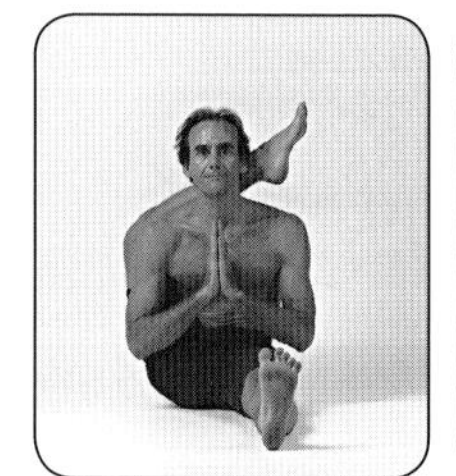
Eka Pada Sirsasana A

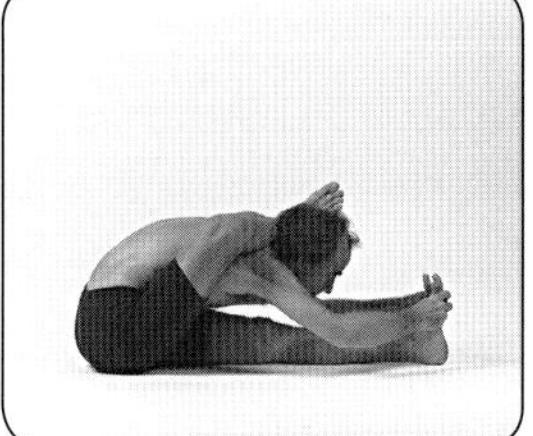
Eka Pada Sirsasana B

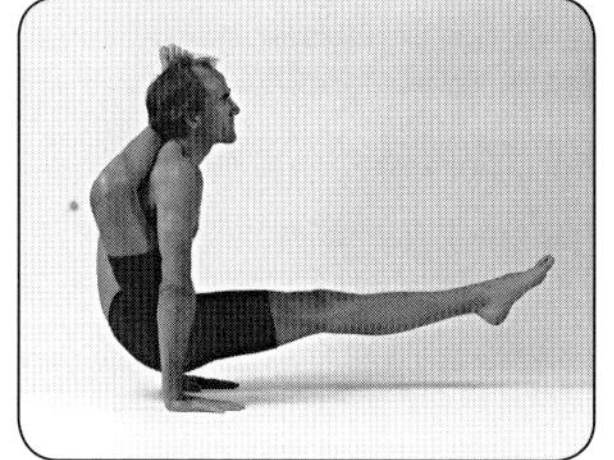
Eka Pada Sirsasana C

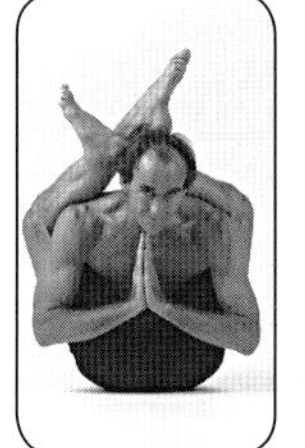
Dwi Pada Sirsasana (A & B)

The Intermediate Series

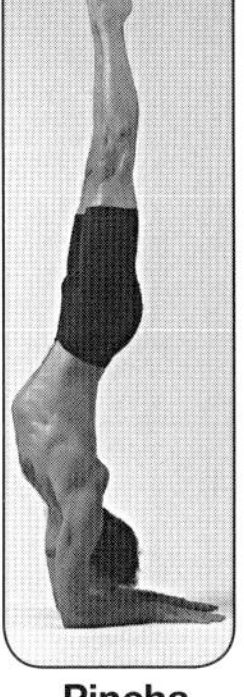
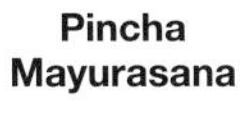

Pincha Mayurasana

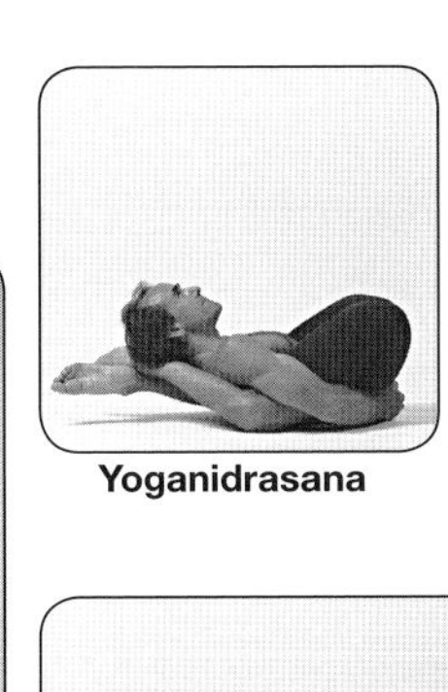

Yoganidrasana

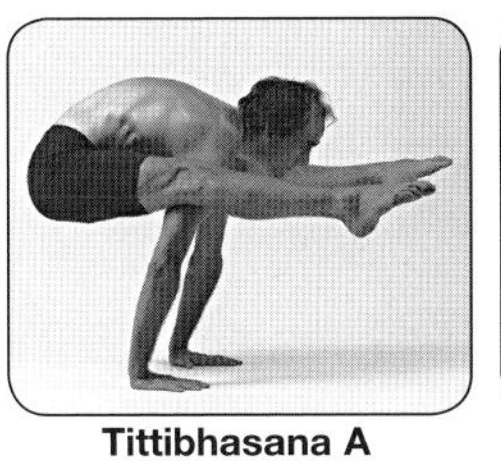

Tittibhasana A

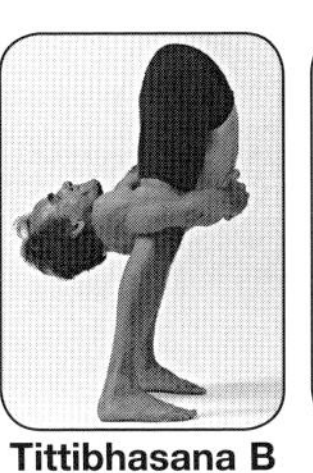

Tittibhasana B

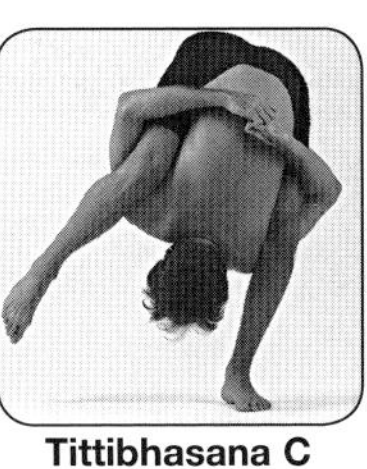

Tittibhasana C

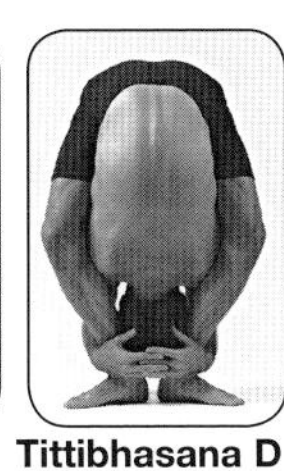

Tittibhasana D

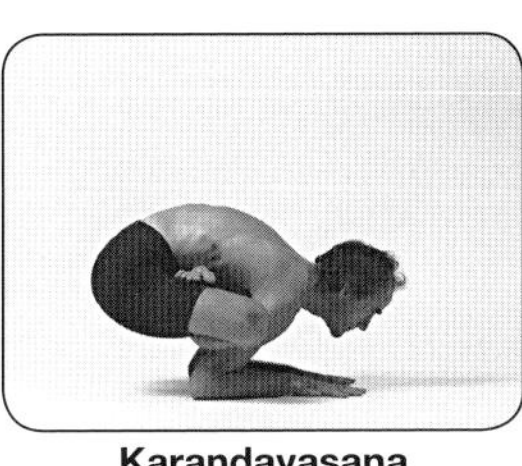

Karandavasana

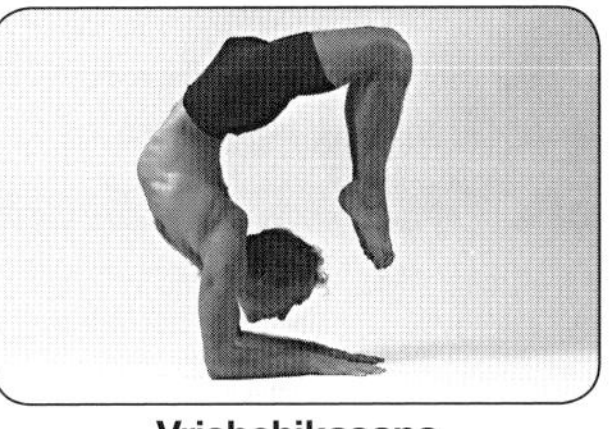

Vrishchikasana

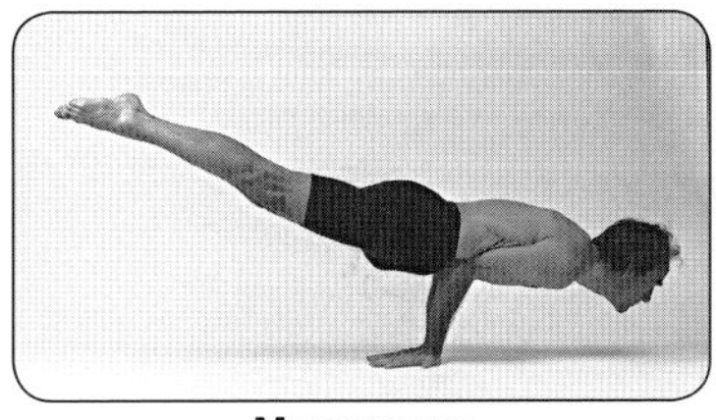

Mayurasana

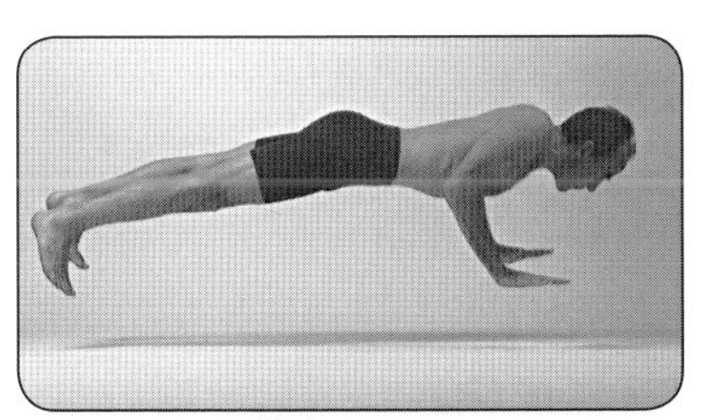
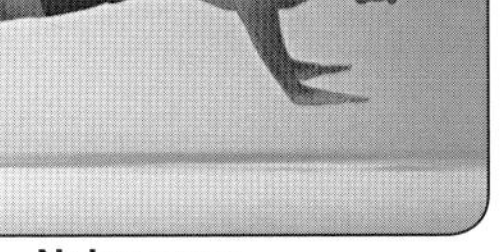

Nakrasana

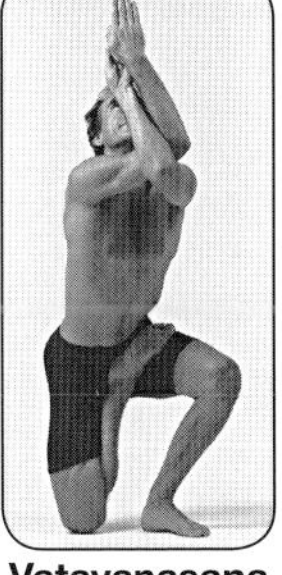

Vatayanasana

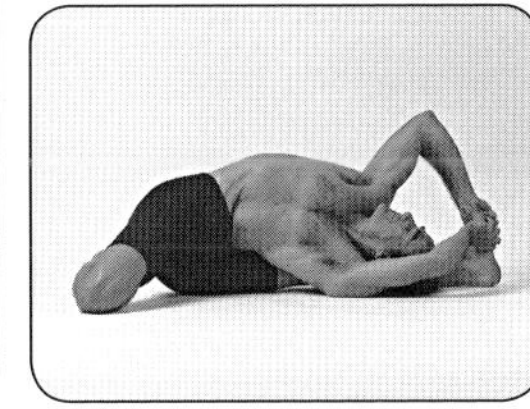

Parighasana

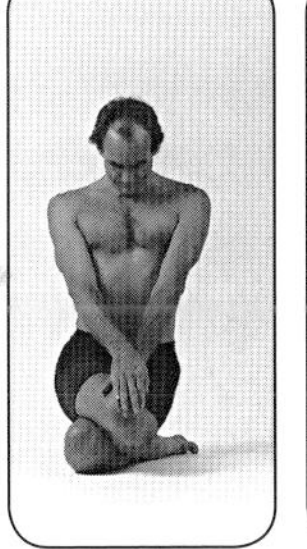
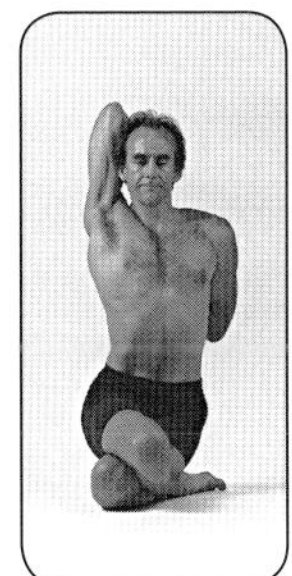

Gomukhasana A & B

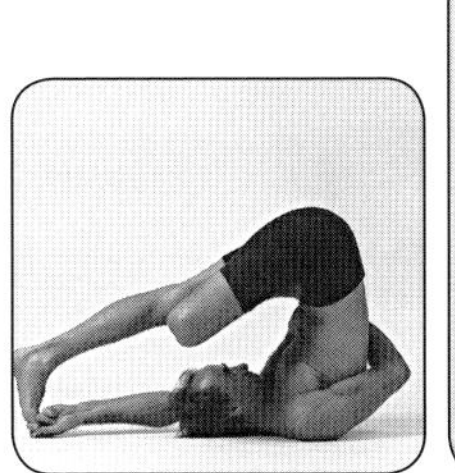
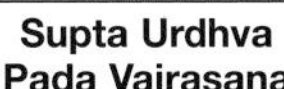

Supta Urdhva Pada Vajrasana

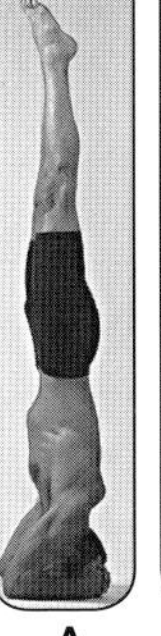

A

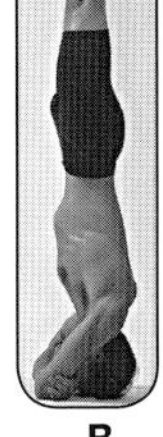

B

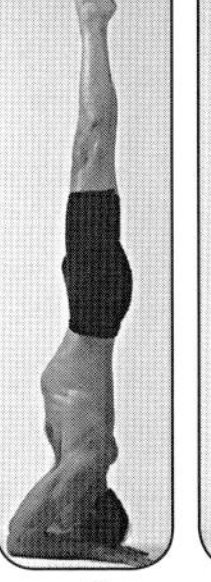

C

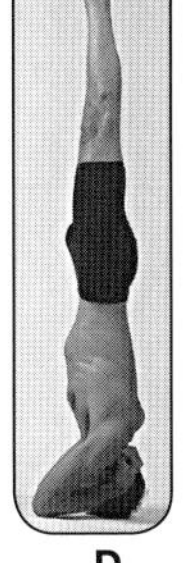

D

Baddha Hasta Sirsasana

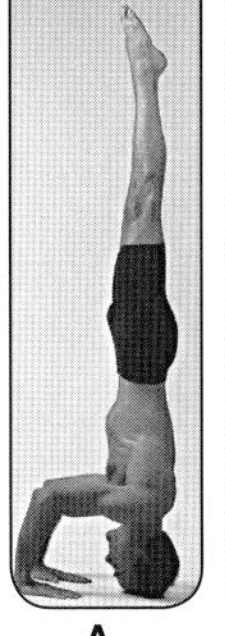

A

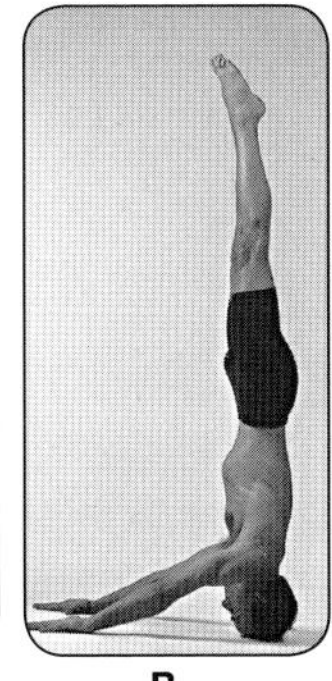

B

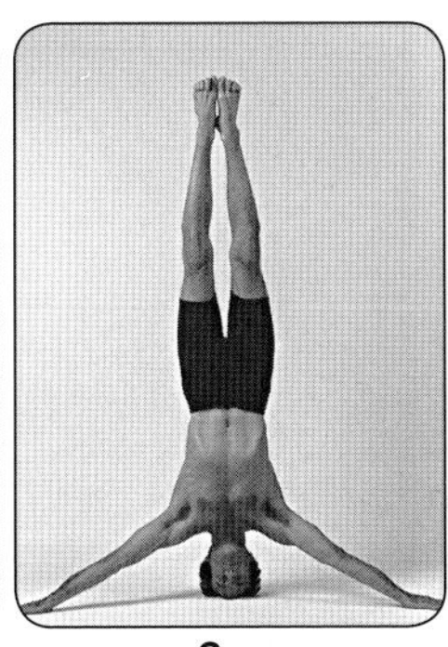

C

Mukta Hasta Sirsasana

The Finishing Sequence

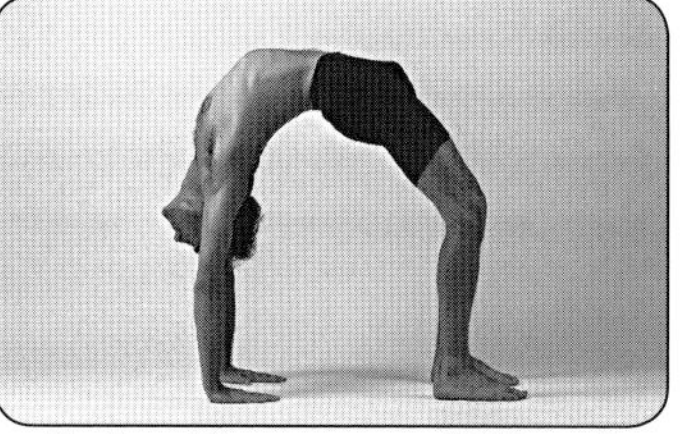

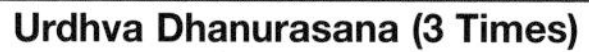
Urdhva Dhanurasana (3 Times)

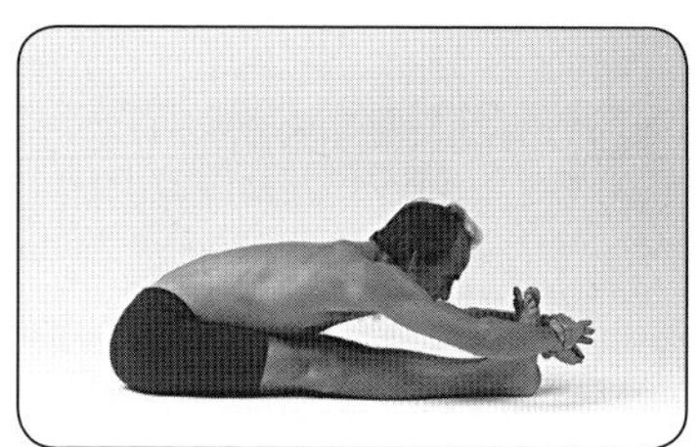
Paschimottanasana

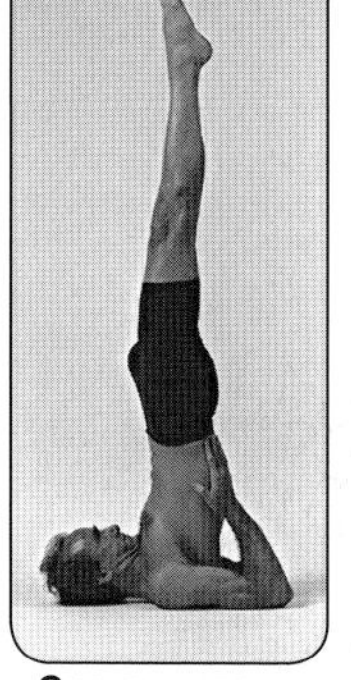
Sarvangasana

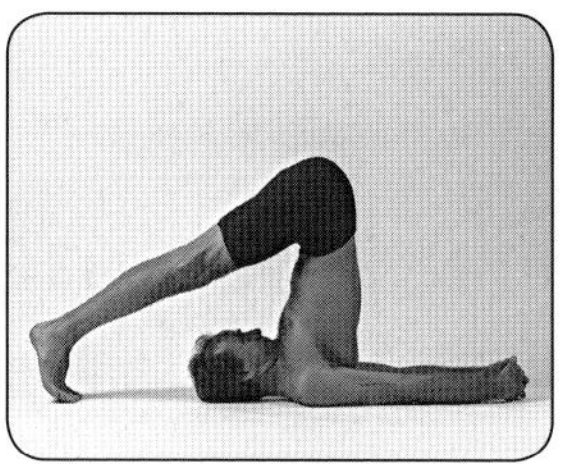
Halasana

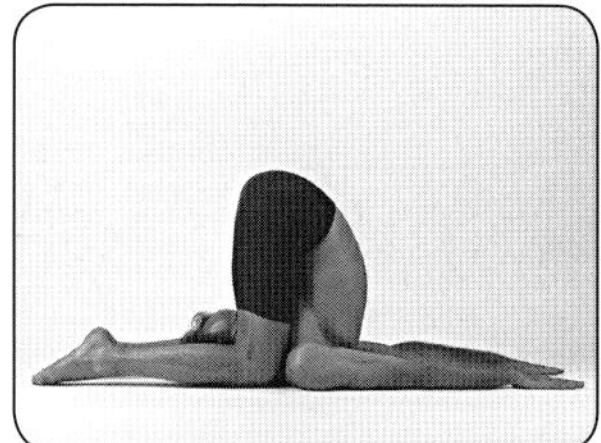
Karnapidasana

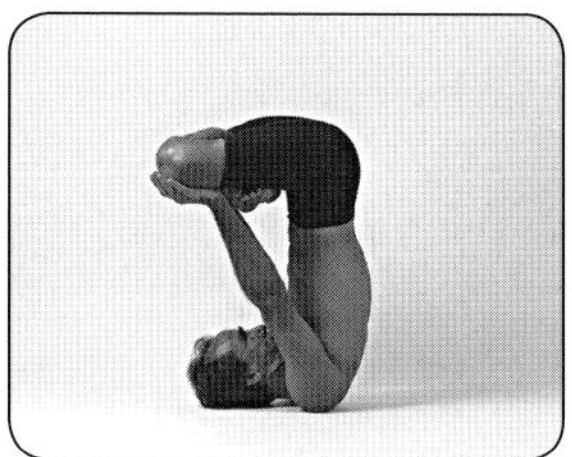
Urdhva Padmasana

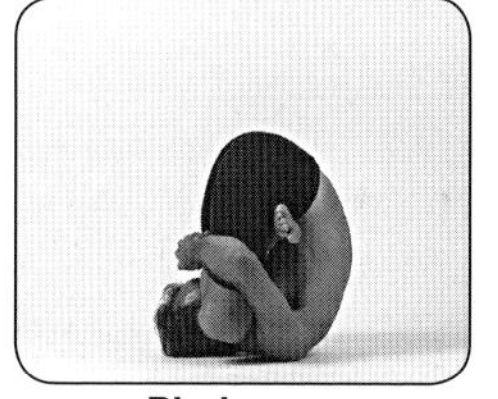
Pindasana

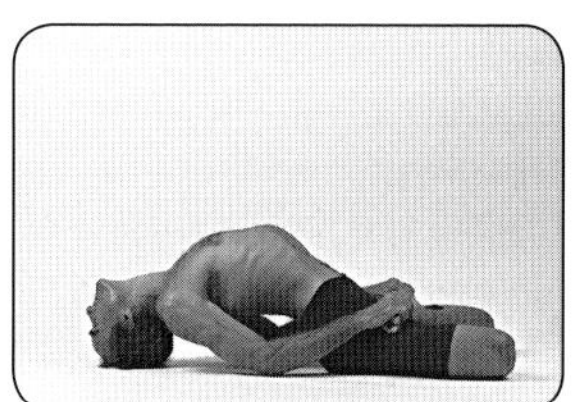
Matsyasana

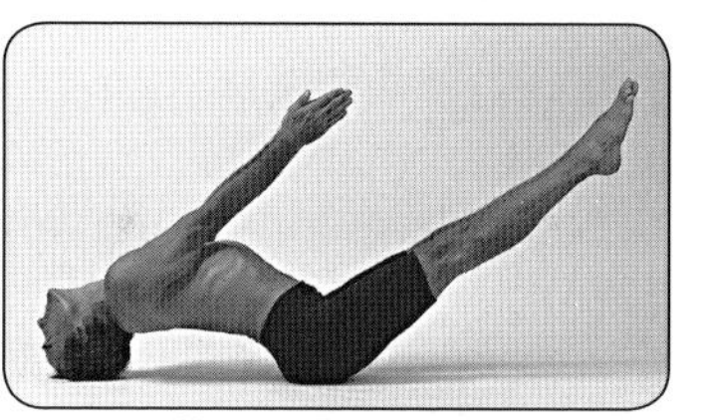
Uttana Padasana

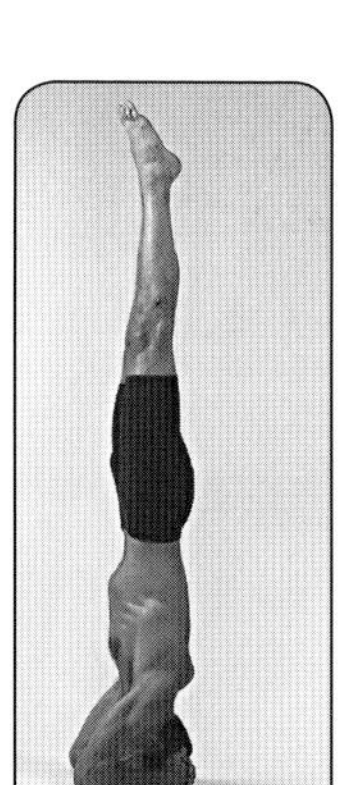
Sirsasana A

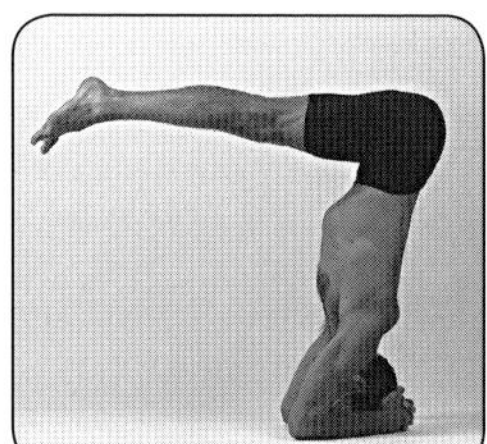
Sirsasana B

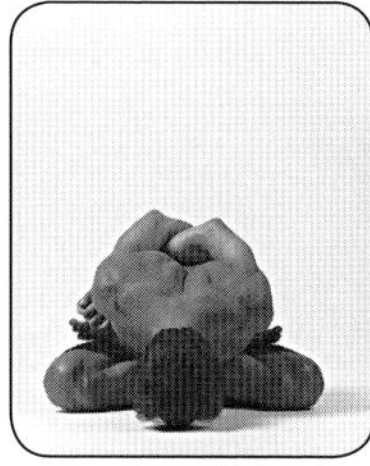
Baddha Padmasana

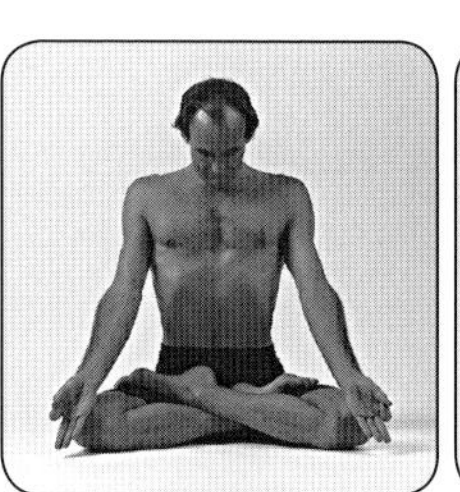
Padmasana

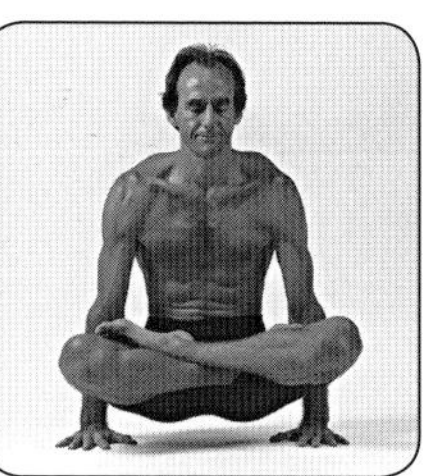
Tolasana

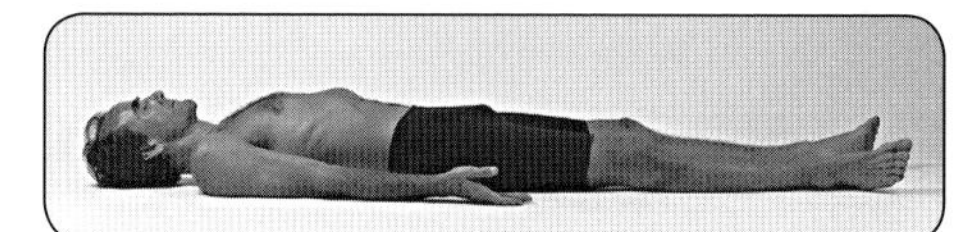
Savasana

Focus

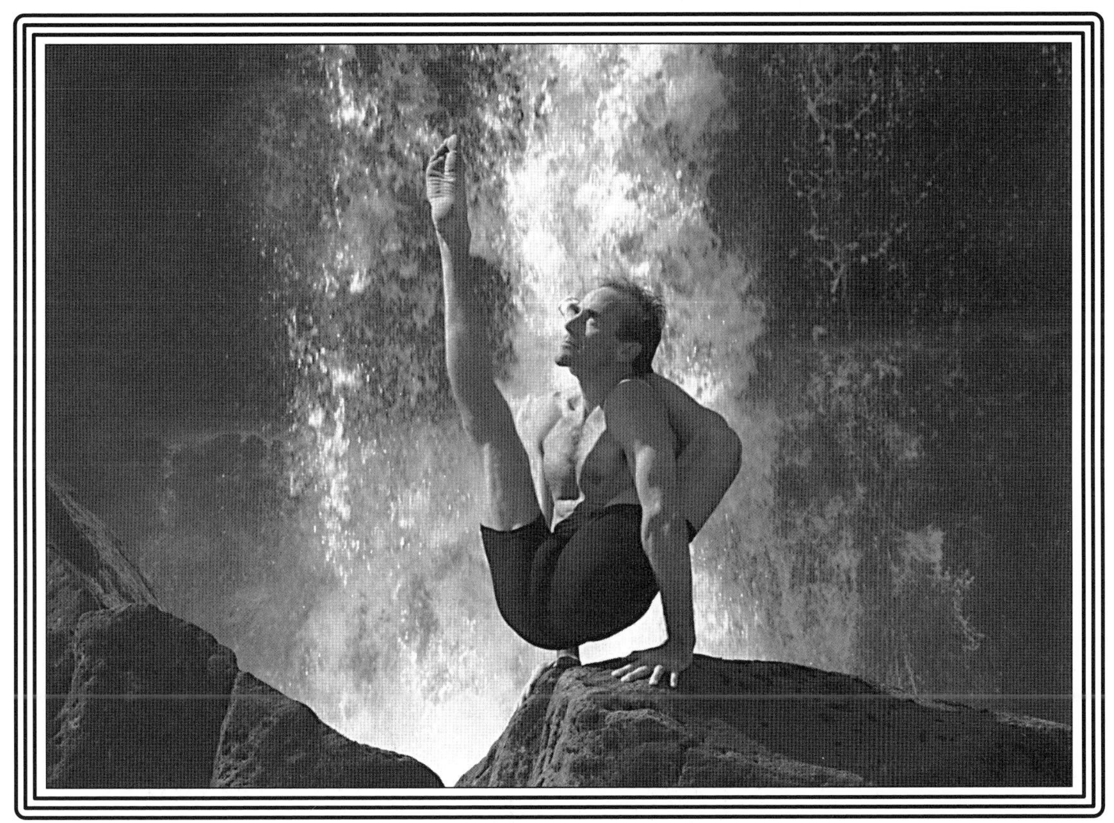

Chakorasana
Advanced 'A' Series
David Swenson ~ Iceland

"When you are inspired by some great purpose, some extraordinary project, all your thoughts break their bounds: Your mind transcends limitations, your consciousness expands in every direction and you find yourself in a new, great and wonderful world. Dormant forces, faculties and talents become alive, and you discover yourself to be a greater person by far than you ever dreamed yourself to be."

Patanjali

Short Forms

"Creating The Time To Practice"

Over the years people have asked me what to do when there is not enough time to practice a complete series. This is a valid question. We live in a fast-paced world. There are fast foods, fast cars and fast computers. All of this speed is meant to give us more free time. Unfortunately, the opposite seems to be the case. With all of the rushing to and fro there is little time left for personal pursuits. It would be easy for me to simply respond by saying one should just make the time by either rising earlier in the morning or taking time away from other activities. For some people this approach may be appropriate, but it is not feasible to expect everyone to apply such a disciplinary regimen. Setting unreasonable goals creates a recipe for discouragement or self-doubt which may lead to giving up the practice altogether. It is much better to practice a small amount rather than none at all.

I have created a set of abbreviated routines which I call "**Short Forms**". They are designed to allow the "**time-challenged**" to have a practice available which may fit into the tightest of schedules. It is much easier to find fifteen minutes or a half-an-hour to practice than it is to find ninety minutes or two hours. These routines are also good to use as stepping stones to approach the full series. It can be overwhelming for the newcomer to Ashtanga to witness the entire Primary Series. I remember my first encounter. I was totally awed by seeing it yet I could not even get through the sun salutations without stopping. These abbreviated sessions are a great way to become familiar with the essence of the practice so that when one has the time or inclination to practice a complete routine it will not be as overwhelming. For many people the shortened versions may also be enough. The important thing to remember is that this is your practice. Create the most suitable routine for your lifestyle. Consistency is more important than quantity in a sporadic fashion. It is much better to practice three days a week for thirty minutes each time than it is to practice one day for two hours and on another day for twenty minutes and then none at all for the next three weeks. Find a routine that you can stick with and the benefits will accrue faster than being sporadic.

Take pleasure in your practice. It is good to finish a session and be looking forward to the next one, rather than making our practice so difficult that we create a loathsome duty out of it. Be relaxed. Enjoy every breath. Feel the magic of moving your body and filling the lungs with air. **The rewards of yoga are personal!** It is an incredibly valuable and diverse tool. My personal experience has been that when I practice yoga, everything else in my life flows more smoothly. I have greater patience and a steadier composure when I practice. We cannot avoid all of the stresses that life offers. Our only real control is how we react to the waves of challenges that are thrust upon us.

Short Form / 15 Minutes

Surya Namaskara A . . . . 5 Times
Surya Namaskara B. . . . . 3 Times

Insert a Vinyasa after each seated asana.
Practice the right side first and then the left side in all bi-lateral postures.
Find alternative options for the asanas in the main text of the Primary Series.

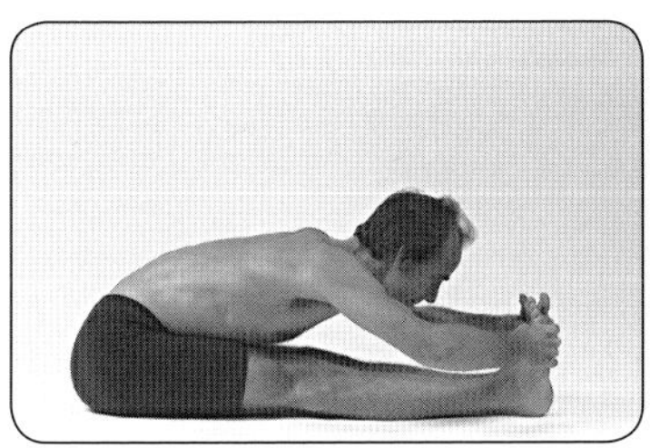

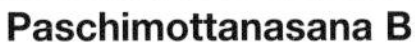

Paschimottanasana B

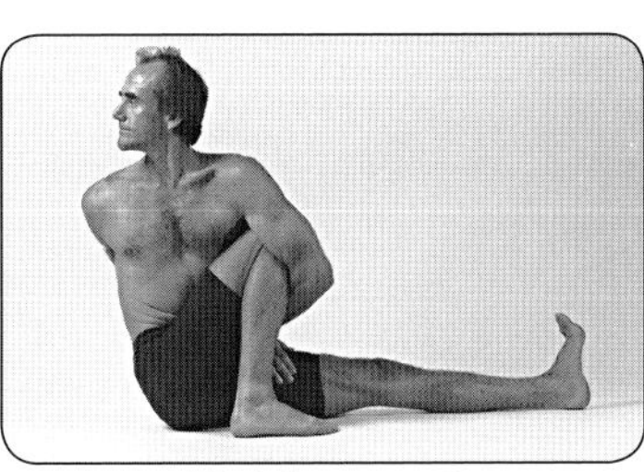

Marichyasana C

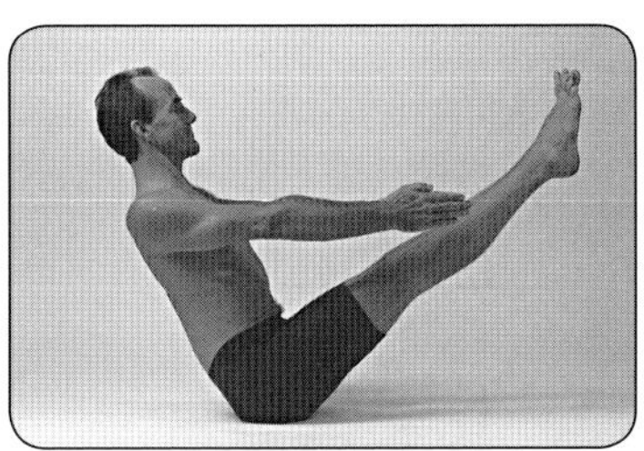

Navasana (Two Times)

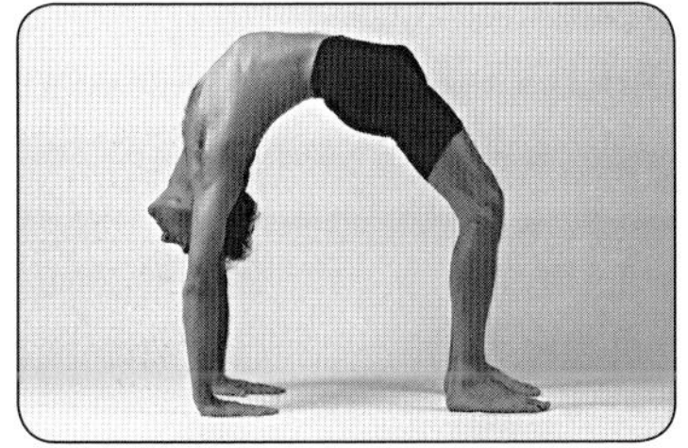

Urdhva Dhanurasana

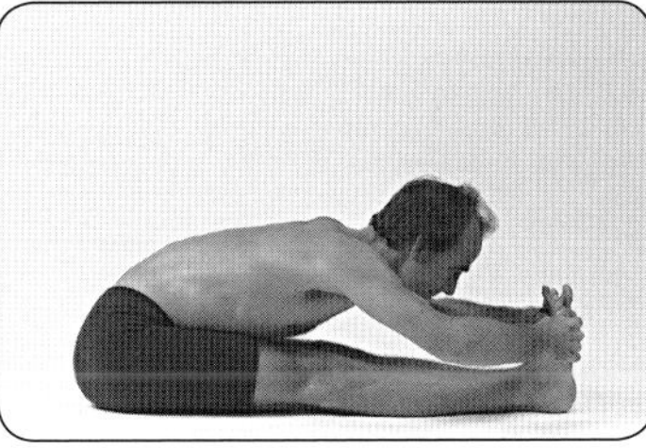

Paschimottanasana B

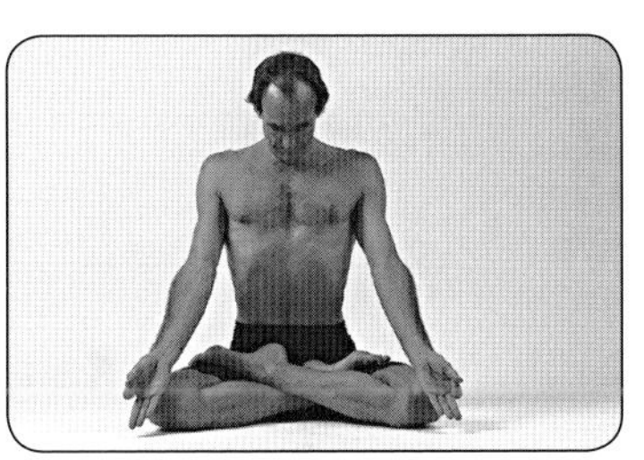

Padmasana

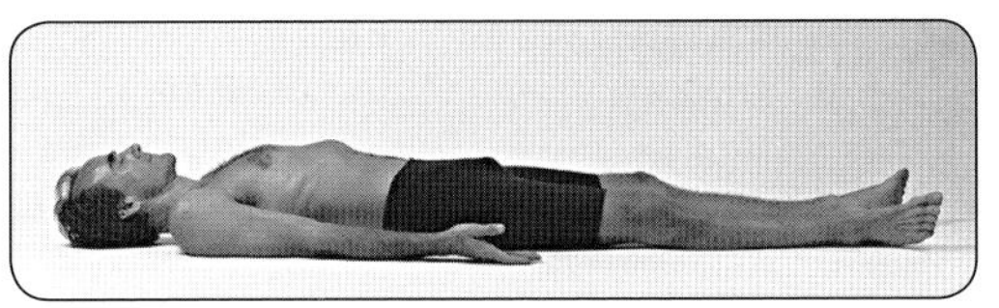

Savasana

"This time, like all times, is a very good one,
if we but know what to do with it."

Ralph Waldo Emerson

Short Form / 30 Minutes

Surya Namaskara A. . . . . 3 Times
Surya Namaskara B . . . . 2 Times

Return to the front of your mat after each standing asana and insert a Vinyasa after each seated asana.
Practice the right side first and then the left side in all bi-lateral postures.
Find alternative options for the asanas in the main text of the Primary Series.

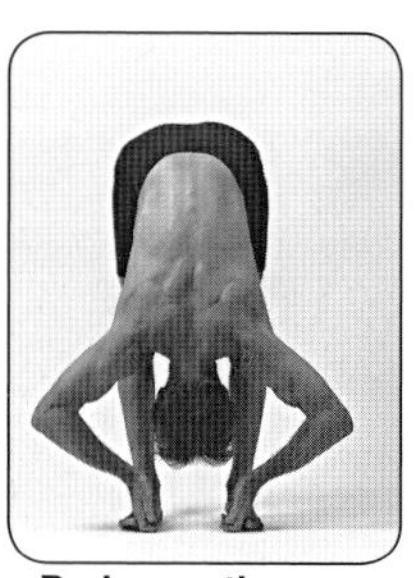

Padangusthasana

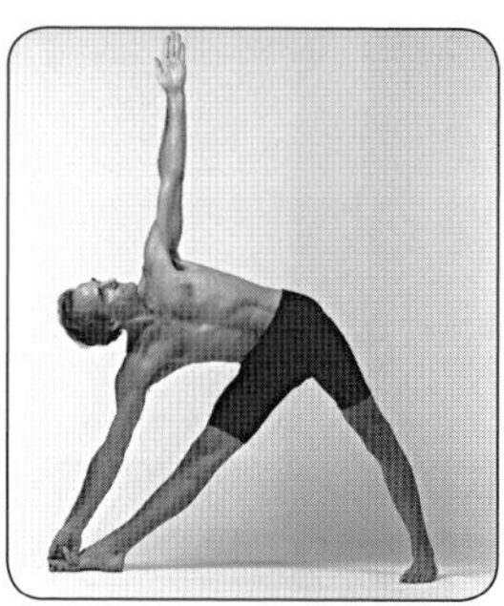

Utthita Trikonasana

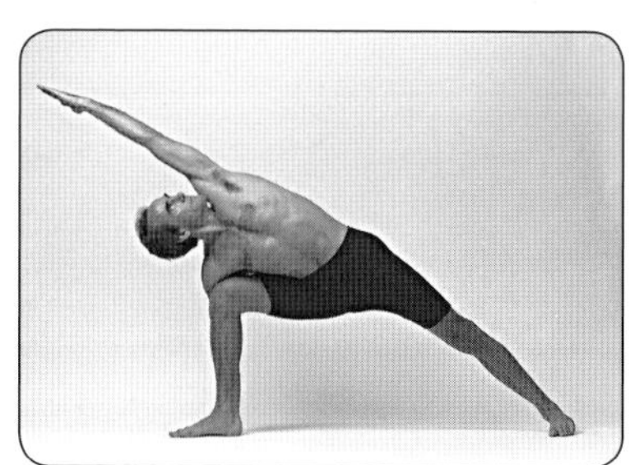

Utthita Parsvakonasana

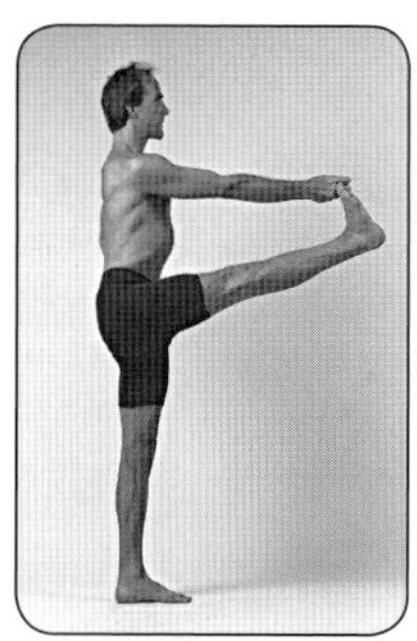

Utthita Hasta Padangusthasana A

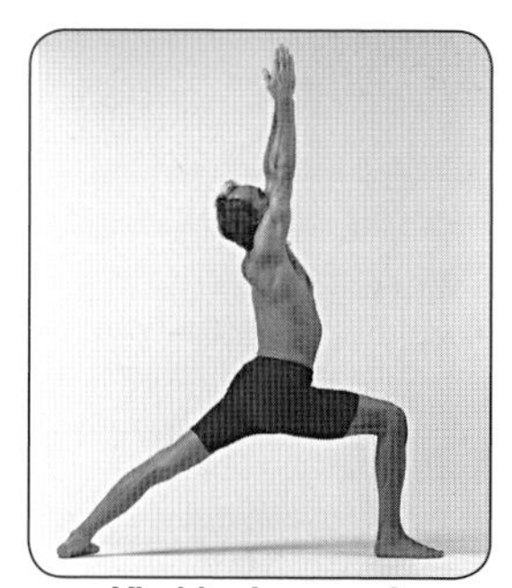

Virabhadrasana A

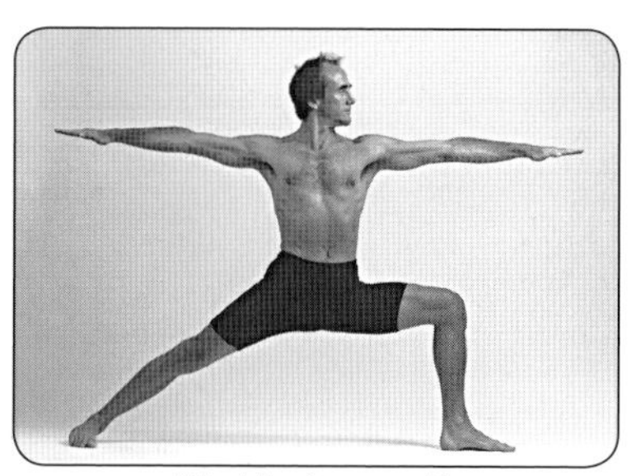

Virabhadrasana B

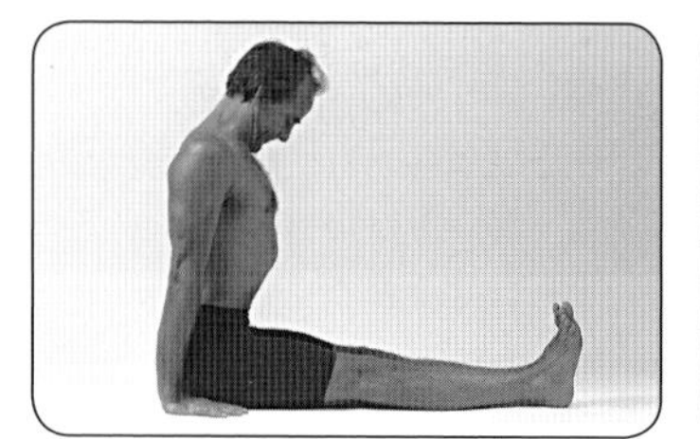

Dandasana

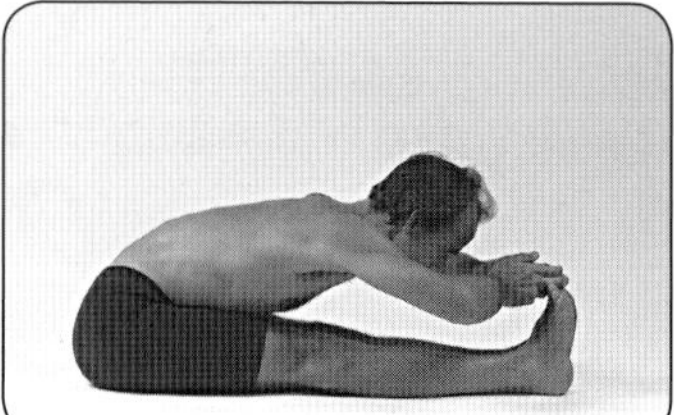

Paschimottanasana A

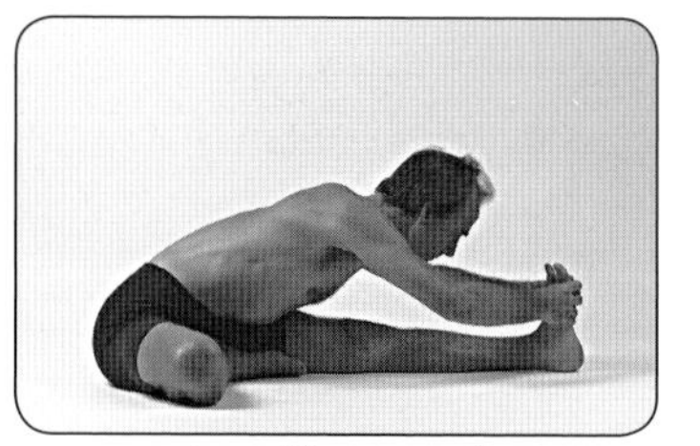

Janu Sirsasana A

Short Form / 30 Minutes

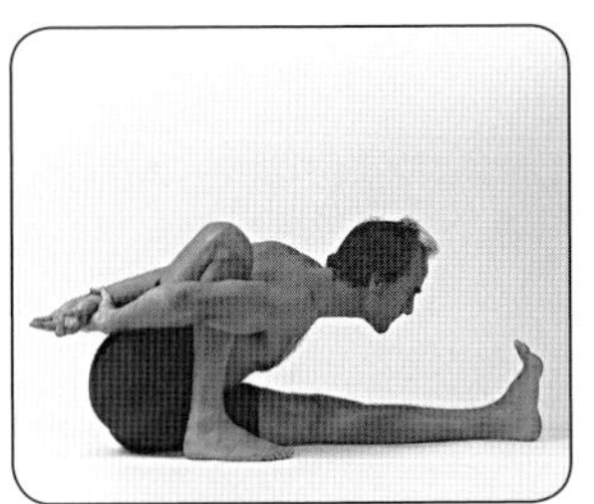
Marichyasana A

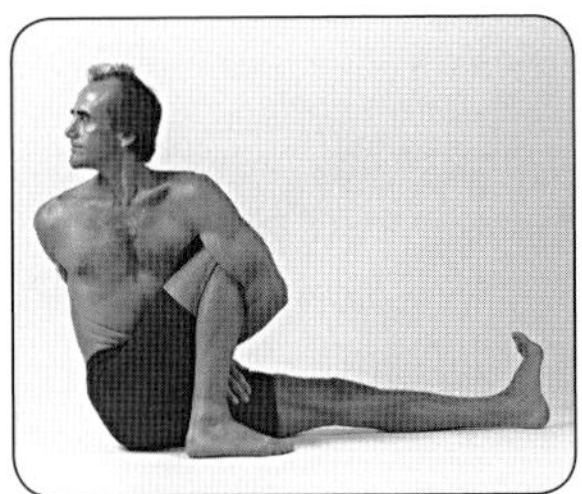
Marichyasana C

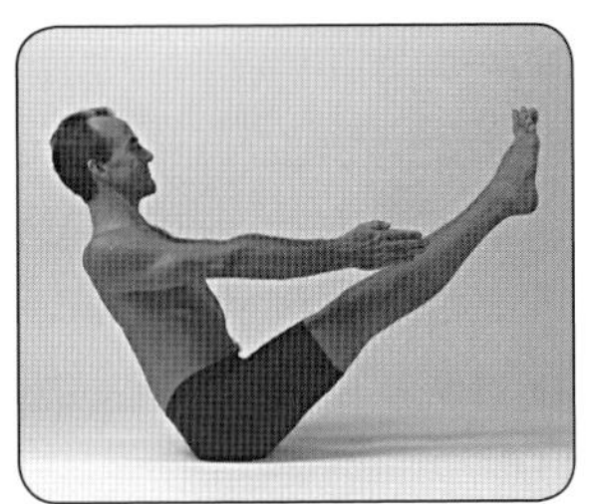
Navasana
(Two Times)

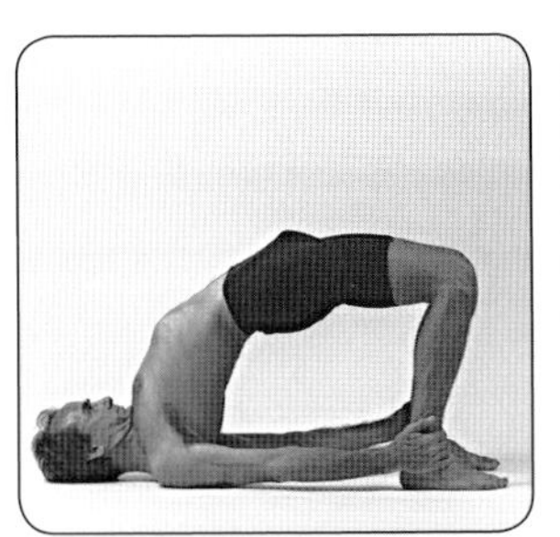
Urdhva Dhanurasana
Modification

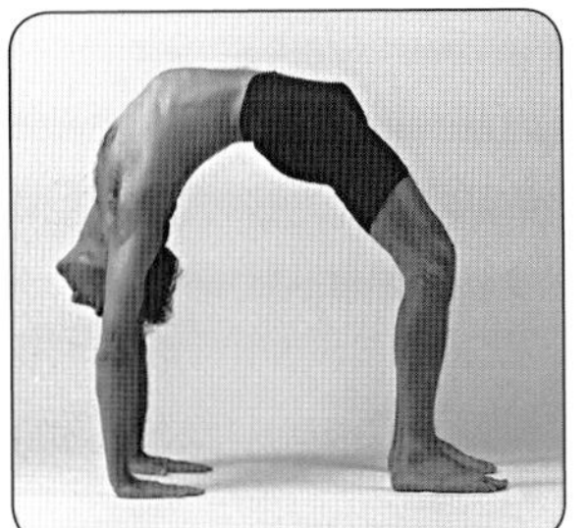
Urdhva Dhanurasana

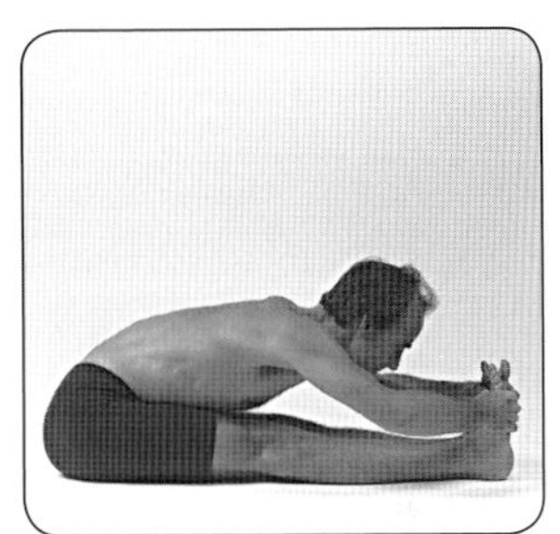
Paschimottanasana B

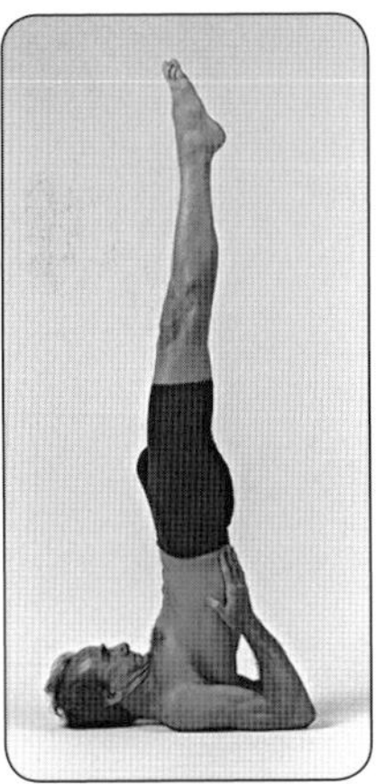
Sarvangasana

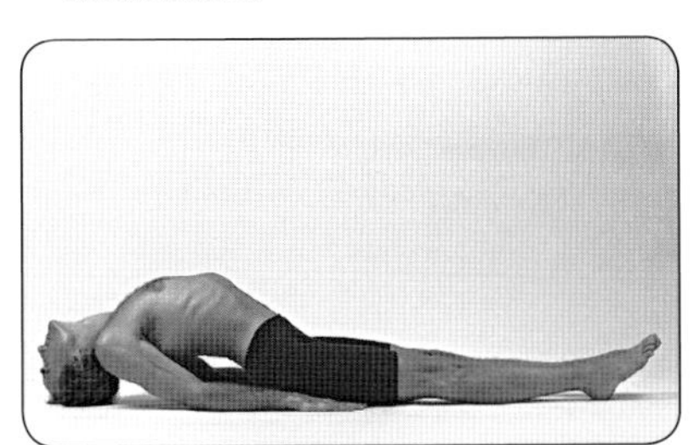
Matsyasana
Modification

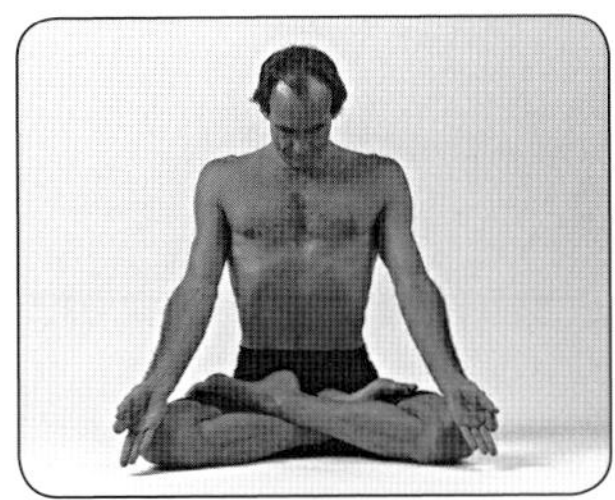
Padmasana

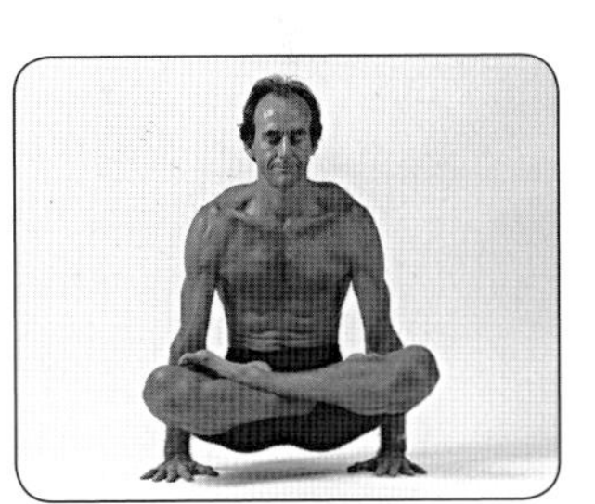
Tolasana

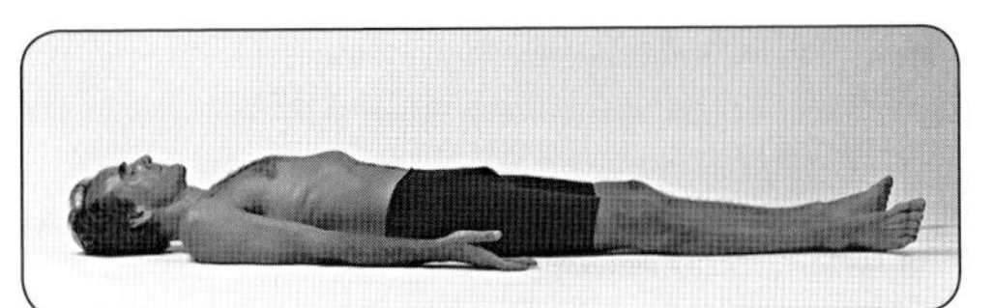
Savasana

Short Form / 45 Minutes

Surya Namaskara A. . . . . 3 Times
Surya Namaskara B . . . . 3 Times

Return to the front of your mat after each standing asana and insert a Vinyasa after each seated asana.
Practice the right side first and then the left side in all bi-lateral postures.
Find alternative options for the asanas in the main text of the Primary Series.

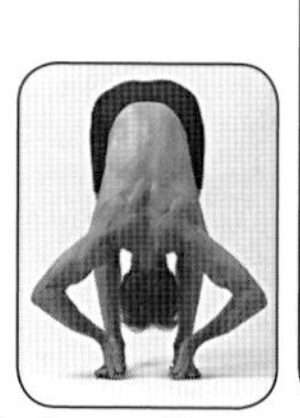
Padangusthasana

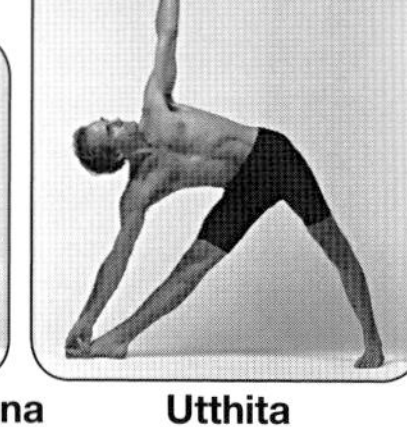
Utthita Trikonasana

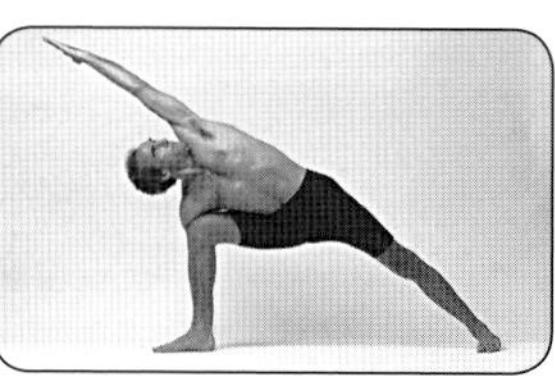
Utthita Parsvakonasana

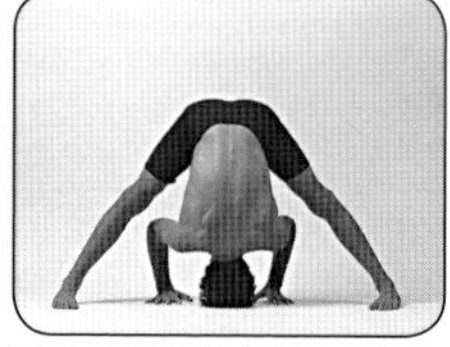
Prasarita Padottanasana A

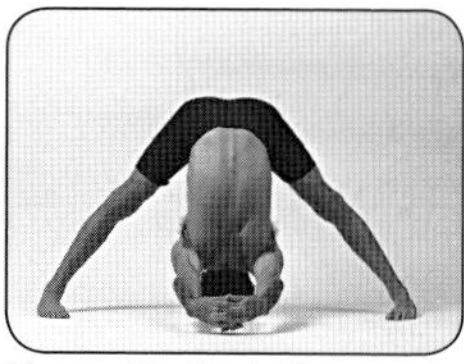
Prasarita Padottanasana C

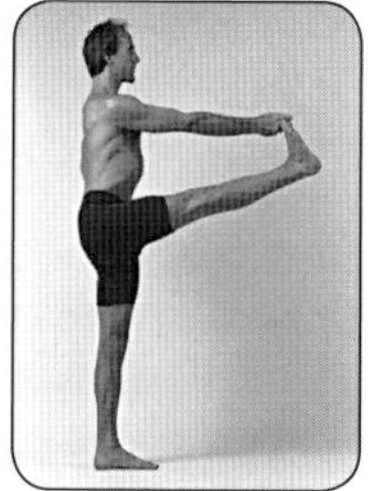
Utthita Hasta Padangusthasana A

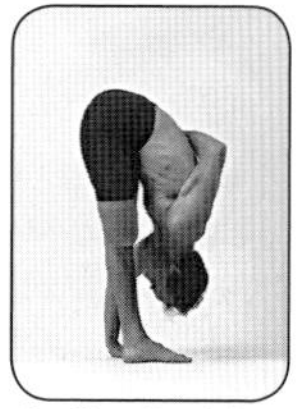
Ardha Baddha Padmottanasana

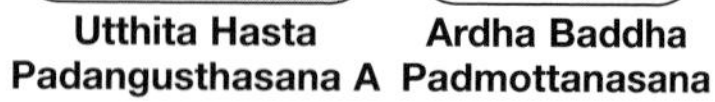

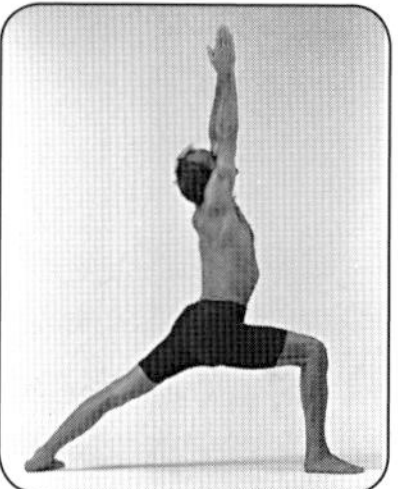
Virabhadrasana A

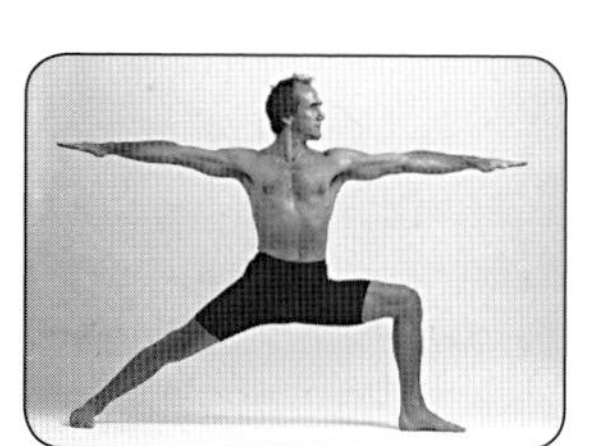
Virabhadrasana B

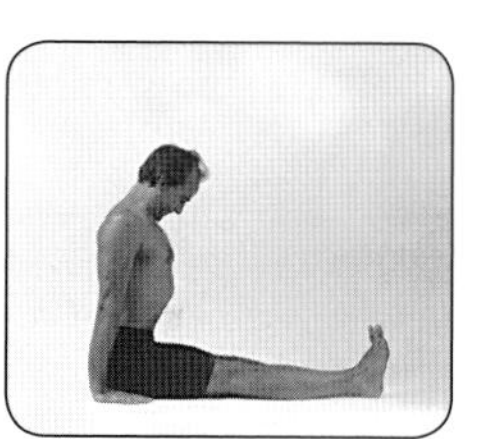
Dandasana

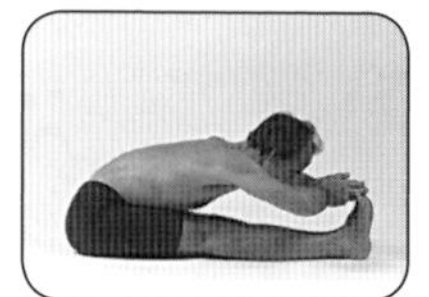
Paschimottanasana A

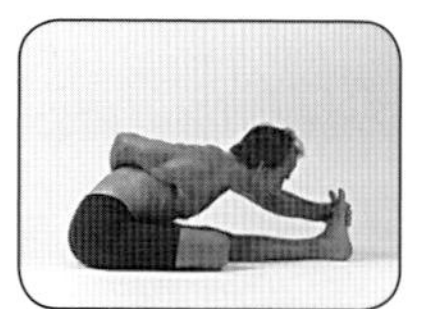
Ardha Baddha Padma Paschimottanasana

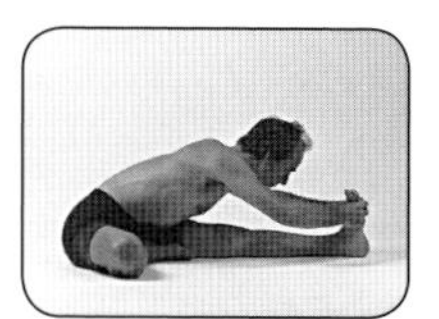
Janu Sirsasana A

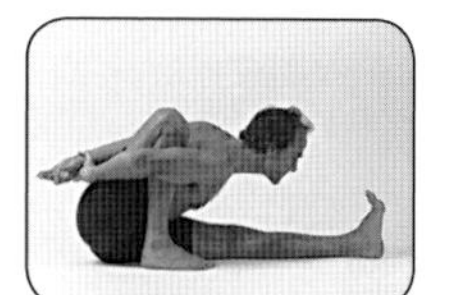
Marichyasana A

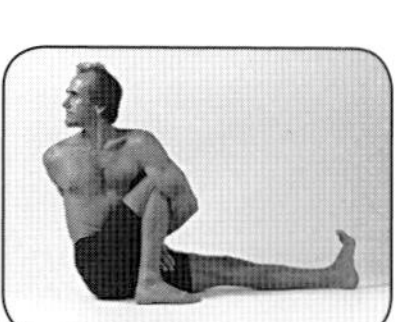
Marichyasana C

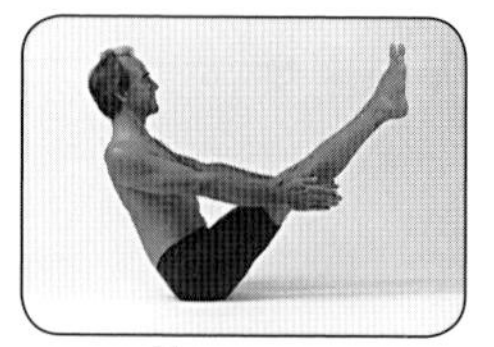
Navasana (Three Times)

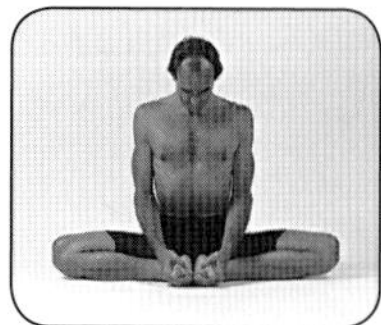
Baddha Konasana A

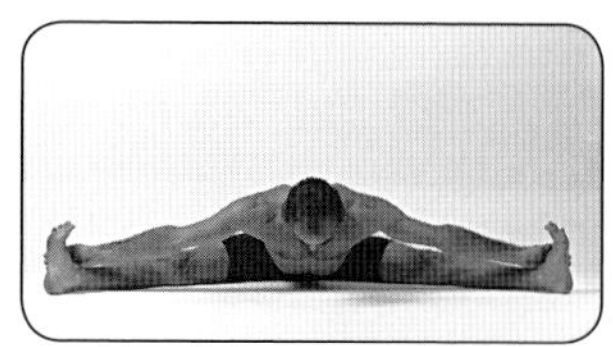
Upavishta Konasana A

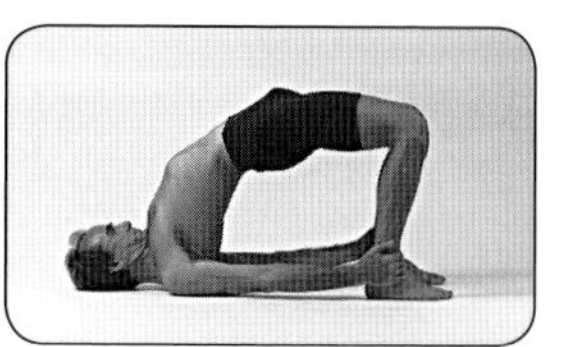
Urdhva Dhanurasana Modification

Short Form / 45 Minutes

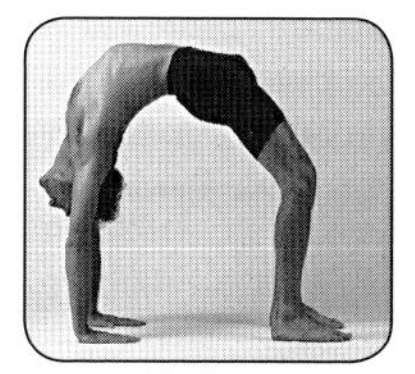

Urdhva Dhanurasana

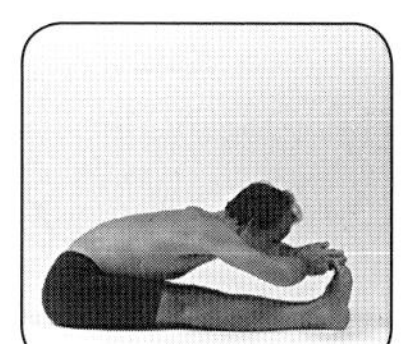

Paschimottanasana B

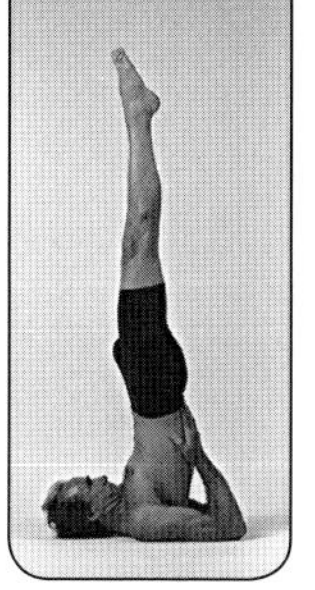

Sarvangasana

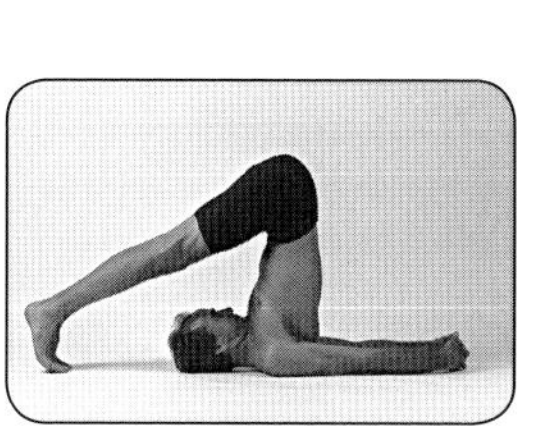

Halasana

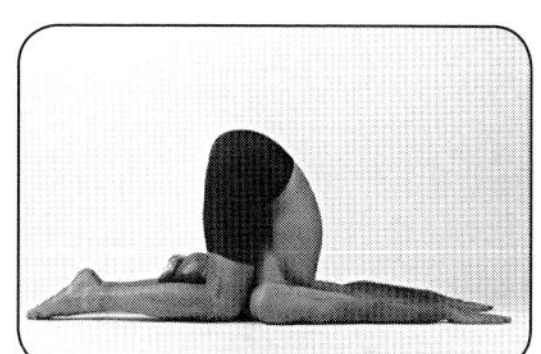

Karnapidasana

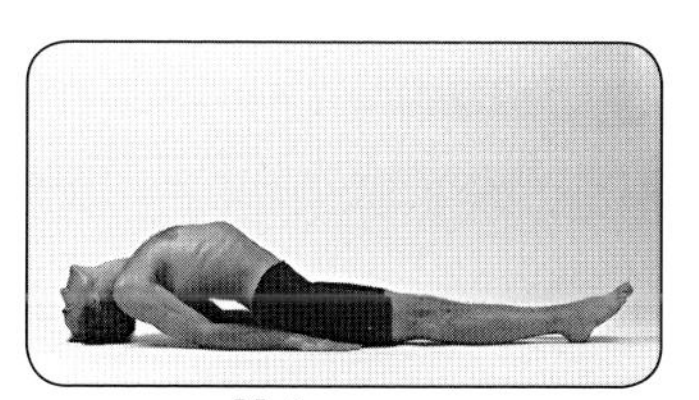

Matsyasana Modification

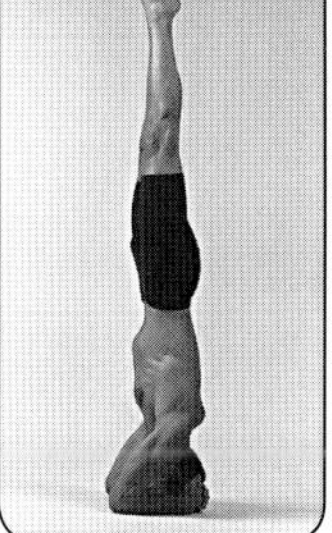

Sirsasana

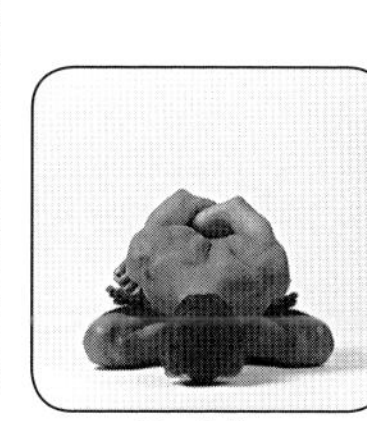

Baddha Padmasana

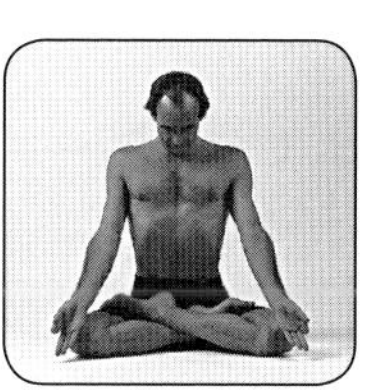

Padmasana

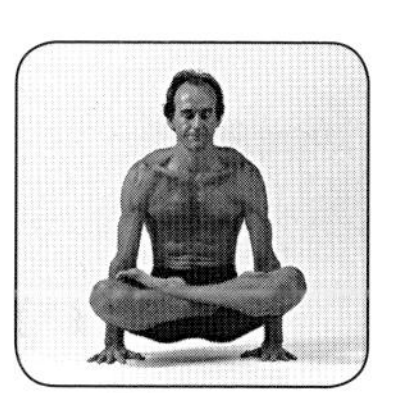

Tolasana

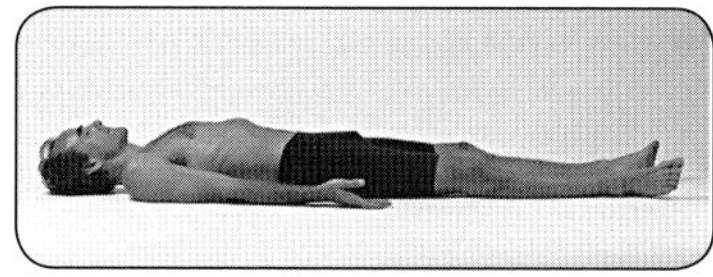

Savasana

"Before Enlightenment
I Chopped Wood and Carried Water;

After Enlightenment,
I Chopped Wood and Carried Water"

Zen Saying

Index

Index

Index

The Strongest Trees in the Forest Grow the Slowest!

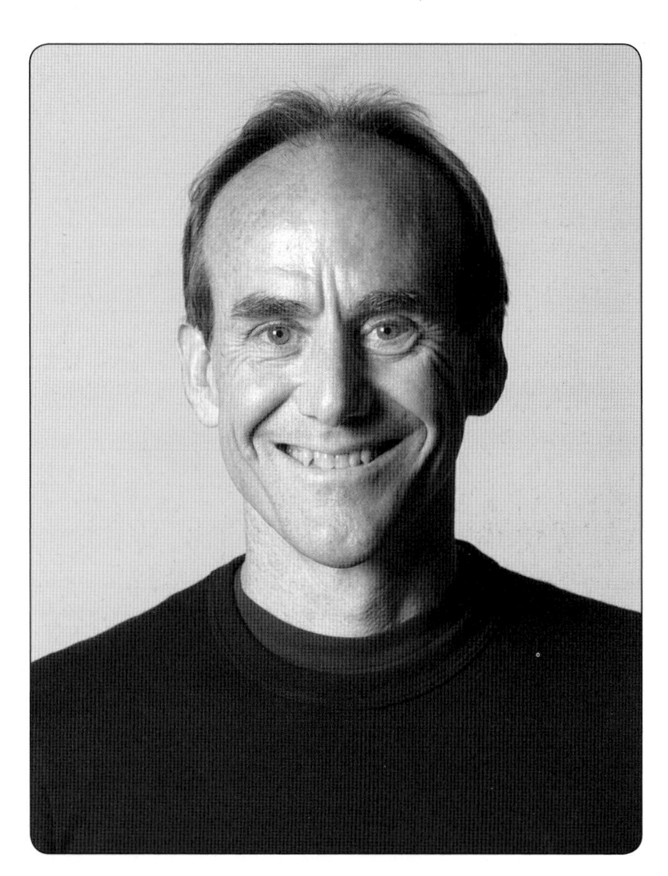

Yoga is a lifelong journey.

We all tend to become lost in the world of immediacy, wanting instant or quick results. The real depth of yoga takes time and patience. It is like a tree growing in the forest. The strongest trees grow the slowest!

Create a realistic practice that fits within the framework of your daily life.

Have Fun Practicing and Enjoy the Journey!

David